THE COUNTRY ALMANAC OF HOME REMEDIES

Time-Tested & Almost-Forgotten Wisdom for Treating Hundreds of Common

Ailments, Aches & Pains

QUICKLY AND NATURALLY

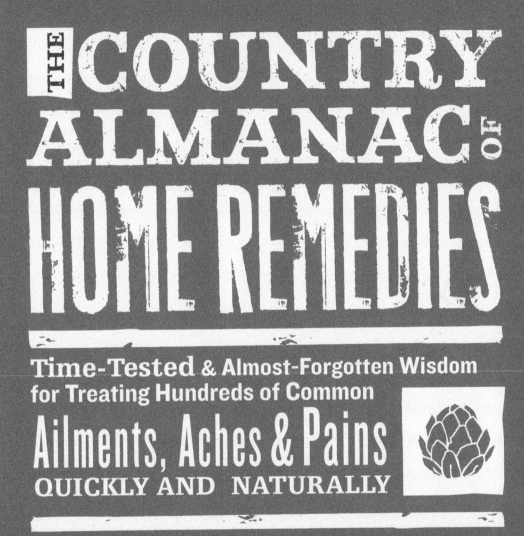

BRIGITTE MARS
AND
CHRYSTLE FIEDLER

FAIR WINDS

Fair Winds Press
100 Cummings Center, Suite 406L
Beverly, MA 01915

fairwindspress.com • bodymindbeautyhealth.com

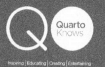

Text © Brigitte Mars and Chrystle Fiedler

First published in 2011 by Fair Winds Press,
an imprint of The Quarto Group,
100 Cummings Center, Suite 265-D,
Beverly, MA 01915, USA.
T (978) 282-9590 F (978) 283-2742
www.QuartoKnows.com

Fair Winds Press titles are also available at discount for retail, wholesale, promotional, and bulk purchase. For details, contact the Special Sales Manager by email at specialsales@quarto.com or by mail at The Quarto Group, Attn: Special Sales Manager, 401 Second Avenue North, Suite 310, Minneapolis, MN 55401, USA.

ISBN-13: 978-1-59233-631-9

Library of Congress Cataloging-in-Publication Data
Mars, Brigitte.
 The country almanac of home remedies : time-tested wisdom for treating hundreds of common ailments naturally / Brigitte Mars and Chrystle Fiedler.
    p. cm.
 Includes bibliographical references.
 ISBN-13: 978-1-59233-446-9
 ISBN-10: 1-59233-446-6
 1. Self-care, Health. 2. Traditional medicine. I. Fiedler, Chrystle. II. Title.
 RA776.95.M27 2010
 610--dc22

                    2010032907

Cover + book design: carol holtz | holtzdesign.com
Photographs: fotolia.com, 24; 39; 55; 72; 143; 158; 182; 200; 206; 241; 250, iStockphoto.com, 93; 113; 164; 192; 222; 257
Illustration: Mike Wanke
Printed in USA

Note: The information contained in this book is intended to educate, delight, and expand your understanding of your health. For any health concerns, first take responsibility for your own health, and then seek the advice of a competent health-care professional when needed.

CONTENTS

CHAPTER 1

NATURAL REMEDIES TO RELIEVE
COLDS, FLU, AND RELATED
ILLNESSES 24

CHAPTER 2

NATURAL REMEDIES TO SOOTHE
EVERYDAY ACHES AND PAINS 39

CHAPTER 3

NATURAL REMEDIES FOR RELIEF
OF BURNS, BUG BITES, AND
SKIN AFFLICTIONS 55

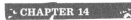

INTRODUCTION

Growing up part time in a small village north of Quebec, folk remedies were a part of my everyday life. My cousins and I all wore little medicine bags filled with garlic and camphor during the cold and flu season to ward off illness. Grandmère had a remedy for everything, it seemed. A cabbage poultice could be applied to a swollen wound, cucumber slices applied to sore, weary eyes to refresh them, and if we did get a chest cold, a mustard footbath would be administered. Though I also spent part of my childhood in upstate New York and my parents quite sensibly took me to the doctor's office for my childhood ailments, I realized that the folk remedies I had been exposed to were often more pleasant and just as effective. (Let's see, would you rather have the honey lemon syrup or the latest drug?)

As an herbalist who has practiced for over 40 years, I know that remedies from nature are safe, time-tested, and often worth trying before resorting to modern drugs. The World Health Organization estimates that between 65 to 80 percent of the world's population use traditional (alternative) medicine as their primary form of health care. Remember, it is the folk remedies that really are the traditional medicine. After all, which has been around longer, Prozac or lemon balm?

Today, in many cases, we also now have the ability to better understand scientifically what millions of people have known all along. For example, garlic really is antimicrobial, cabbage and cauliflower are truly anti-inflammatory, and a mustard footbath does move congestion out of the chest by increasing circulation to the lower part of the body.

With so many people lacking health insurance, it often makes sense to see what nature has to offer. The information you'll find in this book will enable you to cure many common conditions with items you can find in your pantry, kitchen, and garden, without a trip to the doctor. Of course, preventing illness is always best, so good nutrition and a healthy exercise program should be on everyone's agenda.

Often, these treatments cost just pennies, so you'll be saving money, too. By using natural remedies, we also contribute to greening our planet. Of course, if nature's remedies do not give you the assistance you need, it's smart to see your health-care practitioner.

May this book bless you with health, practical knowledge, and consciousness.

Blossom with healthy radiance!

Blessings,
Brigitte Mars, AHG
(American Herbalist Guild)

HOW TO USE THIS BOOK

In the following pages, you'll find common ailments and conditions that can be treated effectively with natural remedies you can find in your kitchen, pantry, garden, and health food store. For each one, you'll find a brief description of the condition, along with its symptoms and causes. You'll learn first about which herbs are best, then any supplements, essential oils, homeopathics, and aromatherapies that are available, before moving on to food do's and don'ts and helpful practices to find relief. Sidebars titled "Cures from Grandma's Kitchen," "Good to Grow!" (for what you can grow yourself), "Thrifty Cures, Skip This!" (for what to avoid), "Good to Know!" (important info), and When to See Your M.D. will guide you as you read.

In this chapter, you'll learn about a few caveats to keep in mind before you begin treating yourself. Please refer to this section often for any safety guidelines and dosage questions. You'll also find helpful information in the appendices. If you have any questions, please consult a qualified health professional for guidance.

Safety First

Before using any of the herbs listed in this book, be sure to consult Appendix A for any contraindications, such as what to avoid during pregnancy or when nursing or taking prescription drugs.

If you're taking prescription medication, don't take any herbs that are not regarded as safe for all persons without first checking with your health-care practitioner. If you're taking medication for a particular ailment, you shouldn't also take herbs for that ailment without first checking with your health-care practitioner. Mixing herbs with prescription drugs can cause exacerbated or unpredictable effects. This is especially the case when you are using an herb for the same purpose as a drug. You may end up with a double dose!

It may be wise to gradually decrease the amount of drugs you are taking while gradually increasing the amount of herbs taken internally over a period of time rather than making any abrupt changes. Separating drugs from herbs for at least three hours can also be wise as many combinations have not been tried or tested.

Dosage Guidelines

Dosages will depend in part on the herbs you are using. If you're using a commercial product, of course you should follow the dosage guidelines on the product packaging. If you've made your own tea or tincture, in general, 1 cup (235 ml) of tea, 1 dropperful of tincture, or 1 or 2 tablets or capsules qualifies as a single dose. For an acute, serious, right-there-in-your-face type of illness, one dose every hour or two would be appropriate. Except while sleeping, of course—rest is good medicine in its own right.

For a chronic health concern, one dose three or four times daily is appropriate. Some herbalists recommend "pulsing" remedies to treat chronic conditions, which means ten days on, then three days off, in a continuing cycle. Pulsing helps the body acclimate and learn to respond even without the herbs. Another pulsing regimen is six days on, one day off, with a three-day break every two or three weeks.

When you are using herbs for therapeutic purposes, continue with the appropriate dosage for at least a week, and then evaluate your progress. If your health concern has been remedied, then you can stop taking the herb formula on a regular basis. However, you might wish to include some of it in your diet from time to time as a "tonic tune-up."

SPECIAL SITUATIONS

The general dosage guidelines discussed above are generally true for adults of average weight. However, dosages may need to be adjusted for different people or different categories of people. For example, large people need more than small people. Women may need less than men. Reduce the dose by one-fourth for those over 65 and by one-half for those over 70.

To figure out a dosage for children, follow one of two rules:

1. **COWLING'S RULE:** Take the child's age at his or her next birthday and divide by 24. The resulting fraction is the amount of the adult dosage the child can have. For example, a five-year-old will be six at his next birthday. The number 6 divided by 24 equals $1/4$; this child should have $1/4$ of the adult dosage.

2. **CLARK'S RULE:** Divide the child's weight by 150. The resulting fraction is the amount of the adult dosage the child can have. For

example, for a 50-pound (23 kg) child, 50 divided by 150 equals $1/3$; this child can have $1/3$ of the adult dosage.

Check with your health-care practitioner if you have any questions or concerns.

FOR HERBS

In general, one cup of tea equals one dropperful of tincture equals two capsules or tablets. If dealing with an acute condition, such as if you are fighting an infection, it may be necessary to use either one cup of tea, a dropperful of tincture, or two capsules or tablets every two waking hours, at least for a couple of days. Then as the condition improves, make those dosages further apart, to a couple of times a day, until no longer needed.

FOR HOMEOPATHICS

Homeopathy is based on the law of similars, or the philosophy that "like cures like." It was developed from the work of Dr. Samuel Hahnemann (1755–1843) who sought an alternative to the barbaric medicinal practices of his time and wanted to offer a safer, more effective form of treatment.

A homeopathic remedy is a tremendously diluted solution of a substance that would, in the body of a healthy person, produce symptoms similar to those of a particular illness. The solution contains an infinitesimal amount of the substance; you might say it contains a pattern replica of the substance. Exposure to the pattern replica, however, triggers a powerful healing response from the body. In other words, by stimulating the body's own healing response, a homeopathic remedy encourages the body to heal itself.

Homeopathic remedies can affect amazingly fast-acting and profound cures. The degree of success, however, depends on selecting the right remedy for a person's constitution. Some basic guidelines for choosing and using homeopathic remedies follow, but you may also benefit from consultation with a professional homeopath to gain insight into the best remedies for your constitution. Note that homeopathy often calls for very small doses of substances that in large doses could be toxic. Do not confuse homeopathic remedies with herbal remedies.

Homeopathic remedies come in the form of small pellets, alcohol solutions, and water solutions. The usual dosage is three or four pellets, or as many liquid drops as the package label recommends, taken under the tongue four times daily. Rather than swallowing the pellets whole, allow them to dissolve slowly under the tongue to be better absorbed by one's mucous membranes. For best results, do not eat or drink for ten minutes before and after taking a homeopathic remedy.

FOR VITAMINS

Check the label for dosage suggestions.

FOR ESSENTIAL OILS

Do not use essential oils internally. For external use, use two drops of pure essential oil to 1 tablespoon (30 ml) of carrier oil such as sunflower oil. Lavender and tea tree oil can be applied undiluted (neat) using no more than five drops at a time. Avoid using essential oils topically during pregnancy, unless you have consulted with your health practitioner.

PREPARATIONS 101: WHAT YOU NEED TO KNOW TO MAKE THE NATURAL REMEDIES IN THIS BOOK

Chances are you have many of the ingredients you need in your kitchen, pantry, or garden to make home remedies. If not, they are easily obtained at health foods stores and even some grocery stores. Once you have everything you need, you can use this section of the book to create beneficial preparations for over one hundred conditions. Let's start with herbal preparations.

Herbal Preparations

For our use, an herb is defined as any useful plant. Herbs are an important component when it comes to treating many of the conditions you'll read about here. In this section, you'll learn how to procure, prepare, and preserve herbs for maximum effectiveness.

BUYING AND STORING HERBS

The first step in making an herbal preparation is to select herbs that are colorful and fragrant and to buy them in bulk. As much as possible, purchase dried herbs that are cut rather than powdered, because powdering causes them to lose their essential oils more quickly.

Growing your own herbal remedies is a wonderful pursuit! Keep in mind, though, if you have fresh herbs in your garden or find them in the wild, you will need to use two to three times the amount listed here, as fresh herbs weigh more than dried herbs. You can also dry your fresh harvest by placing herbs loosely in a clean paper bag and allow them to dry in a shady warm area of the house (such as an attic) or even the backseat of your car.

Whether you are buying dried herbs in bulk from a store or using dried herbs from your garden, store the herbs in a glass jar or non-plastic airtight container. (Plastic is too permeable to protect plant remedies.) Be sure to avoid any moisture on the rims and remove any cardboard inner lid. Ideally, you should not be able to smell the herbs through the container. If you can find amber-colored bottles (I've used recycled bottles that some types of vitamins are sold in), they are great. These dark-colored bottles help keep out light, which will bleach your herbs and cause them to lose their medicinal properties more quickly.

Store herbs in a cupboard where they can be protected from light and heat to better conserve their flavors and therapeutic properties. Many herb books say that leaves and flowers keep for one year and that roots and barks keep for two to three years. However, taste, color, and smell are even better indicators of potency. Nature will provide more herbs the next year, so ideally purchase no more than you are likely to use within the year.

LABELING HERBS FOR USE

Six months from now, it might be difficult to recognize catnip from oregano, so label all of your herbs upon storage. It is also a good idea to write the date of when you purchased or dried the plant material. I also like to write the Latin name of the plant on its container. It helps me learn these beautiful poetic names, which are the same in every language. After writing and saying them a few times, they'll become part of your memory! You'll find the Latin names in Appendix A.

PREPARING HERBS

Grinding herbs is necessary if you are using larger pieces of your own harvested plant material (such as fennel seed, cinnamon sticks, or rose hips) or when you need to bruise whole seeds that are tightly compacted and need help in releasing their flavors. To grind herbs, put the ingredients into a mortar and crush gently with a pestle.

You can also use a blender for grinding herbs, just be sure to do only small batches. If you ever need to grind resinous or sticky herbs, place the herbs in the freezer for a few hours first and they will break up easily in a blender. A coffee grinder also suffices for most dried herbs, but don't use it for coffee too or your coffee will taste like herbs and your herbs like coffee. However you decide to grind your herbs, do it just enough to release some of the aromas from the herbs.

When making herbal products, singing, praying, and offering blessings are always good practices!

You can use herbs in many ways for healing. Instructions follow on how to make a tea, tincture, compress, poultice, eyewash, facial steam, and more. Let's get started!

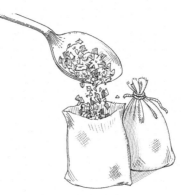

Teas

For centuries, people have enjoyed the benefits of herbal teas. Nothing warms the body and soul like holding a fragrant steaming cup of herbal tea, inhaling its subtle scents as you slowly sip. Why limit ourselves to caffeinated beverages like coffee when the world of herbs can bring us flavor, variety, nutrients, and numerous health benefits?

TEA FOR A TIME-OUT

Another benefit from drinking herbal teas is that it gives us an opportunity in our busy days to take a bit of time for ourselves. Tasting and savoring herbal teas provides us with time for reflection and peace. As we drink herbal tea, we can use the time to think, "I'm nourishing my nervous system" or perhaps "I'm strengthening my immune system," as our brain receives signals from the subtle qualities of the plants.

When using teas for healing, use them for at least one week and then evaluate your progress. If your health concern has gone, then you can stop using the herb on a regular basis and instead include it from time to time as a "tonic tune up."

USE SUSTAINABLE TEAS

Teas that are sold prepackaged in tea bags provide convenience for the go-go-go lifestyle. Yet in order for herbs to be put into these tea bags, they need to be ground into a very fine cut that exposes the surface areas of the herbs thousands of times, thus allowing flavorful and therapeutic essential oils to evaporate more quickly.

Herbs available in loose bulk form make a wider world of herbs available. With the help of a tea strainer, you can bring the benefits of less processed herbs into your life. It can also be less expensive to buy herbs in bulk, and doing so offers you the opportunity to select exactly what herbs you need and want. When fresh herbs are available and abundant in your garden, they are also wonderful to use in herbal tea.

If you must buy prepackaged tea in tea bags, we suggest that you buy from companies that support your beliefs, whether it is organic farming, recycled packaging, hemp tea bags, employing indigenous peoples to harvest herbs and protect the rainforest rather than destroy it, or all of the above.

MAKING THE PERFECT CUP OF TEA

When making tea, start with pure water—distilled (not from plastic bottles as they may contain carcinogens), spring, filtered, or well water. Use one heaping teaspoon (5 g) of dry herbs per cup (235 ml) of hot water. If you are using fresh as opposed to dried herbs, triple the amount as fresh herbs contain high levels of water.

Health food and herb stores offer muslin tea bags and tea balls, which can be filled with herbs and used to steep them to make herbal tea. However, when filling a tea ball, only fill it half way, as tea will expand several-fold as it steeps. If you don't have a strainer or a way to strain out the herbs, know that herbs will eventually sink to the bottom of the cup.

ADDING FLAVOR TO YOUR TEA

Tea can be enhanced with a touch of honey, agave nectar, apple juice (or its concentrate), maple syrup, raw sugar, or a squeeze of fresh lemon, lime, or orange. Raw honey contains enzymes which help reduce inflammation, as well as nourishing minerals and antiseptic compounds. The darker honeys are the more nutritious in terms of mineral content. The lighter-colored honeys tend to have a milder flavor. Remember that honey should never be given to babies under one year of age, as there is a slight danger of botulism. I often add cinnamon extract as a sugar-free sweetener. Some tea drinkers like to use maple syrup.

Licorice root or stevia leaf (an herb from South America) is also added to teas to impart sweetness. Licorice is an anti-diuretic and added to herbal tea blends in Asia to help prevent the herbs from quickly being urinated out. However, use licorice with caution in cases of high blood pressure and water retention. Adding milk to herbal tea usually masks the delicate herbal flavors.

DIFFERENT WAYS TO PREPARE TEA

There are a variety of methods for making tea. Try a few different ones and see what becomes your favorite. Here are a few methods to choose from.

The Teapot Method

Teapots come in a wide variety of shapes and sizes and can delight even the most whimsical of tastes. Prepare your china or porcelain teapot by filling it with hot water and allowing it to stand for a minute or so before you add any tea. This warms the pot so that the tea you pour into it will not cool down quickly and impede the steeping process. Then pour off the water, add loose herbs (1 heaping teaspoon [5 g] for each cup plus 1 extra teaspoon "for the pot"), and fill the pot with boiling water. Cover and allow the herbs and water to steep for 10 to 15 minutes. This also allows the tea to cool to a comfortable drinking temperature. To serve the tea, simply hold a strainer over each cup as you pour.

Hot-Water Infusion

The infusion method refers to teas made from fresh plant material. This is an ideal method for herbal leaves, flowers, and seeds and even roots (such as ginger, osha, and valerian) that have delicate essential oils that would be diminished if boiled. It is best if seeds are lightly bruised using a mortar and pestle to help release their flavor and properties.

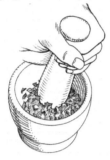

To prepare a hot-water infusion, simply boil 1 cup (235 ml) of water and remove it from the heat. Add 1 heaping teaspoon (5 g) of herb, cover (to prevent the delicate essential oils from evaporating), and allow it to steep for 10 to 20 minutes. When making a more medicinal tea, up to 1 ounce (28 g) of herb can be used per 1 pint (475 ml) of water. Strain the herbs out with a strainer as you pour your tea into a cup before serving.

French Press

A French press is a glass pot protected by a metal frame. Although they are marketed for serving coffee, they work great for herbal tea. Simply add a heaping teaspoon (5 g) of dried herb per cup of water to the press, cover with hot water, and allow the mixture to steep for 10 minutes. The press automatically strains out the herbs, and you can press the herbs with the plunger of the French press to further release their therapeutic value. Note that if you break the glass pot, you can buy a replacement without having to replace the metal frame.

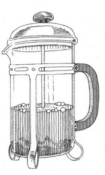

Sun Tea

To make sun tea, place 1 cup (30 g) of herb or herb mixture or 12 tea bags and 1 gallon (3.8 L) of water in a clear glass container. Allow the herbs to sit in sunlight for 4 to 6 hours. It is best to cover the jar to prevent leaves and other items from blowing into the jar. Strain before serving. Note that sun teas work best with leaves and flowers.

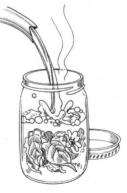

Cold Water Infusion

Cold-water infusions retain more vitamin C and have a brighter color than hot-water infusions. To prepare a cold-water infusion, simply fill a glass pitcher with fresh-picked herb from the list below and cover with spring water. Allow the mixture to steep in the refrigerator for 8 to 12 hours or overnight.

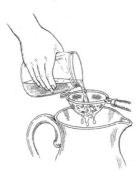

The following are good choices for cold infusion:

- Anise seed
- Bee balm herb
- Catnip herb
- Hyssop herb
- Lavender flowers
- Lemon balm herb
- Lemon verbena herb
- Lilac flowers
- Peppermint herb
- Rooibos herb
- Rose flowers
- Rosemary herb
- Spearmint herb

Cold-water infused tea keeps for up to 4 days in the refrigerator. Should you desire to warm the herbs slightly after the steeping process, do so at preferably no higher than 110° F (43°C) to protect the enzymes. You can also brew tea in the refrigerator for 4 to 5 hours.

Decoction

A decoction is a tea-making method that uses more heat and time and is the preferred method for making teas with roots and barks and some seeds, which are harder, woodier, and require more energy to extract their precious qualities. This is because a decoction helps to draw out the mineral salts of a plant. To prepare a decoction, simmer 1 heaping tablespoon (10 g) of herb in 3 cups (705 ml) of water for about 20 minutes, keeping the pot covered. Be sure to keep the heat very low, as many roots and barks (such as ginger and cinnamon) can evaporate and flavor and medicinal properties can be lost. The herbs can be strained out or left to steep overnight before straining.

Overnight Jar Method

The overnight jar method is an excellent method for extracting the maximum amount of medicinal potential from an herb. It takes time, but it is well worth the effort. This method is more appropriate when the goal of the tea is more medicinal rather than, "Company's coming. Let's have some tea."

Add about 2 ounces (55 g) of root or bark or 1 ounce (28 g) of flower or leaf to the bottom of a clean 2-quart (1.9 L) canning jar. Cover with enough boiling water to reach the top of the jar and put the lid on, allowing the herbs to steep for as long as 30 minutes for seeds, 2 hours for flowers, 4 hours for leaves, and overnight for roots and barks. In the morning, strain the herbs out and enjoy the nutrient-rich brew.

Note that this method is not suggested for licorice root, slippery elm bark, or valerian root, which will simply taste too medicinal or in the case of slippery elm will become too mucilaginous to bear consuming.

RECYCLING HERBS

You can return the herbs that you strain out of the tea to the earth by composting them or by simply throwing the leftover herbs into your yard, garden, or peppermint or whatever patch. Always be conscious of giving something back to the planet rather than just taking from it. An old Hindu saying to remember is, "If you have water to throw away, throw it on a plant."

STORING PREPARED TEA

Tea is full of life force, and any microorganism that enters the tea can multiply. If there is any sign of spoilage, such as bubbles or fermentation, or you a notice a flat flavor, discard the tea and make a fresh batch. Most refrigerated teas will keep for four days in the refrigerator.

Herbal Tinctures

While sipping a cup of tea is lovely, depending on your condition, you may want to use a tincture instead. A tincture is a more concentrated form of an herb. As you read through the book, you'll be instructed on when it's best to use either or both. You can find herbal tinctures at natural food stores or learn to make your own. Here's how:

Tinctures have traditionally been made on the new moon so that the energy of the moon can draw out the properties of the herbs. The herbs you are tincturing are known as the mark. Prepare the herbs by chopping or grinding them. You may tincture several herbs together if you are creating a formula.

Put them into a jar and cover with about an extra inch of brandy or vodka. Alcohol will help to preserve the herbs and extract both the water-soluble and alcohol-soluble properties (any substance used to extract the herbs is known as the menstrum). Keep in mind that alcohol must be at least 50 proof to have good preservative qualities. Vodka is the purest grain alcohol. (Alcohol is also ideal for extracting fats, resins, waxes, and most alkaloids.) Tinctures made in alcohol will last for many years.

Tinctures may also be made using vegetable glycerin rather than alcohol. This is best when making tinctures for those who are alcohol intolerant as well as for children, pregnant women, and nursing mothers. Glycerin is both a solvent and preservative that has an effectiveness somewhere between water and alcohol. It is naturally sweet, pleasant tasting, and helps to extract mucilage, vitamins, minerals, and tannins from plant material. It is good for herbs high in tannins but doesn't extract resins well. It is slightly antiseptic, demulcent, and healing when diluted. Glycerites are usually prepared using 1 part water to 2 parts glycerin. Glycerites have a shorter shelf life than tinctures prepared with alcohol, about 1 to 3 years.

Apple cider vinegar, preferably organic, can also be used as a menstrum. Look for vinegar with 5.7 percent acetic acid or thereabouts for a long shelf life. It is also a digestive tonic and can be used to season food. Warm the vinegar first before pouring over the herbs. Avoid using a metal lid as it may rust, or place a piece of waxed paper between the jar and the lid. This type of tincture will have a shelf life from 6 months up to 4 years.

Regardless of the menstrum used, shake daily and strain after a month, first with a strainer and then through a clean, undyed cloth, squeezing tightly. Pressing the herbs through a potato ricer while still in the cloth can be helpful. Bottle in amber glass bottles. Compost the mark. Label and date. Store away from heat and light. Take tinctures by putting a dropperful in a bit of hot water.

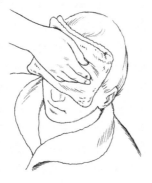

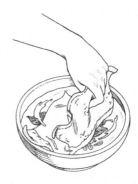

Compresses

You'll hear quite a bit about compresses in this book. That's because compresses are a very effective way to use herbal teas topically to help heal wounds, inflammation, rashes, and skin infections. We absorb what we put on our bodies through the skin. The warmth or cooling properties of a compress can also give comfort. Compresses can also be used to relieve pain, headaches, and menstrual cramps, soothe sore joints and sprains, improve circulation, relieve spasms, soothe bug bites, repair tissue, and stimulate sweat glands and the lymphatic system.

HOT OR COLD COMPRESS?

The best way to determine whether you should use a hot or cold compress is to ask the person needing treatment whether they think cold or hot will offer them the most relief. In general, however, hot compresses are good for backache, arthritis pain, and sore throats. Applying a hot compress to a sluggish area of the body will increase circulation. Ginger compresses are especially warming and pain relieving. Hot compresses should be left in place until the heat has dissipated. Replace with another compress when removing the first one. Three applications are common. After the third hot compress, apply a cool compress to the area briefly.

Cold compresses constrict blood flow and are best for inflamed conditions such as swellings or a headache (you can actually use a hot compress on the back of the neck with a cold compress on the head for relief). Peppermint compresses are especially cooling and inflammation reducing. When a cold compress becomes warm, replace with a new cool cloth. Whenever a compress is done, keep the treated area warm afterwards to avoid chilling the person receiving treatment.

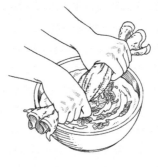

HOW TO MAKE A COMPRESS

Compresses are made by soaking a clean towel (preferably soft cotton or linen) in hot or cold herbal tea or five drops of essential oil per cup of water. Be sure to stir the oil into the water to disperse it. The cloth is then wrung out and applied to the area needing treatment. Covering the wet cloth with a dry towel will help the cloth stay hot or cold. Applying a hot-water bottle can also help the compress retain its heat.

Applying a bag of frozen vegetables or crushed ice over the compress can further enhance a cold compress.

You can hold a compress in place by applying a cut clean sock or pair of tights to hold the compress in place so it doesn't slide off. However, resting while a compress is on is ideal. When the compress temperature changes (the hot cools down or cool warms up), resoak the cloth in the hot or cold tea and reapply. This can be repeated for several rounds if needed.

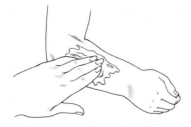

Poultices

A poultice is an herb applied directly to the skin, which can also bring relief from many of the conditions you'll read about here. To prepare a poultice, crush fresh or dried herb, and mix with hot water, apple cider vinegar, or olive or castor oil (the amount depends on what your needs are and what is available) to make a thick paste. The liquid helps to hold the herbs together and in place. If you are using dried herbs, you can add cornmeal or freshly ground flaxseed to thicken the paste, once mixed with water.

HOW TO USE POULTICES

Apply the poultice to the area of the body needing attention, such as a wound, being sure to use enough herb to cover the area. Poultices can be reapplied several times a day or in a succession during one sitting. Either comfrey or plantain leaves or a simple washcloth can be used to hold poultices in place. Poultices are best when moist. Therefore, when a poultice dries out, reapply it. Also, when a cold poultice gets hot or a hot poultice grows cold, remove the spent one and reapply a fresh one if desired.

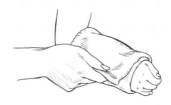

Here are a few of the healing properties of herbs when used in a poultice:

- Cabbage draws out pus and toxins.
- Carrots repair bruises and chapped skin.
- Comfrey leaves or root decrease swelling, sores, and wounds.
- Cucumber cools inflammation and moistens.
- Oatmeal can reduce inflammation and insect bite itches.
- Plantain draws out toxins.
- Potato reduces the inflammation of bruises and sprains.
- Tofu draws out fever and inflammation.

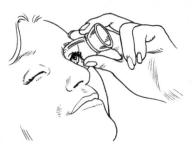

warmed or allowed to reach room temperature before using. Especially in cases of eye infections, it is important to sterilize the eyecup between uses either by running it through the dishwasher with a heat dry cycle or by filling the cup with boiling water for a minute and discarding the water.

Eyewashes

Eyewashes can be used for tired and inflamed as well as infected eyes. Using an eyewash causes the blood vessels of the eyes to contract and then relax. It's the perfect antidote when your eyes are tired from reading or working at the computer. Some even claim eyewashes can improve vision.

HOW TO PREPARE AN EYEWASH

Place 1 scant teaspoon (3 g) of herb in 1 cup (235 ml) of water and simmer at low heat for 10 minutes to assure sterility. Note that eyewashes use herb amounts that are somewhat weaker than tea. Use a very fine strainer to strain the tea to avoid getting particles of herbs in the eyes. Cool the tea to body temperature before administering. Be sure to remove contact lenses before administering any eyewash.

Next, pour the well-strained tea into a sterilized eyecup. Lean back and pour the mixture into the eyes, being sure to blink several times so the eye is well bathed. Lean forward into a sink to catch the remaining solution and repeat with the other eye.

Only use herbs mentioned in the text that have traditionally been used and recommended as eyewashes. Make eyewashes fresh for each day being used to avoid introducing bacteria into the eyes. Whatever is not used in one treatment should be refrigerated and then slightly

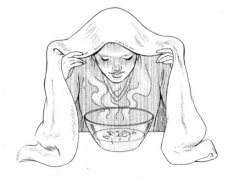

Facial Steams

A facial steam is an excellent way to use herbs to do a deep cleansing, to relax facial muscles, and to improve circulation. It's especially lovely before a party or when you want to look your best, as an invigorating facial steam provides a rosy glow. Facial steams can benefit conditions such as asthma, bronchitis, cough, laryngitis, nasal congestion, and sinus infections by helping to increase circulation and loosen mucus from the respiratory tract.

To perform a facial steam, first wash your face. Next, pour 1 quart (950 ml) of boiling water over a handful of herbs in a heatproof glass bowl. If you have long hair, tie your hair back. Locate your head above the bowl of water and drape a towel over your head. Keep your face about 10 inches (25.4 cm) away from the water source to avoid getting burned as you inhale the sensuous steam for 5 to 7 minutes. If the steam starts to cool down too much, gently blow into the herb pot to cause more steam to rise. Facial steams can be done once or twice a week, or twice daily when congested for 3 to 4 days in a row.

Mouthwashes and Gargles

Mouthwashes and gargles are made by preparing a standard tea and allowing it to cool. Gargle if you want to treat the throat and/or rinse the mouth if that is the place of concern, swishing the liquid around in the mouth and then spitting it into the sink. This can be repeated up to half a dozen times.

Bath Therapy

Merging herbs and warm water can be a great way to incorporate two healing principles, as well as improving relaxation. We absorb the properties of plants through the skin. It is best to bathe at least a couple of hours after a big meal to avoid interfering with digestion. Baths before bed aid sleep as they elevate the body's temperature and the body will compensate by lowering its temperature, thus making us ready for sleep.

BATHING WITH HERBS

To use herbs or substances such as uncooked oatmeal in a bath, simply tie a handful of either fresh or dried herbs or grain into a washcloth and secure with a hair tie. Use a dark cloth so you don't stain your light-colored ones. If you have a stash of clean lost "single" socks, those also work great for bath bags.

You can also make a strong herbal tea with about 1/2 cup (15 g) of herbs. Simmer for 20 minutes, and then strain the tea into the tub. Or simply throw a few ready-made tea bags into the bath. Place the herb-filled cloth or tea bags in very hot running water. As you bathe, use the herb-filled cloth to scrub your body as you deeply inhale the benefits.

When draining the water out of the tub, if you have used something that is floating loose and not enclosed, such as seaweeds or fresh flowers, be sure to use a metal filter over the drain so that you don't clog your pipes. The spent flower and plant material can then be composted.

USING AROMATHERAPY IN THE BATH

An even easier way to prepare the bath is use five to ten drops of pure essential oil (if it's available) as a substitute for the desired herb. For example, you can make a bath with lavender flowers, either in a sock or a tea, or you can simply add 5 to ten drops lavender essential oil to the bath. Add essential oils after filling the tub so that the fragrance does not dissipate and swish the water before getting in so the oil doesn't stick to one part of your body. It can be helpful to close the shower curtain or door to hold in steam. When the bath has cooled to a comfortable temperature, get into it.

Note that if you choose to use any of the citrus products such as lemon peel or orange essential oil, use these at night, as getting exposed to sunlight after bathing in citrus products can make you more photosensitive. Also, if you are using fresh or dried citrus peels, be sure they are organic since they will be coming in contact with your skin.

Following are a few bath ideas for specific conditions. As a rule of thumb, add a couple of handfuls of herbs per bath.

APPLE CIDER VINEGAR BATH: This helps relieve sore muscles, itchy skin, and sunburn. Vinegar helps draw pollutants out of the body. It is an acid medium and contains alpha hydroxy acids. It is also mildly antiseptic, antifungal, and naturally deodorizing. You can even infuse therapeutic herbs—such as calendula, chamomile, lavender, lemon balm, peppermint, spearmint, rose petals, sage, and scented geraniums—into the vinegar to make an herbal vinegar. Add ¹/₄ cup (8 g) herbs to 1 cup (235 ml) vinegar and let steep two weeks to a month. Strain the herbs out before using and rebottle the vinegar.

BAKING SODA BATH: This alkalinizing and detoxifying bath can help calm allergic reactions, chicken pox, eczema, hives, itchy skin, insect bites, poison ivy, sunburn, and fungal infections. Use 1 pound (455 g) per bath.

COLD AND FLU BATH: Try the following bath additions when you want to soothe deep muscle aches that often accompany viral infections: Epsom salts, ginger root, marjoram, mustard seed powder, pine needles, and thyme leaves.

DETOX BATH: Consider using the following cleansing herbs in the bath to help the body get rid of environmental pollutants, internal toxins, and to cleanse the lymphatics: Apple cider vinegar, cypress essential oil, Epsom salts, ginger root, grapefruit, juniper, lavender flowers, lemon peel, rosemary leaves, sage leaves, seaweed (can be bought dried in natural food stores unless you live close to the ocean), and tea tree essential oil.

DRY SKIN BATH: Herbs can have a soothing, lubricating effect from the outside. Moisturize with calendula flowers, chamomile flowers, comfrey leaves, elder flowers, fennel seed, jasmine flowers, lavender flowers, oatmeal, rose buds, and violet leaves.

EPSOM SALTS BATH: This method cleanses the lymphatics, is relaxing for sore muscles, softening to the skin, and detoxifying after bodywork. Epsom salts help to get drugs, chemicals, and pollutants out of body. Those with diabetes, hypertension, or heart disease should rinse off after the bath to avoid absorbing excess sodium from the salt.

FLOWER POWER BATH: Float fresh flowers or orange or lemon peels into the bath water for a refreshing flower power bath. Flower suggestions include lilac, dandelion, daisies, honeysuckle, jasmine, camellia, or lavender. Or, you can trim aromatic leaves (mint, lemon balm, etc.) and put the excess in to the bath.

ITCHY SKIN BATH: To calm itchy skin resulting from insect bites, chicken pox, and poison ivy, use apple cider vinegar, baking soda, chickweed herb, lavender flowers, oatmeal, red clover blossoms, or violet leaf. All of these substances have soothing, anti-inflammatory properties. Essential oils to use in an itchy skin bath include cedar wood, Roman chamomile, lavender, peppermint, and sandalwood.

OATMEAL BATH: Oatmeal calms irritated skin, poison ivy, and dermatitis, and helps lower high blood pressure and alleviate stress. It is rich in minerals like calming calcium, and its naturally occurring mucilage provides a protective balm to sooth the skin. It is very simple to whiz plain uncooked oatmeal in the blender to make a bath powder, or tie ¹/₂ cup (40 g) into a bath bag.

OILY SKIN BATH: Help balance excess oil production in the skin with the astringent properties of basil leaf, lemon peel, or apple cider vinegar.

PREMENSTRUAL BATH: Calms cramps and emotional upheaval with nature's bounty of chamomile flowers, clary sage flowers, or lavender flowers.

SALT BATH: Salt helps to soften the skin and has been used to treat burns. Salt baths are also good after bodywork and for eczema, psoriasis, rashes, and sore muscles. Salt is considered cooling and draws out toxins. Baking soda mixed with salt is suggested after exposure to radiation. Use ¹/₂ cup (120 g) to 2 cups (240 g) of sea salt. People with insulin-dependent diabetes, serious heart disease, and open sores should avoid salt baths as you can absorb the sodium through the skin. Salt can sting on an open cut!

SITZ BATH: Use a baby bathtub for this, if you have one, and sit down in it. Sit so that the water is below the knees and not above the naval. The water should come up about 5 inches (12.7 cm) and the feet should not be submerged. Use cold-water hip baths for back and lower organ problems such as menstrual pain, pelvic inflammatory disease, hemorrhoids, and congestion in the liver and spleen. A cold compress can be applied to the forehead. Sitz baths can be taken as 3 minutes in hot water, followed by 2 minutes in cold water. Alternate, always ending with cold. Keep warm afterwards.

When done bathing, visualize the tension draining out of you, as the water runs out of the tub. Know that you have been soothed by the warm water and Earth Mother. Rise carefully from the bath to avoid lightheadedness. Follow the bath with a cool rinse if desired.

Aromatherapy Preparations

Aromatherapy can be soothing and uplifting. From reducing stress to easing depression, this is one natural remedy you'll want in your tool kit. There are many ways to bring the fragrant beauty of aromatherapy into your daily life. You've already learned about using aromatherapy in the bathtub, but its use definitely does not stop there. Here's how:

FACIAL SPRAY: Add 1 teaspoon (5 ml) of vodka to 1/4 teaspoon (1 ml) essential oil and 4 ounces (120 ml) of distilled water in a clean spray bottle. Shake and mist the face with eyes and mouth closed.

MASSAGE OIL: Mix 1 ounce (28 ml) of your favorite oil with 12 drops total of birch, rosemary, juniper, or lavender oil. Or use 25 drops of essential oil in 1/2 cup (120 ml) of oil.

MOUTH WASH: Add 1 or 2 drops of peppermint or tea tree essential oil to 1/4 cup (60 ml) water. Swish around in your mouth and spit out.

ROOM SCENT: Essential oils are antibacterial and can be used to freshen a sick room and prevent others from catching an illness. To use aromatherapy scents in your home, try putting 20 drops of essential oil and 1 tablespoon (15 ml) of brandy (to keep the oils dispersed rather than floating to the top of the bottle) into a clean spray bottle. Add 8 ounces (235 ml) of water and use as a room spray. You can also place about ten drops of essential oil in a humidifier, on a radiator, or in a pot of water on top of the stove. There are also many aromatherapy diffusers ranging in price that can fill any size room with beautiful fragrance.

SHOWER: Add 8 drops essential oil maximum to a washcloth and use it to vigorously scrub your body.

STEAMING: Add essential oil to a pot of hot water, place a towel over your head, and breathe in the steamy aroma.

TISSUE: Place several drops of essential oil on a tissue and inhale deeply.

TOOTH POWDER: In 4 ounces (115 g) baking soda and 1 ounce (28 g) sea salt, add 15 drops essential oil (peppermint, clove, cinnamon, or tea tree are all good choices).

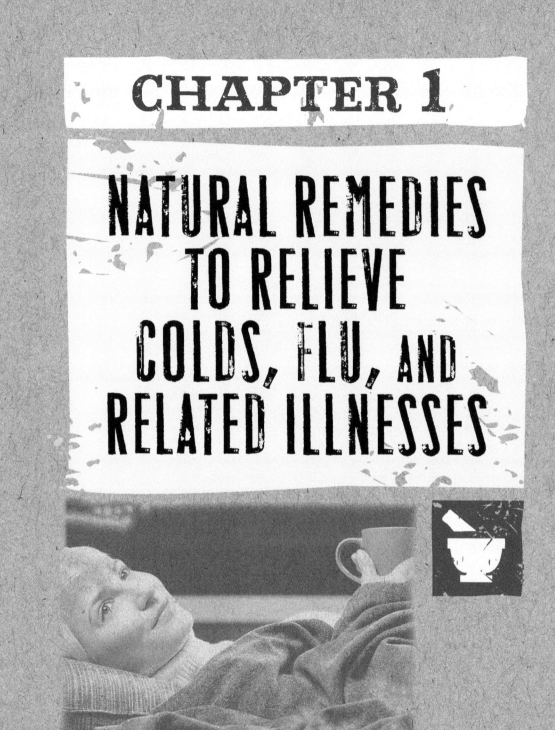

CHAPTER 1

NATURAL REMEDIES TO RELIEVE COLDS, FLU, AND RELATED ILLNESSES

We can't always avoid getting sick. It can even be an opportunity to rest. Here are some ideas to help you get through an illness with a minimum of distress.

Combating Colds and Flu

Colds and flu are both viral infections that often occur in the winter when we are stressed out and stuck inside with lots of people and germs. Viruses enter the body through the respiratory tract and attach to cells lining the nose, throat, and bronchial tubes. Exposure to cold, damp, wind, and rapid temperature change can make us more susceptible to viruses. Colds manifest slowly with cough, nasal congestion, and sore throat, usually without fever. Flu comes on more suddenly with fever, sore muscles, fatigue, and cough. These ailments can last from a few days to about a week, but they can progress into bronchitis, strep throat, or asthma if not properly treated. The sooner one takes action against infection, the easier to minimize its effects. Let's look at some natural remedies you can use to combat colds, flu, and related illnesses.

HERBS FOR COLDS AND FLU

Herbs can help fight infection by stimulating white blood cell production and through their direct antiseptic properties. Many herbs help relieve colds and flu:

Echinacea root stimulates immune-supporting white blood cells, T cells, macrophage, and interferon activity. If you take echinacea at the first sign of a cold, it can ease symptoms according to a study published in the *Journal of Clinical Pharmacological Therapy* in 2004.

When high fever is of concern, boneset is an important immune stimulant and one of the most effective herbs for colds and flu. This is due to its diaphoretic properties, which means it promotes sweating and the release of toxins. It is extremely bitter, so it is best taken as a tincture or in capsule form.

Yarrow leaf and flower also reduce fever through diaphoresis and are antiseptic. Peppermint leaf promotes sweating, has antiviral properties, and is gentle enough for children.

Cures from Grandma's Kitchen

Mix 2 teaspoons (10 ml) of apple cider vinegar and 2 teaspoons (13 ml) of honey in 1 cup (235 ml) of hot water and drink three times daily to break up mucus congestion. Diluted lemon in hot water or berry juices can help relieve fever. These have antimicrobial properties and help to thin mucus secretions.

When nausea accompanies an illness, ginger root, known as the warming herb, warms chills, fights infection, and alleviates stomach distress. Peppermint is also beneficial, being both antiviral and a digestive aid.

Cayenne pepper is rich in vitamin C, warms chills, and decreases congestion. Garlic dilates bronchioles, decreasing congestion and chest colds, and is considered an herbal antibiotic. Thyme leaf expels phlegm and relieves congestion. It is antiseptic and an immune stimulant. You can look for teas, tinctures, or capsules at natural food stores that offer combinations of these herbs, or you can make your own remedies (see "Preparations 101").

With acute conditions such as colds and flu, take a dose of your herbal remedy every couple of hours (when not sleeping), decreasing the dosage as you improve.

CHINESE REMEDIES FOR COLDS AND FLU

Chinese patent formulas, prepackaged herbal combinations that have long traditions of use, can also be effective in treating colds and flu. Yin Chiao is used at the onset of infection to combat fever, sore muscles, chills, dry cough, and sore throat. Gan Mao Ling is used to combat cold and flu symptoms of fever, sore throat, swollen glands, and muscular stiffness. These remedies come in pill form. Follow the directions on the labels as pill size can vary greatly.

VITAMINS FOR COLDS AND FLU

Many people find vitamin C stimulates antibody response. You can take 1,000 mg up to three times daily to shorten the duration of a cold, though it does not necessarily prevent a cold from occurring. This is confirmed by over 30 studies that were analyzed by the *Cochrane Database Systematic Review* in 2004.

Zinc, especially in the form of lozenges, helps prevent viral replication of the cold virus in the throat by stimulating T cell response. Research at Dartmouth College showed that when people took a zinc lozenge every two hours, it shortened sick time to an average of four days. Stay under 50 mg daily unless recommended by a competent health-care practitioner.

HOMEOPATHIC RELIEF FOR COLDS AND FLU

Homeopathic remedies also help colds and flu. Anas barbariae is a homeopathic remedy used for the onset of flu symptoms, nasal discharge or congestion, chills, ear pain, and frontal sinus pain. It is available in health food stores under the name of Oscillococcinum. You can also consult with a homeopath or select the remedy that most closely resembles your symptoms. Homeopathic remedies are usually taken as three to four pellets under the tongue three times daily.

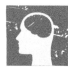

GOOD TO KNOW!

Elderberry can minimize the duration of flu symptoms including catarrh, chills, headache, and respiratory infection. According to a 2004 study published in *The Journal of International Medical Research*, when people were given elderberry syrup, (the brand name is Sambucol), 90 percent felt better after just three days! Elderberry syrup is also delicious! Take a dose every couple of hours you are awake when fighting something off. Decrease as you improve.

FOOD DO'S AND DON'TS FOR COLDS AND FLU

Foods beneficial during illness include chicken soup or miso-vegetable soup. The heat, garlic, and onions (use plenty) help break up congestion. Applesauce with cinnamon is easy to digest and cinnamon has antimicrobial properties. Pureed or baked winter squash and sweet potatoes are easy to eat when you need some nourishment but have no appetite. They are rich in beta-carotene, which helps strengthen the mucus membranes of the lungs. Broccoli, cabbage, carrots, mustard greens, parsnips, and turnips are antioxidant rich. Drink honey-sweetened lemonade as it is high in vitamin C.

SOOTHING PRACTICES FOR COLDS AND FLU

Soaking in a hot bath to which 1 cup (225 g) of Epsom salts and 7 drops of essential oil of eucalyptus or ginger has been added can promote sweating and the release of toxins. This can be done while sipping some diaphoretic herbs such as elderflower and ginger. After, dress warmly and rest.

During recovery time, rent some funny movies. Laughter can help boost immunity. Take time to rest. Be grateful that your body is telling you to slow down and take better care of yourself.

AROMATHERAPY FOR COLDS AND FLU

An aromatherapy diffuser can prevent other household members from getting sick and clear the congested person's sinuses. Essential oils to use include eucalyptus, juniper, lavender, marjoram, peppermint, pine, rosemary, and tea tree. A diffuser creates a fine mist of antimicrobial molecules in the air, which get inhaled.

Relieving Sore Throat or Strep Throat

Sore throats are a real pain in the neck! A sore throat usually develops gradually (one to two days) and may be characterized by cough, headache, tingling around the soft palate, runny nose, mild fever, and swollen neck glands. Strep throat is characterized by its sudden onset, pus in the throat, a temperature from 102 to 104°F (39 to 40°C) and swollen glands. There may be red or white spots on the tonsils; however, this only indicates strep about 50 percent of the time. The good news? Sore throats can be an opportunity for self-healing. You'll find several remedies that bring relief here.

Skip This!

Drinking lots of fruit juices can cause sugar overload, and the acidity of orange and grapefruit juice may further irritate a sore throat. Minimize dairy and wheat products for a few days to curb mucus production.

GOOD TO KNOW!
Propolis, a substance produced by bees from tree resins, helps fight infection and can be sucked in lozenges.

NATURAL RELIEF FOR SORE THROATS

Frequent gargling rinses away microbes and leaves an antiseptic coating on a sore throat. Use 1 teaspoon (5 ml) salt added to 1 cup (235 ml) of warm water or teas of echinacea, goldenseal, or juniper berry or 2 tablespoons (28 ml) apple cider vinegar in water. Gargle every hour initially, and then spit the mixture out. As you improve, gargle every three hours.

The resin propolis, a powerful infection-fighting agent that bees collect from trees to keep their own hives infection-free, helps to strengthen epithelial tissue that lines the throat, creating healthy mucosal tone and treating inflammation. Take a dropperful or two capsules every three hours that you are awake.

Natural food stores carry herbal sprays that contain antiseptic and anti-inflammatory herbs like propolis, echinacea, and myrrh. Spray on sore areas of the throat five to six times daily.

Soothing a sore throat can be aided by licorice root, which soothes irritated mucus membranes and stimulates interferon production. Marshmallow root soothes inflamed mucus membranes including sore throat. Osha root relieves respiratory congestion and improves immunity and also relieves sore throat pain. Note that you should avoid taking osha root during pregnancy as it can stimulate uterine contractions.

To help bring relief and improvement to a sore or strep throat, you can also make a compress. First, brew a strong tea of ginger. Next, soak a face towel in the hot tea, wring, wrap around throat, and cover with a dry towel. When the compress cools, resoak it in the hot tea. Reapply three or four times. You can do the same thing with warmed apple cider vinegar.

Compresses bring increased circulation to an area, moving swelling and toxins, which can then be eliminated more quickly. (See "Preparations 101" for how to make teas and compresses.)

BEST FOODS FOR SORE THROAT RELIEF

When you have a sore throat, it is not unusual to have a decreased desire for food. However, the right food choices can be beneficial. Berries, such as blackberries and mulberries, are cooling to an inflamed throat. Pineapple contains the enzyme bromelain, which helps to digest dead tissue that is permeated with infection. Barley cooked as a grain or added to soup is soothing. Garlic, leeks, and onions are all infection fighters. Leafy greens like kale are alkalinizing and are beneficial for a sore throat. Pureed carrots, sweet potatoes, or winter squash are all rich in beta-carotene and help to strengthen mucous membranes. Light soups and soft foods are ideal.

Thrifty Cures!

Holding a clove of garlic in your mouth is a powerful infection fighter because of its anti-viral and anti-bacterial effects. When tired of holding the garlic in your mouth, slowly chew it up and swallow it.

Salt also helps to relieve pain. Warm some coarse kosher salt in a frying pan and then wrap it in a clean long sock, tied at the end. Wrap it around your neck, secure with a towel, and leave in place for an hour. If you are at the beach, gargle with seawater! You can even suck on a black-pitted olive, which is high in astringent tannins that are also antiseptic.

BENEFICIAL BEVERAGES FOR SORE THROAT

It is important to double or triple your fluid intake when you have a sore throat. Helpful beverage suggestions include herb teas like licorice and slippery elm. Since it's important to consume more fluids, take frequent sips of these herbal teas throughout the day.

In addition, you can boil 1/2 ounce (15 ml) hulled barley in 1 quart (950 ml) of water for 30 minutes with the lid on. Strain, reserving the grain for use in a soup. Drink the remaining barley water.

Apple juice with seven whole cloves (which are anesthetic and antimicrobial) blended into it and strained can also help.

You can also mix 2 teaspoons (10 ml) of honey and 2 teaspoons (13 ml) apple cider vinegar in 1 cup (235 ml) of hot water and sip to curb pain and decrease infection.

VITAMINS FOR SORE THROATS

Vitamins to consider using to treat or prevent a sore throat and strep throat include 1,000 to 3,000 mg vitamin C taken with 500 mg bioflavonoids, which are astringent, tonifying, and infection fighting. (Discontinue if it burns or irritates your mouth.) Vitamin A and/or beta-carotene (10,000 IU once daily) help strengthen the mucous membranes, thereby decreasing susceptibility to infection.

Zinc lozenges inhibit viral replication. They usually contain about 15 mg of zinc per lozenge and up to five can be taken daily for up to a week.

ESSENTIAL OILS THAT SOOTHE SORE THROATS

Essential oils that soothe sore throats include eucalyptus, geranium, lavender, lemon, bitter orange, pine, Clary sage, and tea tree. Add 3 to 6 drops of essential oil to 1 cup (235 ml) of water and use as a gargle or put in an atomizer and spray directly on your throat. You can also add these oils to a vaporizer or aromatherapy diffuser to infuse the air with their antiseptic properties.

GOOD TO KNOW!
The throat is the center of expression and communication. The tendency for people to swallow anger and suppress tears and feelings of fear of rejection may all be contributing factors in sore throats. If you experience this disorder frequently, look at what you can do to bring about better communication in your life.

WHEN TO SEE YOUR M.D.
Strep throat is potentially serious and therefore must be treated with care, either holistically or allopathically. Consult a medical doctor if your throat is sore for longer than 3 days or is extremely red (look with a flashlight), if white spots appear on your throat, if there is blood in your phlegm, if you have a rash or difficulty swallowing, breathing, or opening your mouth, or if you have a fever over 102°F (39°C). When in doubt or if natural remedies do not bring about improvement within 48 hours, contact a competent health-care professional.

ACUPRESSURE FOR SORE THROATS

Acupressure points to stimulate for 30 seconds each several times daily include Lung 1, Large Intestine 4, and Stomach 9. Consult acupuncture books that demonstrate the points, or consult a trained professional.

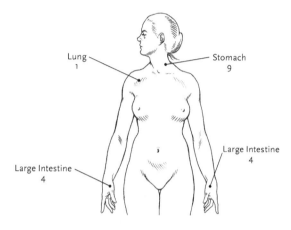

Lung 1

Stomach 9

Large Intestine 4

Large Intestine 4

SOOTHING PRACTICES FOR SORE THROATS

Go outdoors if it is a sunny day and direct some solar rays directly into the throat at the site of pain. Spend three to five minutes getting sunlight right in your throat. Sunlight is one of nature's great antiseptic agents. You can feel the warmth and healing right away! Also focus on breathing more deeply and slowly while you take in the benefits of fresh air.

GOOD TO KNOW!
You can also gargle with 1 tablespoon (15 ml) apple cider vinegar blended with two cloves of garlic and a pinch of salt. Both are soothing and anti-inflammatory.

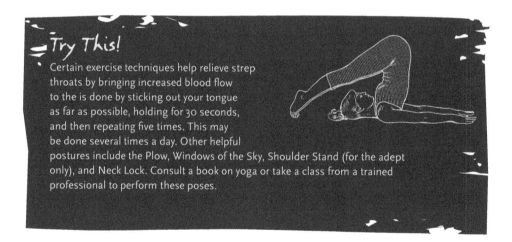

Try This!

Certain exercise techniques help relieve strep throats by bringing increased blood flow to the is done by sticking out your tongue as far as possible, holding for 30 seconds, and then repeating five times. This may be done several times a day. Other helpful postures include the Plow, Windows of the Sky, Shoulder Stand (for the adept only), and Neck Lock. Consult a book on yoga or take a class from a trained professional to perform these poses.

Relieving a Cough

A cough is the body's response to inflammation or irritation in the throat, larynx, bronchial tubes, or lungs. There are two basic kinds of coughs, congested and dry, with each one having different underlying causes. Coughs can be caused by colds, flu, bronchial infections, heartburn, sinus congestion, smoking, and the need to rid the throat of foreign matter such as dust, pollen, chemicals, and other irritants. Let's look at some natural remedies you can use to stop that nasty cough now.

HERBS TO STOP A COUGH

Drink hot wild cherry bark, horehound, or pine needle tea to break up the mucus and open and moisten the airways. You can also chew on a piece of ginger, which helps to disperse mucus congestion.

Cough drops or hard candy often help stop the tickle and moisten the throat if you have a dry cough. Look for herbal lozenges or candy in natural food stores that contain mint, ginger, horehound, hyssop, or wild cherry to calm your cough.

Licorice root, marshmallow root, and slippery elm bark all bind with phlegm and carry it out of the body via the intestines. Use as tea or lozenges as needed, up to a dozen daily.

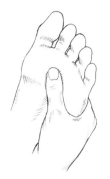

ACUPRESSURE TO STOP A COUGH

The feet contain points that correspond to all parts of the body. By massaging them, you can move blockages in other parts. To affect the lungs, rub the padded area below your big toe in various directions at the first sign of a cough. Also, hold back the toes and press on the raised area with your thumb. This will help relieve chest congestion and corresponds to the lungs according to foot reflexologists.

 WHEN TO SEE YOUR M.D.
See your doctor if you cough for more than three days for no apparent reason or if you have any of the following:

- Shortness of breath or sharp pains in your chest when you cough.
- A fever along with a persistent cough—this could be indicative of a serious respiratory illness. If you have a high fever and difficulty breathing, you may have pneumonia.
- If you cough up blood or bloody mucus or if your mucus is yellow, brown, or green and does not improve in a few days—this may indicate that you have an infection.
- Persistent chills or excessive night sweats
- Laryngitis and a persistent cough that lasts for more than three weeks

BENEFICIAL BEVERAGES FOR COUGH RELIEF

Drink at least eight 8-ounce (235 ml) glasses of water each day to relieve a cough. This is especially important if your cough is due to an illness. Water is the best expectorant you can take and will help thin the mucus and loosen the cough. Drink hot water for the best expectorant effect. Also, keep a glass of water with 2 teaspoons (10 ml) apple cider vinegar in it by the bed. Take a couple of swallows if you wake up coughing.

SOOTHING PRACTICES FOR A COUGH

Breathe in steam from a vaporizer, hot shower, or pan of boiling water. The moist air will soothe the airways and loosen sinus congestion and phlegm in your throat and lungs.

A few drops of essential oil can help fight infection and disperse congestion. Use eucalyptus, cedar, cypress, or pine to help this process.

During the winter, if your house is dry, use a humidifier and a cool-mist vaporizer in your bedroom at night. This will help thin the mucus.

Be sure to thoroughly clean the vaporizer as it can harbor bacteria. Elevate the head of your bed to allow sinuses and nasal passages to drain better.

Thrifty Cures!

To ease that cough, mix $1/4$ to $1/2$ teaspoon cayenne pepper in 1 cup (235 ml) of water and use it as a gargle for a couple of minutes. (You can also gargle a glass of water or juice to which you have added 15 to 20 drops of Tabasco sauce.) Cayenne pepper is antiseptic and rich in vitamin C, helps clear congestion, and draws blood to the throat to fight infection.

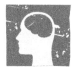

GOOD TO KNOW!

A folk remedy for a cough is to loosely tie a black thread around your neck. It has to be black. Many people vouch for this remedy. We have no idea why it works, but it might be worth a try!

Skip This!

When you have a cough, avoid foods that increase the production of mucus, such as dairy products and wheat.

Cures from Grandma's Kitchen

To relieve a cough, grate one or two cloves of garlic and mix with 1 teaspoon (13 g) of honey, or mix 1 teaspoon (13 g) honey with the juice of a fresh lemon. Not only does honey soothe the tickle, it also has antibacterial properties. Take a dose every three hours if needed.

Fighting Fever

It may not feel like it, but fever is actually your body's ally, causing it to heat up and destroy infection. Trying to suppress fever actually traps the infection in the body and can make it worse. Don't try to lower a fever unless it's higher than 103°F (39°C). If it is, try these tips.

SOOTHING PRACTICES FOR FIGHTING FEVER

First, stay hydrated. Drink plenty of cool water. Next, soak your feet in cool water and apply to your forehead cool-water compresses to which 5 drops of peppermint or lavender essential oil have been added.

You can also mix 2 teaspoons each of apple cider vinegar (10 g) and honey (13 g) in a glass of warm water and drink three times daily. Tea made from ginger, peppermint, lemon balm, and yarrow—all of which are diaphoretic—will help eliminate toxins, heat, and infection from the body. See page 13 for how to make tea or look for herbal tea combinations for colds and fever at natural food stores and use one tea bag per 1 cup (235 ml) of water. Drink three to five cups (0.7 to 1.18 L) daily.

Helping Laryngitis and Hoarseness

When the vocal cords become inflamed, it can be difficult to talk. You can have short-term loss of your voice (acute) or a long lasting problem (chronic). Possible causes include infection, allergens (including smoke and dust exposure), and even heartburn or gastroesophageal reflux disease (GERD). Turn the page to learn how to speak up.

Thrifty Cure!

Apply a raw potato poultice to the soles of your feet to draw heat out of the body.

Cures from Grandma's Kitchen

Did you know that berries have a cooling effect? Strawberries and raspberries both contain anthocyanins, which have an anti-inflammatory effect on the body. Why not blend them together into a honey lemonade? This is better than any lemonade you had as a kid! Here's how to make it:

2 cups (475 ml) water
1 cup (235 ml) peppermint tea
½ cup (120 ml) lemon juice
¼ cup (38 ml) strawberries
1 tablespoon (20 g) honey (not for babies under 1 year old)

Combine all ingredients in a blender and liquefy. Makes 2 servings.
Drink up to a quart (946 ml) daily.

HERBS FOR LARYNGITIS AND HOARSENESS

Eat pieces of ginger or drink ginger tea, which are antibacterial and increase circulation to the chest. Hot peppermint or sage teas will stimulate circulation to the throat and help relax the vocal cords. Drink up to four cups daily.

It's smart to suck on herbal lozenges periodically throughout the day to moisten your throat. Choose moistening slippery elm bark, licorice root, or marshmallow root and bronchodilating ginger, hyssop, or peppermint. Marshmallow root, plantain, slippery elm, and/or violet leaf will also moisten throats. You can use up to a dozen lozenges daily, when sick, but be aware that many contain sugar.

Skip This!

Avoid alcohol and caffeine when you have laryngitis or hoarseness. Both are dehydrating and aggravate the throat.

BENEFICIAL BEVERAGES FOR LARYNGITIS RELIEF

Drink plenty of fluids to keep the larynx moist. Gargle with 1 teaspoon (5 g) of salt or 2 drops of tea tree oil in a glass of water three times daily to combat any infection that might be present.

You can also drink 2 teaspoons (10 ml) of apple cider vinegar (10 g) and raw honey in a cup (235 ml) of warm water 3 times daily for its antibacterial and soothing properties. Cayenne pepper is also effective. Pour 1 cup (235 ml) of boiling water into a cup. Add 1/4 teaspoon of cayenne pepper and a few drops of lemon juice. Stir and sip slowly, the hotter the better.

SOOTHING PRACTICES FOR LARYNGITIS AND HOARSENESS

A steam inhalation can help you feel better fast. Just boil a pot of water and remove from the stove. Add 2 drops eucalyptus essential oil, 3 drops lavender essential oil, and 2 drops pine essential oil. Make a tent over your head and the pot and inhale.

And remember to rest your voice. Even whispering can stress the vocal cords more than talking in a regular voice. Write things down if necessary.

WHEN TO SEE YOUR M.D.

Get medical attention for the following:

- A child who has a fever over 103°F (40°C) that lasts for over 12 hours
- Pregnant women with a fever over 102°F (39°C).
- If you have a fever over 101°F (38°C) that is accompanied by a sore throat.
- If you have a fever over 102°F (39°C) for more than five days.

Improving Your Immune Resistance

The immune system is like a symphony of chemicals, cells, and organs playing together to bring about a harmonious state of health in the body. This 24-hour security system is always on alert, helping the body distinguish between itself and foreign matter (bacteria, viruses, fungi, yeasts, and parasites) and removing damaged, worn-out cells.

We have immune cells throughout our bodies. However, the lymphatic organs—the spleen, thymus, and tonsils as well as the lymph nodes—play a major part. The respiratory system also contains lymph tissue that produces lymphocytes, the digestive system secretes acids that kill pathogens, and the urinary system contains lymph tissue that expels pathogens and maintains the body's pH balance. When stressed, fatigued, and undernourished, the immune system has a difficult time doing its job. Here's how to build the immune strength you need.

HERBS FOR IMMUNE HEALTH

A number of herbs that have been time tested by various world cultures are known to boost immune health. Astragalus is a deep immune tonic, rich in polysaccharides, which strengthen the wei chi (also known as the body's natural defense energy) and increase phagocytosis, interferon, and T cell activity and blood cell production. Baptisia is high in polysaccharides and increases phagocytosis. It is good for lymphatic swelling and deep inflammation.

Echinacea is high in polysaccharides and stimulates interferon production and helper T cells, making cells more resistant to pathogens. Garlic is an antioxidant and an anti-viral that kills a wide range of disease-causing organisms, including viruses, bacteria, fungi, and protozoa. It also increases the body's resistance to infection and protects against epidemics. Ginger improves circulation to all parts of the body and inhibits biochemical pathways associated with inflammation. Reishi mushroom is a deep immune tonic and improves cellular immunity. It also boosts resistance to bacterial, parasitic, and viral infection due to its rich polysaccharide content. Use a dose of herbs in tea, tincture, or capsule form every couple of hours that you are awake.

VITAMINS FOR IMMUNE HEALTH

Nutrients that can help strengthen the immune system include beta-carotene and vitamin A (10,000 IU daily of either), which improve the health of mucus membranes and make them more resistant to airborne and intestinal invaders. These nutrients stimulate the thymus gland to produce T cells needed in the prevention of infection, and vitamin A helps killer cells digest invaders.

Cures from Grandma's Kitchen

Eating black bean soup is a folk remedy for restoring one's voice. Also try eating three cloves of raw garlic a day. Try stuffing one into a pitted date to make it easier to eat!

Vitamin C (1,000 mg daily) is an antioxidant that strengthens the body's resistance to infection. It helps protect white blood cells, boosts macrophage activity, and raises interferon levels as well as thymic hormones and antibody levels. Quercetin, (100 mg three times daily), also part of the C complex, has antiviral capability.

Vitamin E (400 IU daily) and selenium (200 mcg daily) are considered antioxidants. Vitamin E is a free-radical scavenger that increases helper T cells and antibody response. It strengthens the membranes of macrophages. Selenium is necessary for antibody production and potentates phagocytes to kill bacteria.

Zinc (15 mg daily) has inhibiting effects on viral replication. It also helps increase natural killer cell activity in smokers. Zinc also stimulates the production of histamine, which dilates capillaries so that white blood cells can rush to the area of infection.

GOOD TO KNOW!

Every one of the 100 species of common disease–causing bacteria has at least one strain resistant to antibiotics, and that number is rapidly increasing and becoming a major medical threat. The overuse of antibiotics (which literally means "against life") is a contributing factor in weakening the immune system. Antibiotics are effective only against bacterial infections, not viral ones, and they kill off helpful bacteria as well as the harmful.

Probiotics (1 high potency capsule three times daily) inhibit candida and other unfriendly microorganisms, which can contribute to a weakened immune system.

BEST FOODS TO BOOST IMMUNITY

Onions, garlic, scallions, chives, and leeks all contain quercetin, which acts as a powerful antioxidant in your body, scavenging up damaging free radicals. One study in the *Journal of the National Cancer Institute* showed that this family of veggies even lowered the risk for prostate cancer.

Cayenne, chives, cinnamon, garlic, horseradish, leeks, oregano, rosemary, scallions, and thyme all have infection-fighting properties. Also include plenty of cruciferous vegetables such as broccoli, cabbage, cauliflower, kale, and arugula for their sulforaphane content, which is an antioxidant and stimulator of natural detoxifying enzymes.

Vegetables high in beta-carotene, such as carrots, winter squash, green leafy vegetables, and sweet potatoes, protect against carcinogens, induce protective enzyme activity, and suppress cell-destroying free radicals. Fermented foods such as yogurt, miso (made from soybeans), homemade pickles, and unpasteurized sauerkraut help promote healthy intestinal flora and inhibit the growth of harmful bacteria.

Include sea vegetables in the regimen as they provide a wide range of minerals not present in most land-grown food. Seaweeds bind with and carry harmful chemicals and pollutants out of the body and nourish the kidneys, bones, and teeth. Marine vegetables exhibit antibiotic, antiviral, and antifungal properties.

Shiitake mushrooms are immune enhancing, cholesterol lowering, interferon stimulating, and have antitumor activity. Wild and brown rice, quinoa, and barley are immunostrengthening grains.

Every day, eat at least five of these immunosupportive foods. You can use several in a soup or salad easily!

ESSENTIAL OILS TO BOOST IMMUNITY

Immune-enhancing essential oils that have strong antimicrobial properties include cedarwood, cinnamon, clove, Clary sage, garlic, grapefruit, juniper, lavender, lemon, lime, marjoram, orange, oregano, patchouli, peppermint, pine, rosemary, and tea tree. These oils can be diluted in the bath, added to massage oils, or used in diffusers.

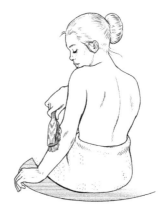

LIFESTYLE CHANGES THAT BOOST IMMUNITY

Practice dry brush skin massage daily. You can find this kind of brush at your health food store. Stroke the brush over your skin (gently!) toward

Skip This!

Excess sugar and fruit juice can contribute to hypoglycemia and suppress T cell activity and phagocytosis. Caffeine and alcohol, when consumed in excess, cause depletion of nutrients, especially calcium and B vitamins. Excess alcohol consumption can suppress lymphocyte development and their ability to produce antibodies. A high-fat diet slows down macrophage ability to destroy infection-causing invaders. Excess fat can also lead to shrinkage of the thymus gland and lymphoid tissue.

Chemical additives such as artificial food colorings, nitrates, and preservatives stress the kidneys and liver. Eating food to which one is allergic is a stress, causing the body to focus on neutralizing the allergen rather than healing. Eating less animal food minimizes contact with pesticides and other chemical additives. Choosing organic foods minimizes exposure to harmful chemical additives.

Finally, during inclement weather dress warmly. Protect the kidneys, head, and feet from overexposure to wind and temperature extremes.

your heart to rev up circulation and the release of toxins. Then shower and end your shower with cold water if you are feeling brave! This constricts blood vessels on the surface, sending blood deeper into the body, facilitating the removal of toxins, and increasing T cell production. A far infrared sauna can be an excellent (and more enjoyable) way of removing toxins from the body. Be sure and get one from a reputable dealer to ensure it is built to last.

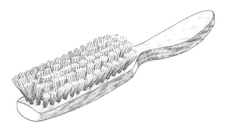

Stay active. Get outside and enjoy sports or just tromp around. Yoga, chi kung, and tai chi can be done indoors during any kind of weather. Be sure to get adequate sleep as well. We need our zzzzzs to produce sleep immune specific chemicals, as during rest is when much of the body's repair work is done.

Meditation, prayer, deep breathing, and inspirational readings are all good ways to reduce stress. Practice right living, positive thinking, and healthy relationships for a healthy immune system. Beware of negative thoughts and minimize stress. Have creative outlets and a job you enjoy. Avoid disciplines that stress you out.

We can't always avoid every cold, flu, or sore throat that comes our way. Once in awhile we should give ourselves the opportunity to rest, recover, and be nurtured. Maybe have someone else make us soup. Practice visualization. See yourself in good health!

Cures from Grandma's Kitchen

One effective and pleasant way to incorporate a number of immune-stimulating foods and herbs in your diet is to make an "Immune Soup."

First, sauté garlic and onions in a bit of olive oil. Then add some chopped vegetables like broccoli, cabbage, or carrots. Include several sliced shiitake mushrooms. Add 2 or 3 pieces of astragalus (you won't eat it but it will impart its therapeutic qualities to the broth) or codonopsis. Add enough water to make it the consistency you desire. Adding a small handful of sea vegetables will provide a host of minerals.

If you are not vegetarian, you can simmer a hormone-free chicken (with the skin removed) in your soup. It's also possible to add previously cooked beans or whole grain quinoa or brown rice to the still simmering soup.

After a couple of hours, measure out 1 teaspoon (5 g) of miso for every 1 cup (235 ml) of water that you used in the soup. Make a paste by mixing the miso with a bit of the soup broth and then add it into the soup. Miso is high in lecithin and helps break down fatty deposits in the body. You have now made a very nutritious and delicious Immune Soup!

CHAPTER 2

NATURAL REMEDIES to SOOTHE EVERYDAY ACHES and PAINS

All it takes is one small part of your body to experience pain to cause you to feel out of sorts. Here are some remedies to get to the source of the pain and improve your body's response to it so you feel better fast.

Alleviating Arthritis

The word "arthritis" comes from the Greek word arthron, meaning "joint," and itis, meaning "inflammation." When the condition is acute, joint swelling, pain, heat, and redness may be present. As a chronic condition, joint pain, stiffness, lack of mobility, and eventually bone deformity can occur. Rheumatoid arthritis is an inflammatory condition and autoimmune disease. Osteoarthritis affects the weight-bearing joints (knees, hips, and spine). Here's how to ease pain and discomfort.

TOPICAL HERBS FOR ARTHRITIS RELIEF

Ginger compresses can be deeply comforting. Just dip a clean washcloth into 1 cup (235 ml) of hot (not scalding) ginger tea and apply it to the aching joint in question. Cover with a dry cloth to help hold the heat in until it's cool. Replace as needed.

You can also apply cayenne pepper cream (available at health food stores and some pharmacies), using enough to cover the afflicted area to decrease the amount of a neurotransmitter, called substance P, which relays pain messages to the brain. The key ingredient in cayenne pepper is capsaicin. A study published in the *Journal of Rheumatology* in 1992 showed that capsaicin is effective in relieving the tenderness and pain associated with osteoarthritis. It can be applied 2 or 3 times daily.

To make your own liniment (a tincture applied to the skin) for topical use to alleviate arthritis pain, steep 1 tablespoon (5 g) cayenne pepper in 1 pint (475 ml) of apple cider vinegar for two weeks, shaking daily. Strain. Apply gently to the skin but wash your hands afterward and avoid getting it close to your eyes, which would sting.

Cures from Grandma's Kitchen

Use a cabbage leaf poultice (see page 19) to help draw out the pain and inflammation associated with arthritis. Another folk remedy that many people swear by is drinking a mixture of 2 teaspoons (13 g) raw honey and 2 teaspoons (10 ml) unpasteurized apple cider vinegar in 1 cup (235 ml) of warm water. The high potassium content of the vinegar dissolves calcium deposits around the joints. Potassium also promotes the growth of cells and tissues. This can be taken up to three times daily.

VITAMINS AND NUTRIENTS FOR JOINT HEALTH

Take 1,000 mg daily of calcium for healthy bones, as well as 400 mg magnesium and 1,000 IU vitamin D daily so that the calcium is properly absorbed into the body. Magnesium also relaxes tight muscles and inhibits the action of hyaluronidase, which can destroy synovial fluid and joints.

Glucosamine sulphate is essential for the formation of mucopolysaccharides, necessary for connective tissue. This nutrient reduces inflammation, helps to repair traumatized tissue, and cushions joints, so it is particularly helpful in relieving osteoarthritis. Glucosamine also thickens synovial fluid and stimulates the production of new cartilage and connective tissue. Take 250 to 500 mg three times daily.

Bromelain, an enzyme that comes from pineapple, also reduces inflammatory prostaglandins. Take 500 mg daily.

BEST FOODS TO FIGHT ARTHRITIS

Arthritis is an inflammatory condition, so anything you can ingest to "cool off" the body is important. Essential fatty acids found in fish oil can reduce inflammation, lubricating the joints. Take one to three fish oil capsules daily. For the same reason, include at least a couple of servings weekly of fatty fish like salmon, mackerel, herring, sardines, and halibut in your diet. Chia seeds, hemp seeds, and flax seeds can also be consumed on a daily basis for their quality lubricating oils.

Other beneficial foods for arthritis include nutritive and anti-inflammatory almonds, avocados, barley, brown rice, carrots, celery, kamut, quinoa, millet, oatmeal, black beans, artichokes, beets, burdock root, endive, kale, okra, parsley, parsnips, sweet potatoes, watercress, winter squash, yams, and pecans.

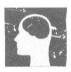

GOOD TO KNOW!

A deficiency of copper can contribute to osteoarthritis. Copper bracelets are reported to be beneficial by many people who suffer from arthritis. This may be because our skin is porous enough to absorb trace amounts of copper, which can stop free-radical damage to the tissues.

GOOD TO GROW!

Did you know that you can get relief from arthritis by stinging the afflicted area with nettles? That's right. This sort of therapy is called urtication. Just cultivate a nettle patch or find some growing wild and wriggle any arthritic area in the plants, getting stung several times. Nettle sting contains formic acid, which stimulates a natural antihistamine reaction. Although the sting is less than pleasant, the technique provides excellent relief. My friend's grandfather in Germany would roll naked down a nettle-covered hill to treat his arthritis!

Raw string beans have long been considered a therapeutic food for arthritis because of their ability to eliminate uric acid, which can contribute to joint pain. Celery seed as a condiment helps eliminate uric acid in the body too.

Cherries, hawthorn berries, and blueberries are rich sources of anthocyanidins and proanthocyanidins, which are water-soluble colorful pigments in food that have antioxidant activity and help prevent collagen breakdown.

Use turmeric in food for its anti-inflammatory properties. Drinking a shotglass of aloe vera juice 10 minutes before each meal also reduces inflammation. Look for it at natural food stores.

SOOTHING PRACTICES FOR ARTHRITIS

Bathing in warm water to which 1 pound (455 g) of Epsom salts has been added is very pain relieving. Add 5 to 10 drops of essential oils of coriander, eucalyptus, fir, ginger, lavender, pine, rosemary, or wintergreen. All of these herbs help improve circulation, and wintergreen even contains salicin, a pain-relieving compound. If you are feeling bold, practice dry brush skin massage and alternate hot and cold showers (ending with cold).

Exercising in water can be a soothing way to stay in shape, and such exercise has less impact on the joints. Swimming and bicycling are beneficial exercises that are less likely to cause stress on the joints. If it's too much to be active every day, alternate one day on, one day off. Don't exercise beyond feeling "good tired." Otherwise, you will be wiped out the next day!

Easing Backache Pain

When you have a backache, it's difficult, if not impossible, to function effectively. I know. I was in a private plane crash years ago. We came down hard and my back ached for years afterwards. A chiropractor friend suggested the book, *Somatics* by Thomas Hanna. I followed the exercises in there and within a week, the pain I had harbored for more than a decade was gone. This is a great place to start. These cures can help you too.

Skip This!

Minimize foods rich in oxalic acid, such as beet greens, rhubarb, Swiss chard, and spinach, which can contribute to irritating crystals forming in the joints. Nix foods in the nightshade family like tomatoes, eggplant, potatoes, green pepper, paprika, and tobacco because they contain solanine, which is a neuromuscular toxin.

Thrifty Cures!

Interestingly, there is a popular folk remedy that suggests those who suffer from arthritis should carry a raw potato in their right pocket until it shrivels up, at which time it is replaced with a new one. It is believed that the potato absorbs inflammation. In fact, ladies of days gone by even had special potato-carrying pockets sewn into their dresses for this purpose.

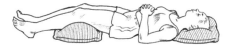

NATURAL CURES FOR AN ACHING BACK

A hot ginger tea compress, or a salve containing wintergreen (a natural analgesic) and capsaicin (made from cayenne pepper, which blocks the brain's perception of pain) can help soothe a bad back when applied topically to the painful area.

Eat black beans and chia seeds, which are high in minerals that support the kidneys. The kidneys, when weak, can cause lower back pain.

GOOD TO KNOW!

Sleeping in a position known as "Lazy S" is often the best for a sore back. It entails putting a pillow under the head and upper neck, keeping the back flat on the bed, with a pillow under the knees. This keeps the hamstring muscles from pulling and exerting pressure on the lower back. Roll carefully out of bed. Stretch to move circulation. Be sure you have a supportive mattress too! Waterbeds are not helpful.

SOOTHING PRACTICES FOR AN ACHING BACK

Soaking in a tub to which 1 pound (455 g) Epsom salts has been added is soothing for an aching back. The magnesium content of the salts helps relax sore muscles.

Soothing yoga postures include the cobra, backbend, locust, plow, bow, full twist, alternate leg pull, and elbow to knee. Swimming is an excellent exercise that does not stress the back.

Wear the color blue to help your back heal. Blue is considered cooling and anti-inflammatory. It is perceived by the brain as calming.

And finally, try to brace yourself when sneezing to prevent further misalignment.

Pain in the upper back corresponds to the heart, pain in the midback can correspond to issues of digestion and emotional security, and pain in the lower back can indicate kidney issues or feeling a lack of support.

 ### WHEN TO SEE YOUR M.D.

Get medical attention for a backache in the following situations:

- That comes on suddenly with no apparent cause.
- That is accompanied by other symptoms, such as cramps, chest pain, fever, stomachache, or breathing difficulty.
- That lasts more than two weeks without relief and/or if the pain radiates down the leg to the foot.

Helping Heal Headache

Oh, your aching head! Headaches are one of the most painful and debilitating afflictions. Vascular headaches result from dilation of the blood vessels in the head, whereas non-vascular, or psychogenic, headaches result from stress. Many headaches are caused by neuromuscular skeletal imbalances. Low blood sugar can also be a cause.

Migraines are considered a vascular condition. They are often preceded by auras in which objects appear surrounded in light. Strange smells, numbness, and difficulty with speech may also occur. Blood vessels can constrict and then over dilate, which causes pain. The pain can be general or local, but it is usually on one side of the head, in the frontal or temporal region. Migraines may also manifest as numbness, tingling, nausea, vomiting, and diarrhea. The pain may shift from one side of the head to the other. Attacks may last less than a day, up to three days, and in some cases weeks. Migraines may occur cyclically or from a particular food allergy. Yeasted breads, gluten-rich foods, citrus fruits, and processed meats can also bring on migraines. Menstrual cycles and birth control pills also may be factors.

Stress, poor posture, and lack of sleep can all contribute to tension headaches. Tension headaches are more likely to occur as one's day becomes increasingly stressful. Neck pain often goes along with tension headaches. The pain may be on one or both sides. Here's how to find relief from headache pain.

HERBS FOR HEADACHES

A number of herbs can help reduce the frequency and intensity of headaches. Look for capsules containing the following herbs at natural food stores and take as directed:

- Butterbur, also known as petasites, has a potent anti-inflammatory/anti-allergenic effect, which has been shown very effective in reducing headaches, specifically migraines. Two-thirds of participants in a study published in the medical journal, *Headache* (2005) had more than a 50 percent reduction in migraines when taking butterbur.
- Feverfew stops blood platelets from releasing too much serotonin and histamine, both of which can dilate blood vessels and lead to headaches. A review of research about feverfew published in the medical journal, *Public Health Nutrition* in 2000 showed that it was safe and effective at preventing migraines. Feverfew works best as a preventative taken on a daily basis rather than when a headache is already in progress.
- Ginger inhibits biochemical pathways associated with inflammation and prevents blood platelet aggregation. It also increases oxygen utilization and blood flow to the brain.

Cures from Grandma's Kitchen

An Irish folk remedy for curing headaches is to loosely tie a bandanna around the head and slip slices of raw potato between the head and bandanna. Place the potatoes where the pain is, over the temples or eyes. Lie down in a quiet room. After an hour, the potato slices should be warm and the headache relieved. Slices of apples or peeled aloe vera can be used in place of the potatoes.

- White willow inhibits prostaglandin production, which can contribute to inflammation. It contains salicin, a forerunner of aspirin, but it is much milder.

You can also try making a compress of tea of lavender, peppermint, or rosemary. Soak a cloth in the hot tea and apply it to the forehead and back of the neck. Chilling the tea and making a cold application may feel even better. You be the judge.

Thrifty Cures!

Eating two apples a day can help prevent headaches by providing sufficient anti-inflammatory enzymes. Go for tart apples, as the sour flavor will help move liver stagnation, which according to Asian medicine is a contributing factor in headaches.

Skip This!

Caffeine causes blood vessel constriction, so caffeine consumption and withdrawal can cause headaches. It is best to gradually decrease caffeine rather than remove it from your diet all at once. Nicotine can also cause headaches by constricting blood vessels. Other foods that can trigger headaches include chocolate, wheat, citrus, corn, tomatoes, apples, bananas, peaches, peanuts, onions, and red meat. These are common allergens and thus cause inflammation. Minimize excess spicy foods, chocolate, fats, and fried foods, and avoid ice-cold foods and drink. Ice-cold foods cause constriction in the blood vessels, which can cause the head to feel tight and painful.

Foods high in the amino acid tyrosine, such as aged cheese and wine, can cause migraine headaches. The class of chemicals known as vasoactive amines can also cause headaches in some people. This includes the following:

- Histamines in aged cheese, eggplant, spinach, tomato, chicken liver, and wine
- Tyramines in avocados, bananas, cheese, citrus, red wine, peanuts, fermented, pickled and smoked foods, plums, sourdough bread and baker's yeast
- Phenylethylamine in chocolate and cheese

Also avoid chemical food additives such as sulfites, nitrates, nitrites, and red and yellow dye. Chewing gum can also stress muscles, leading to a headache.

SUPPLEMENTS FOR HEADACHES

Throbbing in the eye area (caused by vasoconstriction) can be eased by 100 mg of niacin, which is a vasodilator. Don't be afraid of the ten-minute hot prickly rash this may produce. It will not last and will not harm you.

Magnesium (500 mg daily) relaxes muscles and can help migraine and tension headaches. Essential fatty acids such as those found in fish, flax, and hemp seed oil can also help by reducing the inflammation associated with headaches. Take 1 teaspoon (5 ml) daily or follow the directions on the bottle of capsules you choose.

The supplement 5-hydroxytryptophan (5HTP) is a precursor to serotonin, and those with low levels of this brain chemical are more susceptible to pain. Taking this supplement according to the bottle's dosage guidelines may help as well.

BEST FOODS TO HEAL HEADACHES

Eat smaller, more frequent meals to keep blood sugar levels on a more even keel and to prevent headaches. Foods to eat more of include black sesame seed, carrots, celery, and scallions. They are all rich in important trace minerals and improve liver function which promotes optimal health.

Eat raw cabbage to cure any headache, and use radish to cure headaches in the back of the head. Both help energy move downward in the body, rather than rising to the head. If you're in the kitchen, also try inhaling deeply from a jar of mustard! It helps improve circulation to the head via the nasal passages.

Skip This!

Electromagnetic pollution can be a factor in headaches. Do you live near major power lines? Is your bed near an excessive number of clocks, a TV, stereo equipment, or computer ware? Do what you can to minimize any of these factors, such as moving the bed or electric paraphernalia.

Avoid exposure to hot sun, which can bring on headaches. Wear a hat when outdoors.

Cures from Grandma's Kitchen

A simple folk remedy to cure a headache is to sit with your feet in hot water. Add 1 teaspoon of ginger (2 g) or mustard powder (3 g) to each gallon (3.8 L) of water. While doing this, apply a cold compress to the back of the neck at the base of the skull for five minutes.

Another folk remedy is to dunk both hands into hot water (within reason) for 1 minute.

SOOTHING PRACTICES FOR A HEADACHE

Try unwinding in an aromatherapy bath of lavender, peppermint, or rosemary. Stuffing a sachet full of aromatic headache herbs like peppermint, rosemary, and lavender can make an aromatherapy headache pillow. Take it to bed with you. Breathe in the comforting aromas.

Pay attention to how you hold yourself. When muscles are tight, circulation throughout the body is impeded, often resulting in pain. Do you clench your jaws or hold your neck tight? Biofeedback training can teach a headache-prone person to relax more and can also improve circulation. When dealing with a headache, lie down, do deep slow breathing, and practice tensing then relaxing each part of your body.

For tension headaches, try yoga. Pranayama, meditation, and neck rolls can all relieve headaches, but avoid excessive forward bends and backbends.

One hydrotherapy technique for alleviating headaches is to sit on a waterproof stool in the shower with your legs apart, bending forward with your hands clasped in back of your neck. Allow your elbows to fall between your knees so your upper back muscles get stretched. Aim a spray of warm or hot water toward the back of your head for 5 minutes. Turn off the water, dry off, and then soak a face towel in very cold water. Apply it to the same area you were spraying with hot water. Leave in place for half a minute. Some find that spraying a cold jet of water directly onto the soles of the feet constricts blood vessels and relieves headache too.

You can also take ten deep inhalations from a bottle of essential oil of rosemary to alleviate a headache. Visualize breathing in the colors violet, blue, or green, which are cooling to inflammation.

OTHER REMEDIES FOR A HEADACHE

An Asian folk remedy for curing a headache is called Li-Shou. It is done by standing with your feet about 20 inches (50.8 cm) apart. Rub your hands together to warm them and then gently stroke your face 30 times from the forehead to the chin in the same direction. While doing this, partially close your eyes and look down at your toes. Then extend your

 WHEN TO SEE YOUR M.D.
Sometimes headaches require medical attention. See your health-care practitioner for the headache in the following situations:

- Was caused by a blow to the head.
- Gets worse when you cough, sneeze, or vomit.
- Is accompanied by fever, memory loss, double vision, or speech or hearing difficulties.
- Is accompanied by sexual, bladder, or menstrual problems
- Appears suddenly in a patient who is elderly and if arteries on the side of the head are engorged.
- Is accompanied by sweating and fever.
- Begins after taking some kind of medicine.

Rather than simply blocking out the pain of a headache, it is important to determine the cause and change it.

arms in front of you at waist level with your fingers touching, swinging them back and forth 100 times. This helps to divert blood from the head to the hands as well as stimulate endorphin production.

The acupuncture point hoku can be stimulated with the fingers to give headache relief. It is located in the fleshy mound in the hand just above where the thumb and forefinger bones come together.

Many who suffer from headaches have also been helped by hypnosis, which can help you let go of emotional patterns that contribute to head pain. Craniosacral work is also very helpful in releasing stored tension in the head, neck, and spine. Some people even find that if they can have a bowel movement at the onset of a headache, the headache will diminish because the body is eliminating toxins.

Easing Hemorrhoid Discomfort

Hemorrhoids are considered "varicose veins in an unfortunate place." Hemorrhoids, also known as "piles," are enlarged veins located in the lower rectum or anus that are caused by blood blockage in the veins of the hemorrhoidal complex. The hemorrhoids begin above the internal opening of the anus and may become large enough to protrude. The subsequent squeezing of them while sitting brings on pain.

If you suffer from hemorrhoids, check to see if you've been consuming too much coffee, alcohol, or fried or extremely spicy foods that may be irritating the liver and thus the anus.

Hardened stools and constipation are primary causes of hemorrhoids. Constipation may be caused by diet, lack of fluids, and certain medications, among other things. When someone is constipated, the wavelike motion (*peristalsis*) that moves the bowels through the intestines is nearly nonexistent, and the straining to have a bowel movement causes hemorrhoids. For more information, see the chapter on constipation. For now, here's what you can do to ease hemorrhoids!

HERBS FOR HEMORRHOIDS

Good herbs to use internally include collinsonia, witch hazel, white oak bark, and plantain. Collinsonia is an astringent that especially affects the liver, veins, and colon. Witch hazel and white oak bark are astringent, which helps tighten prolapsed tissue, and plantain is soothing and anti-inflammatory.

Thrifty Cures!

Strange as it may seem, I have had excellent results treating hemorrhoids using a whittled out suppository-shaped piece of raw potato. Insert the suppository (lubricated with a bit of oil) high into the rectum at night before bed. Do this for three nights in a row, inserting a fresh one each night. Don't try to remove it, as it will come out in your stool the next day.

A compress of chilled witch hazel extract can also be applied topically to hemorrhoids to reduce swollen tissue due to the presence of astringent tannins in the witch hazel.

Bleeding hemorrhoids will stop if you take 2 teaspoons (10 ml) of apple cider vinegar in a glass of water at every meal. You can also take $1/2$ to 1 teaspoon (1 to 2 g) of cayenne pepper in a glass of water at every meal for several days until the hemorrhoids are gone, then once or twice a week for a good maintenance dose. Cayenne can also be taken as 1-capsule doses. This will clear up hemorrhoids and keep them from reoccurring.

Studies done in Europe found that horse chestnut helps to increase blood flow, strengthens connective tissue, tightens veins, and decrease redness and inflammation. One of its compounds, escin, has been found to close the small pores in the walls of the veins, making them less permeable, stronger, and reducing leakage of fluid into the surrounding tissues. Take horse chestnut capsules 2 to 3 times a day. Avoid horse chestnut if you have liver or kidney disease or if you are pregnant or breastfeeding.

Health food stores usually carry some sort of topical herbal salve you can apply to hemorrhoids. These salves often contain astringent herbs such as white oak bark, horse chestnut, and yarrow; soothing anti-inflammatory herbs such as plantain and comfrey; and antiseptic herbs such as yellow dock and goldenseal. You can also apply apple cider vinegar (which is antiseptic and astringent), aloe vera gel (which is soothing and anti-inflammatory), and vitamin E (which promotes tissue regeneration) to hemorrhoids. Apply any of these healing and astringent substances externally to hemorroids up to three times daily, especially before bed.

HELPFUL NUTRIENTS FOR HEMORRHOIDS

Blueberries, blackberries, cranberry, raspberries, and cherries all contain flavonoids that strengthen the walls of veins. It is also often helpful to take a supplement of 500 mg of bioflavonoids plus rutin daily to strengthen the capillaries.

SOOTHING PRACTICES FOR HEMORRHOIDS

Though it takes a bit of effort, a sitz bath (hip bath) can bring great relief to hemorrhoids. Simply fill two baby bathtubs—one with a hot tea of witch hazel, white oak bark, comfrey, and plantain, the other with ice water. Sit your bottom into the hot tea bath for three minutes. Then go immediately to the ice cold bath for one minute. Alternate from one to the other. Always start with the hot bath and end with the cold one. Dry off, apply some healing salve to the inflamed hemorrhoids, and then dress comfortably.

EXERCISE FOR HEALING HEMORRHOIDS

One of the most helpful techniques for healing hemorrhoids is Kegel exercises. Simply tighten and relax the anal sphincter. This helps to strengthen and tone the area rather than it becoming flaccid and giving out as time passes. Sets of 21 flexes 3 times a day is a good goal.

Yoga postures such as the fish, plough, and shoulder stand are also helpful as a hemorrhoid preventative as well as for treatment.

Avoiding Jet Lag and Other Traveling Pitfalls

Flying long distances is stressful for the body and can lead to jet lag. A plane's environment is often lower in oxygen than the regular atmosphere and also quite dry, which may cause you to become dehydrated. Once you arrive at your destination, you may also encounter unfamiliar bugs and parasites that can wreak havoc on your system. But you can arrive refreshed and stay healthy. Here's how.

NATURAL REMEDIES FOR BEFORE YOU GO

Before taking your trip, load up on antioxidant vitamins A (10,000 IU), E (400 IU), and the mineral selenium (50 mg) daily for a week before departure. This will help protect you against free-radical damage caused by radiation during the flight. Also take an anti-stress high-potency B-complex (50 mg) vitamin with 1,000 mg of time-release vitamin C once daily while on your trip.

GOOD TO KNOW!
Rescue Remedy is a combination of five Bach flower remedies. It is available in natural food stores. It is good for helping you deal with all sorts of stressful situations that can occur when traveling, such as fear of flying, lost luggage, or stolen passports. Bring some along to stay calm just in case you encounter a crisis along the way. Take three drops under the tongue or in a half glass of water as needed.

Diarrhea is a common traveling ailment. Start taking a high potency probiotic supplement a week before leaving and during the trip to help establish friendly intestinal flora. Look for the types that don't require refrigeration. Take 1 capsule three times daily. Take three garlic capsules daily to prevent dysentery if traveling to areas where that is a problem. If you can, bring your own activated charcoal water filter. Look for one that will remove giardia.

NATURAL REMEDIES FOR WHEN YOU ARRIVE

During the flight and afterward, be sure to drink plenty of fluids, especially water, to rehydrate your body. If you land during the day, get some sunlight to recharge your batteries. This will help you adjust to the new time zone.

The hormone melatonin is manufactured in the brain during periods of darkness to promote sleep. It helps reset your body clock and facilitates deep and restful sleep. The level of melatonin in the body decreases with age, making people over the age of 50 more susceptible to jet lag. If you are traveling across time zones, take up to 8 mg of melatonin 30 minutes before bedtime at your destination. Take for four days after arriving to make you less sleepy, more efficient at work, and less moody. Also, try to sched-

GOOD TO KNOW!
Whenever possible, try to keep your feet above your head. For example, when lounging on the couch, support your legs and back and drape them up over the top of the couch. Inverted postures help divert circulation from the area of inflammation and elevate the area needing inflammation reduction.

ule your arrival before 9 PM so you can get a rejuvenating night's sleep. A drop of lavender oil on your pillow can also help you sleep in a new environment.

Once you depart, take ginseng or eleuthero, as both are considered adaptogens, an agent that helps the body adapt to different environments, climate changes, altitudes, and stress. Use ginseng or eleuthero twice daily in capsules or tincture, following the dosage guidelines on the bottle.

A lavender or rosemary aromatherapy bath and a clay mask followed by a quick cold shower can have you feeling refreshed and alive in no time. There is also nothing wrong with allowing some time to get your feet back on the ground before beginning a whirlwind schedule. Stay put for a day or two before "le grand tour" if possible.

The Chinese patent formula Cerebral Tonic Pills can also be used to help overcome jet lag. Take as directed on the packaging.

A few homeopathic remedies that can help alleviate jet lag by balancing the body's energy are as follows:

- Arnica: Helps alleviate the shock and stress of changing time zones
- Cocculus: Helps alleviate irritation, weakness, fogginess, nausea, and faintness
- Nux vomica: Helps alleviate nervous debility with trembling, lack of appetite, irritation, and constipation
- Phosphorus: Helps alleviate dizziness, sluggishness, absentmindedness, nausea, and fogginess

Natural food stores carry many homeopathic combinations that help overcome jet lag. Usually three to four pellets are dissolved under the tongue three or four times daily.

GOOD TO KNOW!
Bring along a bottle of versatile lavender, peppermint, or tea tree essential oil. Your spray mister can serve a double purpose. On arrival, spray the bedding to deter bed bugs.

If you get a cut in a tropical climate, apply tea tree oil directly to prevent the nick from becoming major jungle rot. Even bathing in contaminated water can be a problem. Every time you wash, add one drop each of tea tree, eucalyptus, and lavender essential oil to a sink full of water.

Skip This!
Avoid caffeine and alcohol when flying as they will dehydrate you.

FOOD DO'S AND DON'TS WHEN YOU TRAVEL

Salads washed in unsafe water can transmit parasites, so stick with peeled or cooked vegetables. Vegetables need to be washed in purified water if uncooked. Eat only fruit that can be peeled like bananas, papaya, and pineapple. Papaya and pineapple both contain natural digestive enzymes and make an excellent way to end a meal. Papaya seeds have anti-parasitic properties and can be consumed in doses of 1 teaspoonful (3 g) daily. Both pomegranates and cranberries also have anti-parasitic properties.

Liberal use of raw garlic and onions also helps prevent unfriendly microorganisms (and even bug bites!). Squeeze lime or lemon juice on as many things you eat as possible as such juice has detoxifying and anti-infection properties.

Freezing does not necessarily kill parasites, so think twice before eating that popsicle or ice cream, no matter how refreshing it sounds. If you do eat meat, make sure it is well cooked and eaten hot; otherwise, potential parasites make this is another good reason to avoid meat. Raw seafood can carry hepatitis. Avoid eating with unclean hands.

Be aware that ice cubes are often made with parasite-infested water (ice tends to create more thirst and hinder digestion anyway).

When buying bottled water, make sure the bottle is properly sealed. If in doubt, order beer or soda in moderation. Wine is considered safe and even antibacterial. The rule to remember is, "If you can't peel it, boil it, or cook it, forget it."

IF YOU DO GET SICK

Should you find yourself with diarrhea, you can make an electrolyte-rich beverage to replace lost nutrients by mixing 8 ounces (235 ml) of clean water with $1/4$ teaspoon baking soda and $1/4$ teaspoon salt. Another formula to replace lost nutrients is made by combining 1 quart (950 ml) of boiled water with $1/2$ cup (120 ml) lemon juice, 2 tablespoons (13 g) honey, $1/4$ teaspoon sea salt, and $1/4$ teaspoon baking soda. You may also want to tuck a few packets of electrolyte powder into your travel first aid kit. Homeopathic Arsenicum can help diarrhea that is the result of eating tainted food.

Ume concentrate made from the umeboshi plum can also stop diarrhea, prevent parasites, treat food poisoning and digestive upsets, relieve a hangover, as well as prevent typhoid. It truly is one of those "Don't leave home without it" remedies. It can be purchased in pills or as a paste. Charcoal capsules are another excellent for stopping even a severe case of the runs. Take two capsules three of four times daily.

GOOD TO KNOW!
A high-protein meal will increase alertness and the ability to think clearly. A high-carbohydrate meal will make it easier to sleep either on the plane or at your destination.

Skip This!
Avoid alcohol at high altitudes for the first couple of days as its diuretic effects will contribute to the body's loss of minerals and to making you dehydrated.

Research the areas you will be traveling to better equip yourself for the trip. Know before you go. Tourist and resort areas, though less adventurous, are usually at lower risk for disease. Check with health officials to find out if malaria, dysentery, cholera, encephalitis, or other health bugaboos are a threat where you are going and be prepared.

People often find it difficult to sleep in an unfamiliar environment, no matter how exhausted they are. Consider bringing along some herbal sleeping potions such as valerian capsules or chamomile tea bags. You might also want to travel with an herbal sleep sachet stuffed with hops and catnip to place in your pillow.

A wise traveler should bring along an extra set of prescription glasses. No point in sightseeing if you can't see! If you are on medication, be it herbal or otherwise, keep it with you should your luggage get lost. It is also wise to have the Latin names for any herbs you are on (they are the same in every language) or generic names for any medication you are using should they need to be replaced.

Ideally, travel with few enough possessions so that you can keep your luggage with you rather than checking it. The wise traveler brings twice the money and half the clothes one would expect to need. Make copies of your passport and credit cards and leave them with someone you trust. Keep a separate paper with you that lists your passport number, date, and place of issue. Only exchange currency at official places such as banks and stations. Have a solar calculator to keep track of exchange rates accurately. Treat the local people with respect. Traveling is supposed to be different from home. That's why we do it. Have an adventure!

Preventing and Treating Hangover

Hangovers tend to occur because you have consumed more than your liver has been able to cope with. The drinks most likely to cause hangovers include bourbon, brandy, champagne, cognac, rum, rye, whiskey, and red wine. Vodka, gin, and white wine are less likely to cause hangovers. In general, the less flavor a substance has, the less likely it is to cause a hangover. Mixing several kinds of drinks increases hangovers and so does the use of carbonated beverages, which enter the system quickly. Symptoms of hangovers include irritability, depression, headache, nausea, and dizziness. Let's look at some folk remedies for hangover prevention and treatment.

NATURAL CURES FOR HANGOVER

Take 2 to 6 teaspoons (13 to 40 g) of honey every 20 minutes upon waking, depending on the severity of the hangover. Continue with the honey until you start to feel better and then take 4 teaspoons (27 g) with your first meal. The potassium in the honey helps counteract the effects of the alcohol and will decrease the cravings for it.

Thrifty Cure!

Eat a banana! Bananas are rich in the important electrolytes magnesium and potassium, which are severely depleted during heavy drinking.

To help ward off a hangover, take a 100 mg B complex vitamin before bed and again upon arising to break down alcohol in the body. B vitamins are water soluble and get washed out of the body by the diuretic effects of alcohol.

Hangovers are produced by dehydration (alcohol is a diuretic) and hypoglycemia (alcohol is full of sugar). So drink plenty of fluids before and after drinking to prevent dehydration. Aim for twice as much water or non-alcoholic beverage to each drink you take. Sports drinks, which are high in electrolytes, help replenish what the kidneys have excreted during drinking. Take before bedtime. In the morning, a glass of orange juice or tomato juice can help dispel a hangover more quickly, as can teas of anise, mint, or chamomile.

Eat before imbibing. That's because when the stomach is full, alcohol absorption is slowed.

Fruit juice contains natural sugars, which help the body metabolize alcohol faster. Elevating blood sugar levels by eating a snack of fruit before bed can help prevent a hangover. Eating oily foods like cheese or nuts before drinking and starchy foods while drinking also help prevent a hangover. Eating a few dates in the morning or a grapefruit will also elevate blood sugar levels, making you feel better.

KEEP IN MIND

A Siberian folk remedy to sober up is to have the person lay on their back while someone briskly rubs their ears in a circular motion. Don't rely on this or any of the other methods discussed here to still drive.

GOOD TO KNOW!

Take one tablet of activated charcoal per drink while you are drinking. The charcoal absorbs the impurities in the alcohol, which are the cause of the hangover. However, note that the charcoal also absorbs important nutrients, so if you are a heavy drinker, don't use this remedy daily as you will end up with nutritional deficiencies.

Thrifty Cure!

Try a compress of water on the head to which a few drops of geranium oil have been added to soothe a hangover-induced headache.

Skip This!

Coffee has long been used to sober folks up. However, it is a strong diuretic that can cause further dehydration so it should be avoided.

CHAPTER 3

NATURAL REMEDIES FOR RELIEF OF BURNS, BUG BITES, AND SKIN AFFLICTIONS

Whether we are indoors or outside, life sometimes presents challenges. It helps to know what to do so that a little problem doesn't have to become a big one. Here are some suggestions for relieving burns, bug bites, and skin afflictions naturally.

Healing Animal Bites and Scratches

A dog bite or a cat scratch can be distressing for both man and beast. Fortunately, there are plenty of simple things you can do to heal wounds fast, from healing herbs to homeopathic remedies.

HERBAL FIRST AID FOR BITES AND SCRATCHES

Bleeding will clean out a wound or scratch, but you'll also need to wash it with antiseptic soap and hot water. Allow the water to flush the wound by running over the bites for 10 minutes. Next, apply a few drops of lavender or tea tree essential oil, echinacea tincture, or hydrogen peroxide topically to further disinfect the wound.

You can also apply some goldenseal powder, a plantain leaf compress, or charcoal poultice over the wounded area, using enough of the moistened remedy to cover the area. (See "Preparations 101" on page 18 for information on how to make a compress.) After applying the poultice, apply a sterile dressing.

Take an extra 500 mg of vitamin C for kids and 1,000 mg for adults and a dropperful of echinacea tincture several times daily internally to prevent infection for at least three days afterwards.

 WHEN TO SEE YOUR M.D.
Get medical attention in any of the following circumstances:

- A bite occurs from a human or wild animal.
- The bite is on the face, which can leave scarring.
- A child who has allergic tendencies has been bitten.
- The bite results in a bluish discoloration at the bite site, indicating nerve or blood vessel damage.
- Signs of infection appear.

Cures from Grandma's Kitchen

Treat second- and third-degree burns by blending ¹/₂ cup (120 ml) wheat germ oil with ¹/₂ cup (170 g) raw honey and ¹/₂ teaspoon lobelia powder. Store in a clean glass jar in a cool place. When needed, add enough chopped or blended comfrey leaves to make a paste. Apply gently with a new clean paintbrush! Don't clean off the paste, just keep painting on additional layers 2 or 3 times daily to regenerate new skin. Comfrey contains allantoin, which stimulates tissue regeneration.

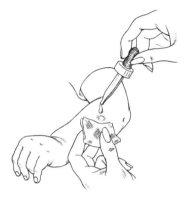

HOMEOPATHIC FIRST AID FOR BITES AND SCRATCHES

Give homeopathic Ledum if the wound is deep, especially if the area is swollen, red, and feels cold. Give homeopathic Apis if the wound is hot and stingy and if cold applications bring relief. Homeopathic Lachesis is a remedy specific for dog bites, whereas homeopathic Acetic acid is for cat bites. In all instances, take 3 to 4 pellets under the tongue 4 times a day if needed.

PRACTICE THIS

Teach children to avoid petting animals they do not know and to not approach wild animals. Wild animals that allow themselves to be petted are more likely to be sick. Large dogs can cause the most serious bites. Do not leave children alone with animals and avoid interfering with animals that are mating, fighting, or eating.

Relieving Burns

Burns are a nasty surprise. First-degree burns leave a red painful mark without blisters and often occur from mild sunburn or brief contact with a hot object. Only the first layer of skin is affected. Second-degree burns cause blisters and swelling. This can happen when you are splashed with boiling water or even from severe sunburn and can cause scarring. Third-degree burns may look white and charred and may occur from prolonged contact with hot objects or severe electrical shock. Such burns can involve all the skin layers, including the subcutaneous tissue, and often damages muscles and other tissues.

To help alleviate pain from any type of burn, elevate the burned area above the heart to slow circulation. Avoid breaking blisters or removing tissue. An insulated dry cold pack can help relieve pain and so can these tips.

NATURAL REMEDIES FOR HEALING FIRST- AND SECOND-DEGREE BURNS

Fill a basin with cold (not freezing) water and submerge the burned area in it for as long as it takes for the pain to subside. If water is scarce, rinse gently with milk or beer or apply clean water compresses. Never apply anything to a burn before doing this as you can actually seal in the heat, causing more damage. Soaking burned areas in salt water, especially kosher salt, is also beneficial.

Calendula salve, grated carrot, comfrey poultice, cucumber slices, raw honey, tofu, wheat grass, plantain poultice, raw potato or potato juice, vinegar, yogurt, or cooled damp black tea bags can all be applied topically to first-degree burns after the heat has been soaked out of them. These all will have a cooling and anti-inflammatory effect.

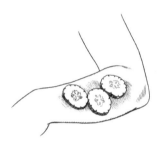

After soaking the burn, apply undiluted lavender or tea tree essential oil to the burned area. Give 2 drops Rescue Remedy under the tongue to minimize the trauma of the situation.

Topical application of Saint John's-Wort oil is also an excellent burn remedy and helps repair nerve damage. Apply any of these remedies three to four times daily. Protect any burned areas from the sun. Avoid applying anything with cotton balls, which have irritating fibers that can stick to the burn. Use clean fingers, a clean piece of cloth, or even a clean new paintbrush.

If you burned your mouth, rinse it with cold water. Then take 2 teaspoons (10 ml) of olive oil and slowly swish it around your mouth. Sucking on ice cubes also helps.

HOMEOPATHICS FOR HEALING BURNS

Homeopathic Urtica urens can be given for first-degree burns. Homeopathic Hypericum is used internally to help repair nerves damaged by burns. Homeopathic Arsenicum album is for burned skin that appears seared, scaly, red, swollen, and is sensitive to touch. Take homeopathic Cantharis, Hypericum, or Causticum for second-degree burns. Homeopathic

Thrifty Cures!

If you burn a fingertip, place your thumb on the back of your earlobe and the burnt fingertip on the front. Press firmly for a minute for relief.

Cures from Grandma's Kitchen

Try drinking this beneficial tea to help the body heal from a burn:

2 parts comfrey leaf
1 part red clover blossoms
1 part nettles
1 part skullcap
1 part marshmallow root

Drink $^1/_2$ cup (118 ml) every 2 hours along with 1 capsule comfrey root to promote cell regeneration and 1 capsule echinacea to prevent blood poisoning and infection.

Urtica can be given for pain that feels like stinging. Homeopathic remedies are used as 3 to 4 pellets dissolved under the tongue 3 or 4 times daily as needed.

NUTRIENTS FOR HEALING BURNS

Eat lots of healing chlorophyll-rich super foods such as spirulina, chlorella, and blue-green algae. These are available in capsules; take up to two capsules three times daily. Also recommended is eating soothing oily avocados, olives, and olive oil to help burns heal and to keep the skin moist.

Burn victims are prone to candida, as injured tissue provides a breeding ground for opportunistic infections. Use an acidophilus supplement to minimize fungal overgrowth, one to two capsules between meals three times daily.

For the recovery phase of burns, take an antioxidant vitamin supplement that contains 1,000 mg vitamin C, 400 IU vitamin E, and 15 mg zinc to promote healing and minimize scarring.

GOOD TO KNOW!

Remove rings or tight clothing in the area of the burn; if swelling does occur, these items may be difficult to remove later.

GOOD TO KNOW!

A Chinese patent herbal formula for burns is topical application of Jing Wan Hong (also known as Ching Wan Hung), which can be applied directly to the skin after cleaning or onto clean gauze and then applied to the skin.

Drink plenty of fluids when burned to help replace lost fluids. However, never give an unconscious person anything to consume. Turn an unconscious person on their side to allow body fluids like vomit or saliva to drain to prevent choking. Raise the opposite side of the body with a supportive pillow or cushion.

GOOD TO GROW!

Aloe is naturally cooling and anti-inflammatory, so keep a jar of aloe vera in the refrigerator to use for topical burn application. Aloe plants benefit from having their outer leaves cut, so use the inner gel from older, lower leaves on first- and second-degree burns and reapply several times daily.

WHEN TO SEE YOUR M.D.

Second-degree burns covering more than 15 percent of an adult and 10 percent of a child and all third-degree burns should receive medical attention. In addition, burns that increase in pain more than two days after the incident, discharge pus, or cause problems in moving the joints, or occur with a high fever should be seen by a health professional. Burns on the face may result in blockage of the respiratory tract; get prompt medical attention if swelling occurs or breathing becomes impaired. If there is shock that doesn't improve, seek medical attention.

Healing Hives

Hives are hot and itchy and can make you want to hide. First, try to figure out the cause of the hives. Are you very stressed? Are you using a new lotion, bubble bath, makeup, or detergent? Are you eating a food you're allergic to? If possible, change whatever you suspect may be a cause. Next, try these remedies.

HERBS FOR HEALING HIVES

Drink two to three cups of either a single herb or a combination of the following: calendula, chamomile, dandelion leaf and root, nettles, plantain, and red clover tea to help the body's normal channels of elimination such as the kidneys, liver, and lymph. Natural food stores carry pre-made detoxifying herbal tea blends.

Soak in the bathtub with a couple of handfuls of oatmeal tied into a washcloth. Pat the soothing oatmeal mucilage that exudes from the cloth on the skin. Or bathe with a pound (455 g) of alkalinizing baking soda.

After you dry off, apply cooling and soothing aloe vera juice or cooled chamomile tea with clean fingers or a soft cloth as an anti-inflammatory agent to the affected area.

Skip This!

Avoid spicy foods like ginger and cayenne, as they tend to bring toxins to the surface of the skin by powerfully increasing circulation. Foods likely to cause rashes, as they are common allergens, include citrus fruit, strawberries, mangoes, tomatoes, shellfish, nuts, and chocolate.

COOLING PRACTICES FOR HEALING HIVES

Eat a bland diet including alkalinizing celery, cucumbers, and kale and other green leafy vegetables. Wear cooling blue rather than red or orange.

Getting Rid of Lice, Crabs, and Scabies

These three parasites can make those infected with them very uncomfortable. Head lice are prolific, and females lay between 50 and 300 nits in their life cycle. Nine days later, the eggs hatch. Nits are tiny yellow ovals that attach themselves firmly to the hair shaft and survive by biting and sucking blood. They can live up to two days without a host.

Pubic lice are also known as crabs. Crabs are generally transmitted by sexual contact. They are hard to see but look like tiny black- or rust-colored spots clinging to the base of pubic hair. Using a magnifying glass can help them be more visible. They are treated in the same manner as head lice.

Scabies, also known as body lice, infest the body, especially in areas of the wrists, finger webs, hands, elbows, underarms, waist, feet, scrotum, and nipples, burrowing into skin and causing itching. Scabies can live in the seams of clothing, migrating to the body for their twice-daily feedings.

Parasites are more likely to invade those in poor health, so a lifelong practice of good hygiene and sound nutrition is wise. Strengthen your energy shield! If you do get infected, here's how to stop the itch.

ESSENTIAL OILS TO GET RID OF LICE

To make a natural lice shampoo out of herbs, add 5 drops each of essential oils of tea tree, rosemary, lavender, peppermint, and eucalyptus to a base of 5 teaspoons (28 ml) of pure olive oil. Add a small amount of regular shampoo to the mixture and put this all over the hair to the ends. Leave on an hour under a shower cap to prevent drips. Rinse and shampoo the hair.

You can also add 20 drops of these same essential oils to $1/2$ cup (120 ml) apple cider vinegar and an equal amount of water. Shampoo, rinse, and pour the solution over your head. Leave on for 20 minutes before rinsing out. Avoid getting any essential oils in your eyes or mouth. Repeat in 10 days.

Another remedy is to blend 12 cloves of garlic in 1 pint (475 ml) of water and work the solution into the hair and scalp. Cover the head with a plastic shower cap, leave on one hour, and then wash your hair. Repeat treatments again in 10 days. After shampooing, rinse the hair and scalp with vinegar. This loosens the glue that holds the nits onto the hair shafts. Rinse with hot water—but not so hot that it burns. Follow the same procedure as with the mayonnaise (see page 62) to remove remaining nits.

KEEP IN MIND

Every person in the household will need to be checked. Human lice do not live on animals (and vice versa). And it is only polite to let the parents of any children your child was in contact with know that they should inspect their own children. This sounds embarrassing, but it's not a great idea to let other children get more and more lice before their parents notice. Also, you do not want any of these children giving lice back to your child! It is especially important to inform the school office and your child's teacher.

NATURAL REMEDIES TO DETER SCABIES

Eat lots of garlic and seaweed to make the parasites dislike the taste of your blood. Also consume liver-cleansing foods such as carrots, beets, burdock, dandelion greens, and barley. Drink blood-purifying teas such as cleavers, dandelion root, echinacea, and red clover blossoms three times daily. By detoxifying the blood, you'll make the parasites less interested in you and more apt to seek out a less healthy host.

Use a salt rub on your skin by moistening salt with water and rubbing all over the body. Leave on for $1/2$ hour. Soak deep in a hot bath scented with tea tree oil for 30 minutes to an hour. Then friction dry. Take a sauna. Scabies can't survive in temperatures of 120°F (49°C) for more than 5 minutes.

After the heat treatment, apply undiluted tea tree and lavender oil to infested areas of the skin to deter the critters, who won't like the taste and will leave. Itching can persist for several days, even after the parasites are dead.

Parasite invasion symbolizes letting others have power over you. Reclaim your body and life. You are stronger and smarter than they are. Don't allow things to get under your skin.

Ṛ Pregnant wmen or infants should consult with a competent health-care professional before following any of the remedies for treatment of parasites. Essential oils can be too strong for young skin, and essential oil use during pregnancy has not yet been well researched.

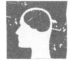

GOOD TO KNOW!
If there are any nits on the eyelashes or eyebrows, coat them thoroughly with Vaseline. Reapply four times a day.

Thrifty Cure!

Head and public lice can be killed quickly, easily, cheaply, and safely with mayonnaise. Buy a new jar of real mayonnaise as one in the refrigerator may be too cold and old. Grab several handfuls—enough to cover all the hair, being sure to get behind the ears and down the neck a bit. Cover with a disposable plastic shower cap to keep the mess to a minimum. Leave the mayonnaise on for two hours to smother the lice and developed eggs. Remove and dispose the shower cap, wash the hands well, and shampoo. It may take two or more shampoos to get the hair clean.

The mayonnaise may not kill the newest nits since the unborn lice inside may not have developed enough to need air yet. To deal with nits left behind, under good lighting (such as natural sunlight), comb out any remaining eggs with a fine-toothed metal comb. Nits are usually found near the scalp. Check the hair by tiny sections, especially around the edges of the hair, at the neck, and behind the ears. Put each nit or hair into a bowl of vinegar. Flush away any contaminated tissues. Boil the comb for three minutes in water or throw it away after use.

Repeat the smother-the-hair-with-mayonnaise-technique seven to ten days after the first application to kill any survivors. Continue to check the hair daily for a few weeks since you or your child may still be around others who are infected.

Disinfect Everything!

Your hair or your child's hair is not your only worry. All of the clothing that you or your child has worn and towels used for the last week should be washed in hot water. If there is some item that will shrink in the washer, you can put it through the dryer on the hot cycle for 30 minutes without washing it first.

All bedding (sheets, blankets, pillows, pillowcases, comforter, mattress cover) needs to either be washed in hot water, dried dry on the hot cycle, or put into a plastic bag and left sealed up. (They say that lice can only live away from the human host for 48 hours or so, and the nits can survive 7 to 10 days without a host, but keep the bags sealed for at least two weeks—just in case—and because more eggs could hatch during this time period or new lice could be brought home.)

Bagging will also be necessary for stuffed animals, hats, throw pillows, barrettes, ponytail holders, hair ribbons, helmets, necklaces, and anything else that has come in contact with you or your child or combs and brushes. Vacuum the mattress, couch, chairs, rugs and floors, car seats and backs, car rugs, and upholstered church pews thoroughly then dispose of the vacuum bag.

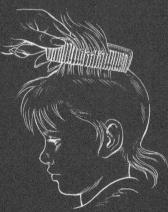

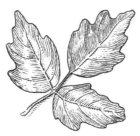

Ditching the Itch of Poison Ivy and Poison Oak

Poison ivy and poison oak are a hot mess. And it's not the type of hot mess you see on Project Runway! It's the kind that is red and itchy. Poison ivy is more abundant east of the Rocky Mountains, with poison oak growing west. Both plants are very similar, with poison oak having more lobed leaves, similar to that of an oak tree. The toxic principle in both is called urushiol. It is one of the most potent external toxins on earth. Usually within 6 to 72 hours, the skin may burn, itch, and look red. Small blisters that look similar to fleabites will appear first. Later, a crust may form.

Not only can you get this nasty itch from touching the plant, you can also get it from touching clothes, pets, sporting equipment, car seats, tools, or anything else that has been in contact with the plant. People with delicate or fair skin who are very sun sensitive are considered the most susceptible. A number of home remedies can help comfort and speed healing of "the awful itch."

℞ **WHEN TO SEE YOUR M.D.**
Seek medical attention for cases of poison ivy or poison oak occurring near the eyes, mouth, genitals, covering more than half the body, or causing a high fever.

HERBAL REMEDIES FOR POISON IVY AND POISON OAK

Herbs that have shown the most success as far as bringing relief when applied topically are made from teas of the following plants: burdock leaf and root, calendula, goldenseal root, grindelia, myrrh, plantain leaf, and white oak bark. They all have blood-purifying and soothing properties.

To make a tea for topical application, put 1 cup (30 g) of any of these herbs or a combination of them in a half-gallon (1.9 L) canning jar. Fill the jar with boiling water or hot apple cider vinegar. Cover and let stand 12 hours. Strain the tea and apply the liquid by patting it on gently to the afflicted area.

Another excellent herb for topical use is jewelweed (*Impatiens* spp.), which is rich in natural tannins. However, rather than making a tea of this plant, the fresh juice is preferable. (You can simply run the fresh herb through a juicer.) Since jewelweed is available only during the summer months, and poison ivy is around longer, you can freeze the jewelweed juice into ice cubes and store them in plastic bags in the freezer. Apply the juice or frozen cubes directly to the skin.

Thrifty Cures!

Once you have poison ivy or poison oak, cleanse your system by drinking teas three times daily of burdock root, dandelion root, nettle herb, and red clover blossom. You can also make a poultice of green clay and apple cider vinegar and apply to the itchy area.

HOMEOPATHIC HELP FOR POISON IVY AND POISON OAK

Many people find that homeopathy can help them better resist poison ivy. Homeopathic Rhus tox (which is actually made from poison ivy) 12x or 30c potency (homeopathy is measured in x or c doses), where 3 pills are taken every 2 hours, can be used before or after exposure.

KEEP IN MIND

If you do get poison ivy, avoid washing with a washcloth as this will cause it to spread. You may find that bathing helps to bring some relief. Add 1 cup (235 ml) of apple cider vinegar, oatmeal (80 g), or baking soda (221 g) to the bath.

Keep your nails short and change and wash clothing daily. Try to avoid sweating or getting too much sun.

Learn to identify the plant and avoid it. Wear gloves and clothing that covers you well before going out in infested areas. If you think you have contacted poison ivy or poison oak, remove and launder your clothing. Wash your body within 10 to 30 minutes. It is important to use an alkaline soap without an oil base to avoid spreading the urushiol.

Skip This!

Burning poison ivy or poison oak can cause dangerous smoke that irritates the eyes and lungs. Don't do it!

Skip This!

Avoid citrus and tomato products during a poison ivy or poison oak outbreak as these foods can exacerbate the rash due to their high acid content. Also avoid foods in the Brassicaceae family such as cabbage, broccoli, cauliflower, and mustard greens. They are so cleansing that they will cause the rash to spread during an outbreak.

GOOD TO GROW!
A folk remedy for poison ivy and poison oak prevention is to rub fresh artemesia leaves on exposed skin when going out. It grows wild in many parts of the country.

Cures from Grandma's Kitchen

Make a paste of water or apple cider vinegar mixed with baking soda, oatmeal, or Epsom salts. Aloe vera juice, tofu, and watermelon rind all provide cooling relief. One pint (475 ml) of buttermilk to which 1 tablespoon (18 ml) of sea salt has been added is also helpful.

Remedying Ringworm

Ringworm is a fungal infection that can affect the scalp, body, feet, and nails. The name comes from a characteristic red ring of small scales that appears on the infected person's skin and has nothing to do with worms, thank goodness. Though it is not dangerous, it is contagious. As a first step, you need to practice excellent hygiene, washing clothing, bedding, and towels in hot water followed by a dryer cycle. Avoid sharing towels. Next, use these natural cures.

HERBAL REMEDIES FOR RINGWORM

Apply 3 to 5 drops of essential oils of lavender or tea tree topically to the area. You can also use echinacea tincture, goldenseal tincture, and/or myrrh tincture simply by applying enough to cover the affected area three times daily.

You can also rub a crushed garlic clove briefly over the area several times daily, but don't leave the garlic clove on the skin as it can burn. Garlic oil, a major anti-fungal agent, can also be used internally (take three capsules daily). In addition, take one dropperful of black walnut tincture (a powerful antifungal agent) three times daily and a probiotic supplement three times daily to help the body better resist fungal overgrowth.

KEEP IN MIND

Fungi thrive in warm, moist areas, such as locker rooms and swimming pools and in skin folds. Avoid sharing clothing, sports equipment, towels, or sheets. Add 1 cup (235 ml) of apple cider vinegar to the final rinse water of your laundry.

Wear loose-fitting natural clothing and use natural fibers in bedding so the skin can breathe and fungal infections will not thrive.

Skip This!

Cut out sugars, alcohol, and fruit juices when you have ringworm as all of these foods nourish fungi.

Thrifty Cures!

A traditional folk remedy for ringworm is to place a copper penny in vinegar until the penny turns green and then rub the wet green penny on the affected area. Another folk remedy is to make a paste of apple cider vinegar and salt and apply to the affected area. Repeat three times daily.

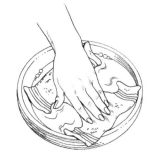

Soothing Sunburn

Spending too much time in the sun can leave you feeling overdone. Excessive sun exposure can contribute to premature aging, wrinkles, and even skin cancer. Prevention is the key. But if you do get toasted, here's how to feel better fast.

NATURAL REMEDIES FOR SUNBURN

After excess sun exposure, take a cool shower or soak in a tepid bath to which you have added 1 cup (235 ml) of alkalinizing apple cider vinegar or 7 drops of cooling and anti-inflammatory peppermint or lavender essential oil. Black or green tea bags are high in pain-relieving astringent tannic acid and can be moistened and applied to the skin or made into a tea and added to the bath water.

Another soothing bath for sunburn is $^1/_2$ cup (111 g) of baking soda and a small handful of sea salt. Tepid oatmeal baths (use 1 cup [80 g]) are also soothing and cooling.

After your bath, apply 1 cup (235 ml) aloe vera juice with 10 drops of lavender oil to soothe the skin. Use just the amount needed to cover afflicted areas. Store remaining portions in the refrigerator in a clean, labeled glass jar.

Drink peppermint tea to cool you from the inside. Drink plenty of water to help rehydrate the skin.

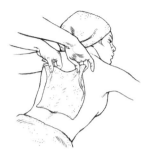

KEEP IN MIND

Look for natural sunscreens at health food stores and apply 30 minutes before exposure. Wear a hat that gives shade to the back of the neck and drink plenty of water.

Soothing Boils

Boils, also known as *furuncles*, are a sign of excess heat in the body. These tender pus-filled areas are often dark red or purplish in color. Symptoms include itching, mild pain, and localized swelling. Boils are most likely to occur on the face, scalp, buttocks, legs, and underarm area and can be caused by food sensitivity, poor hygiene, infected hair follicles, and weakened immunity. Here's how to bring things to a head.

HERBAL REMEDIES FOR BOILS

If possible, elevate the site of infection so that it is above the heart. To draw a boil to its head, which will draw the toxins to the surface and thus out of the body, apply a hot ginger tea compress. (See "Preparations 101" on page 12 for information on how to make a hot ginger tea compress.)

Skip This!

Avoid further sun exposure until symptoms have subsided. Do not break blisters. Avoid midday sun. Be aware that you can get burned through light cotton clothing.

Cures from Grandma's Kitchen

Look in your fridge for sunburn relief. Blend up some yogurt and cucumber and apply directly to the skin or apply a grated potato poultice. Or you can even apply a compress of cold milk! For sunburned eyes, apply cucumber slices, grated raw potato or apple, or chamomile tea bag poultices.

Alternatively, you can soak the afflicted area in a hot Epsom salt solution (1/2 cup [115 g] of salt to 1 quart [950 ml] of hot water). You can even apply a hot black tea bag!

Next, mix red clay with enough apple cider vinegar to make a thick paste and apply directly to the affected area. Leave it on until it dries. This helps to dry the boil and draw toxins to the surface. Do this several times a day.

After the boil breaks, apply echinacea extract or lavender oil to the area several times a day. You can also take echinacea, red clover, violet leaf, and burdock root as a tea, tincture, or capsules, as all of these herbs are considered alterative, or blood purifying.

Soothing Blisters

Breaking in a new pair of shoes or just walking too much can lead to a blister. A blister is a small pocket of fluid within the skin's upper layers, often caused by friction, burning, freezing, chemical exposure, or infection. Most blisters are filled with a clear fluid called serum or plasma. However, blisters can be filled with blood (known as blood blisters) or pus if infected. Here's how to feel better.

 WHEN TO SEE YOUR M.D.
Seek medical help for a boil:

- **If red streaks appear to radiate outward from the boil site.**
- **If the patient is an infant or very elderly.**
- **If the boil is on the upper lip, nose, scalp or outer ear (all are too close to the brain).**
- **If the boil is in the armpit or groin or on the breast of a nursing mother.**
- **If a fever over 100°F (38°C) persists.**

HERBAL REMEDIES FOR BLISTERS

Keep the area clean and relieve any pressure on the blister. It is best to leave blisters unbroken. Treat blisters as you would an open wound.

If you must pop a blister, first, make a small puncture at the base of the blister using a sterilized needle. Next, wash with soap and water and apply a plantain poultice, echinacea tincture, or essential oil of lavender or tea tree topically. Cover with a breathable Band-Aid.

KEEP IN MIND

Consider wearing two pairs of socks to prevent foot blisters. Wear gloves or wrap hands when handling tools.

Preventing Insect Bites and Easing Itch

Bug bites result in itchy welts that you shouldn't scratch, even though you really want to! Such welts appear when the saliva injected by a mosquito, bee, or ant causes a histamine response. Here's how to prevent bites and treat them too.

Essential Oil Remedy to Ward Off Insects

To ward away insects, try this herbal insect repellent:

- 2 ounces (60 ml) almond oil
- 5 drops essential oil of eucalyptus
- 5 drops essential oil of lavender
- 5 drops essential oil of tea tree
- 5 drops essential oil of citronella
- 5 drops essential oil of rosemary

Mix together and apply liberally, avoiding the eyes and mucus membranes.

To create a more bug-free environment, consider diffusing essential oils of citronella, eucalyptus, geranium, lavender, rosemary, and tea tree. You can also make a room spray by combining water with a few drops of the oil. Hanging a bouquet of dried tomato plant leaves in the room also wards off insects. Perhaps some insects just don't like the aroma.

Here are a few ideas to keep bugs from finding you an easy target:

- When heading out, tuck in your hair and shirts and socks so bugs have less access to your skin.
- The best colors to wear are white, tan, and light green, which are less attractive to bugs.
- Avoid floral prints (you don't want to look like a flower), loose clothing, the color blue (the preferred color of mosquitoes), hair spray, perfumes (you don't want to smell like a flower either), sandals, and shiny jewelry (which can also attract attention from the bug world).

GOOD TO KNOW!
Taking 3 or 4 garlic capsules a day will also make you an unappetizing host. 100 mg (50 for kids) of vitamin B complex taken orally creates a smell that many bugs don't like. Taking homeopathic Staphysagria also may prevent you being bitten. Essential oils such as cedarwood, citronella, lavender, and tea tree can be applied topically to pulse points such as the wrists, behind the knees, and behind the ears every hour or so.

FOR ANT BITES

You can treat ant bites topically with any of the following:

- Apple cider vinegar (or a paste of baking soda and apple cider vinegar)
- Green clay
- Cucumber juice (or just rub a slice of cucumber over the area)
- Essential oil of lavender

All of these will help neutralize any venom and dry up the itching and stinging chemicals left by the ants.

FOR BEE STINGS

Remove the stinger by dragging the edge of your fingernail or a credit card across it. Wash the area with soap and water. Make a paste by adding water or vinegar to meat tenderizer, which is made from papain, the enzyme derived from papaya. This helps break down the inflam-

℞ WHEN TO SEE YOUR M.D.
For some, insect bites have the potential to be dangerous. Watch for skin flushing, severe coughing, wheezing, anxiety, blurred vision, and vomiting. Rush to the nearest emergency room if you or others experience any of these symptoms when bitten.

GOOD TO GROW!
Include aromatic plants such as artemesia, lavender, or rosemary in your garden. You can rub them on your body to prevent insect bites!

matory properties of the venom. Baking soda mixed with water and applied directly to the stung area also provides relief.

Take a dropperful of echinacea several times during the day to reduce swelling. Taking 100 mg of bromelain (an enzyme derived from pineapple) and quercetin (a flavonoid with anti-inflammatory activity) orally every 4 hours will also help reduce inflammation.

Skip This!

Stay off of meat and spicy, oily, and heavy-protein foods. You want your body to focus its energy on healing, not breaking down foods that are difficult to digest. Avoid sugar too as sugar provides food for bacteria.

 GOOD TO KNOW! Insects are attracted to people who eat lots of bananas, so curb your banana intake. Alcohol consumption causes blood vessel dilation, thus making you more desirable for mosquitoes.

Homeopathic Apis is ideal for stings that are swollen. Take 4 pellets under the tongue 4 times a day. If you have some vitamin C handy, take about 1,000 mg to reduce swelling.

If you are allergic to bee stings, carry an emergency kit with you or seek medical attention immediately.

FOR BLACK FLY BITES

Apply tea tree oil, lavender essential oil, or witch hazel to bites by dabbing a few drops from the bottle with your fingers. You can also apply a paste of powdered charcoal. Just open a capsule or two and mix with enough water or apple cider vinegar to get it to stick. All of these substances help relieve pain and itching due to their anti-inflammatory actions.

FOR CATERPILLAR/CENTIPEDE BITES

Brush off a caterpillar or centipede in the direction they are traveling or irritating hairs may remain in your skin. Apply essential oil of lavender to the bite as needed. Echinacea tincture can be used topically and internally. Repeat these treatments three or four times daily until you have relief.

Cures from Grandma's Kitchen

If you've been bitten by a bug, soak in a bathtub with 1 cup (235 ml) apple cider vinegar or 1 pound (455 g) baking soda. (Use half as much for children.)
Or try adding 1 gallon (3.8 L) peppermint tea or ½ cup (235 ml) of sea salt.

FOR MOSQUITO BITES

Wash the bitten area and apply three to five drops essential oil of lavender or some apple cider vinegar. Apply ice. Other helpful things to apply topically include mud, plantain leaf poultice, witch hazel, lemon juice, and baking soda mixed with enough apple cider vinegar to make a paste and moistened with vitamin C powder. Essential oils that can be applied directly to a bite include peppermint, lavender, and tea tree.

FOR TICKS

When removing a tick, use disinfected tweezers, grab the tick as close to the head as possible, and pull straight out. Wash the bite area and your hands well with antiseptic soap, dry and then apply a few drops of Echinacea 3 times daily.

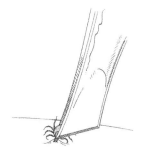

FOR WASP STINGS

For wasp stings, apply apple cider vinegar, damp tea leaves, garlic, an onion or potato poultice, and baking soda as a paste. Take homeopathic Vespa 30x internally. Taking 1,000 mb of vitamin C and 100 mg of panothenic acid for 3 or 4 hours helps provide a natural antihistamine effect, thus reducing swelling.

Soothing Painful Shingles

Shingles, also known as Herpes varicella-zoster virus, can be very painful. Shingles occur when the chicken pox virus (which lays dormant in the body after you get it) is reactivated by stress, fatigue, or another illness. Shingles can cause pain along the nerves, and is first signaled by a burning or shooting pain, pricking, or tenderness. The nerves on the chest, face, back, neck, arms, and legs are most often affected. The pain is due to the swelling of the blisters, though pain may persist even after the blisters heal as the nerves have become irritated. Attacks have been known to last from a week in younger folk, though older people may suffer as long as two months.

NATURAL REMEDIES THAT EASE INFLAMMATION AND STRESS

Choose anti-inflammatory and antiviral herbs such as black walnut, dandelion root, echinacea, licorice root, lomatium, Oregon grape root, and yellow dock. These can be used in teas (1 cup [235 ml] of tea), tinctures (1 dropperful) or capsules (1 to 2) three times daily.

Propolis tincture and aloe vera juice can also be used topically to provide antiviral properties. Use enough to cover the affected area.

The Chinese patent formula Chuan Xin Lian is also anti-inflammatory and antiviral. Look for it at natural food stores and follow the directions on the label.

Homeopathic Rhus tox can speed recovery by stimulating the body's immune response. Take four pellets four times daily.

Hops, passionflower, oatstraw or seed, skullcap, and valerian help calm pain and stress. Look for an herbal tincture containing some of these relaxing herbs at health food stores and take a dropperful three to four times daily.

SOOTHING SALVES THAT EASE PAIN

Salves used topically often help shingles. Look for a salve that contains antiviral substances such as the amino acid lysine and the herbs calendula, chaparral leaf, comfrey leaf or root, echinacea root, goldenseal root, licorice root, marshmallow root, plantain leaves, tea tree oil, and Saint-John's-Wort.

Peppermint essential oil can also be applied topically to numb the pain. Peaceful Mountain makes a product called Shingles Rescue that many have said is helpful. Get these in the health food store and apply three to four times daily.

SUPPLEMENTS THAT PROMOTE HEALING

Take a daily dose of vitamin A (10,000 IU), vitamin C (1000 to 3000 mg), and vitamin E (400 IU) to help fight infection and promote healing. Take a good B-complex vitamin (50 mg) as well as calcium (1,000 mg) and magnesium (500 mg) daily to help your body deal with the stress of this illness. Lysine can help keep the virus from replicating by inhibiting its growth. Take 500 mg up to six times daily for up to 2 weeks.

BEST FOODS FOR SHINGLES

With an inflammatory condition like shingles, you'll want to eat foods to cool the blood, mostly fruits and vegetables. Mung beans, apples, beets, carrots, cucumbers, lemon, and water can all be taken. Drink $1^{1}/_{2}$ quarts (1.4 L) of beet, celery, or cucumber juice daily (unless pregnant) to alkalinize the body and cool inflammation internally.

SOOTHING PRACTICES FOR SHINGLES

Color therapy can help you feel better. Color is energy, and the last colors in the spectrum have a calming and cooling effect. Use green (generally healing) for the acute stage and violet for painful nerves. Blue helps calm pain. Wear those colors or spend time under lights of those colors.

 GOOD TO KNOW!
Taking an extra B12 (500 mcg) every hour for the first day and 200 mcg a day thereafter can help relieve pain and speed healing of the blisters.

CHAPTER 4

NATURAL REMEDIES TO THE RESCUE FOR INJURIES AND FIRST AID

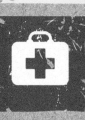

Knowing what to do in an emergency is essential so you can act quickly. This section will help you know just what to do when an injury occurs. If you are in doubt, call your doctor or go to your nearest emergency room.

Treating Cuts and Wounds

You might have been slicing a vegetable, opening a can of cat food, or tackling that home improvement project when you got cut. A superficial cut is called an abrasion. If the wound is deep, it is a laceration. If the wound is deep or was caused by something rusty, seek medical attention. Also if infection develops pus, if there is swelling or excess redness, if foreign material is embedded in the wound, or if you have a fever, get thee to a health care professional. If not, use these tips to heal thyself.

HERBAL REMEDIES FOR WOUNDS

Wash the injured area with soap and water. Rinse and blot dry. If there is visible dirt, use sterile gauze to wipe it out. However, do not use cotton balls, which can leave fibers in the wound.

Next, apply a calendula herbal salve (available at natural food stores), honey, or lavender or tea tree essential oils, which are all soothing and antibacterial.

You can also take echinacea tincture orally to help prevent infection.

For a paper cut, which can be painful yet too tiny for a bandage, moisten the wound and apply some powdered cloves for their anesthetic properties.

It is best to leave a wound exposed to air so it can breathe. However, if your kids like to play in the dirt, cover the wound with a bandage or sterile gauze to keep it clean. Use a butterfly bandage if the wound is large; this will help the wound "knit" back together more easily.

HOMEOPATHIC REMEDIES FOR WOUNDS

Homeopathic remedies for cuts include Hypericum, especially for wounds where there are many nerve endings, such as fingertips, or for wounds manifesting as sharp shooting pain. Homeopathic Ledum is for deep puncture wounds, especially if the area is swollen, reddish, and numb or cold. Take as directed.

Cures from Grandma's Kitchen

Grate raw potato and apply it directly to soothe the bruised area. Or try using cabbage leaf, which is improved by breaking up the cabbage by rolling the leaf with a rolling pin! Witch hazel and castor oil both cool, soothe, and reduce inflammation as well.

Bettering Bruises

You may have knocked your shin on a coffee table or bumped into your desk. You get a bruise when the skin is struck with force yet the skin is unbroken and blood rushes to the damaged tissues below the surface. As a first step, elevate the area that is bruised. Apply an ice pack to reduce swelling. After the first 24 hours, heat can be applied after swelling and inflammation have subsided. These tips can help you feel better too.

 WHEN TO SEE YOUR M.D.
A serious bruise may indicate underlying injuries. Head bruises could be a sign of skull fracture and may require medical attention. If pain from a bruise is worse after 24 hours, get checked out to make sure there is not a broken bone. If bruises occur without any evidence of trauma (such as bumping into things), they may be an indication to get checked for anemia, leukemia, or a deficiency in vitamin C with bioflavonoids or vitamin K.

GOOD TO KNOW!
If you bruise easily, take a supplement of vitamin C with bioflavonoids and rutin to help strengthen collagen production and the capillaries. Look for a combination remedy that contains about 1,000 mg vitamin C and 250 mg bioflavonoids daily.

NATURAL REMEDIES TO REDUCE INFLAMMATION

Bromelain, an anti-inflammatory enzyme derived from pineapple, can reduce swelling and inflammation. Take 500 mg two or three times daily.

You can apply an herbal salve, like comfrey, to a bruise or essential oil of lavender (no more than 5 drops) can be applied as it is a powerful anti-inflammatory agent.

Chinese patent formulas that help bruising include Zheng Gu Shui, Dit Dat Jou, and Tiger Balm. Gently apply them to the bruised area three or four times daily.

NATURAL REMEDIES TO IMPROVE CLOTTING ABILITY

Consume plenty of vitamin K–rich foods, such as green leafy vegetables, which improve your blood-clotting ability. Nettle tea is also high in vitamin K. Drinking 1 quart (950 ml) daily can help if you bruise easily.

HOMEOPATHIC REMEDIES FOR BRUISES

Usually 3 or 4 pellets of the following homeopathic remedies are slowly dissolved under the tongue 3 or 4 times daily for bruise relief:

- Homeopathic Arnica soothes deep bruises. You can take this by mouth and topically, in the form of a salve, oil, or gel, but only on unbroken skin.
- Homeopathic Ruta graveolens helps pain caused by a blow and for one who feels as if the bone is bruised. Ruta is most often used when it is the elbow, kneecap, or shin that has been bruised.
- Use homeopathic Hypericum for bruises to sensitive areas such as fingertips, lips, nose, or eyes.
- Homeopathic Bellis is taken for bruising with swelling that is worse from pressure and better from motion and rest.

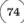

- Homeopathic Ledum is the remedy for bruising with extreme tenderness that is made better by cold and rest and worse from warmth and motion.
- Homeopathic Rhus tox is good for swelling and inflammation around the soft tissue and when the joint feels better after having moved a bit.

Easing Black Eye Inflammation

You can think of a black eye as a bruise around your eye. It happens when blood and other fluids collect in the space around the eye, resulting in swelling and dark discoloration. Here's how to feel better fast.

HOMEOPATHIC HELP FOR BLACK EYE

Use homeopathic Ledum for black eyes when cold applications help. Homeopathic Hypericum can help excessive pain. Homeopathic Arnica can help if there is injury to the soft tissue above or below the eye. If there is injury to the eyeball, use homeopathic Symphytum.

Stopping Bleeding

Bleeding, technically known as hemorrhaging, is the loss of blood from the circulatory system. When a wound bleeds, it can be scary. But what's important is taking control immediately and calling for help if you need it. These solutions can also help.

WHEN TO SEE YOUR M.D. Most black eyes are minor injuries and heal on their own in a few days; however, they may signify a more serious injury. Seek medical attention if vision problems develop.

BLEEDING FIRST AID

Lay the victim down and keep the person calm. Stress can elevate blood pressure and increase blood loss. Cover with a clean cloth and apply pressure directly unless there is a large object embedded in the wound. Maintain continuous pressure for 5 to 10 minutes. If the wound is large, squeeze the sides of the wound together firmly but gently. Raise the wounded area above the heart to help control bleeding unless a fracture is suspected.

To stop bleeding in the lower part of the body, press on the femoral artery against the pelvic bone. It helps to have the victim lay flat on their back as you place the heel of your hand on the crease of the thigh and groin. These two pressure points are to be used only if pressure and raising the limb don't stop the bleeding. Discontinue the points once bleeding has ceased. They should not be pressed for longer than five minutes.

GOOD TO GROW! Shred up some plantain leaves, mix with a bit of water, and apply topically as a poultice. It will draw out any remaining debris and soothe and protect the injured area.

GOOD TO KNOW! One of the most common things that sends people to the emergency room in my town is trying to slice frozen bagels with a sharp knife. It's important to thaw them first!

WHEN TO SEE YOUR M.D.

If an object is deeply embedded in the victim, seek medical attention. Bleeding occurring from the ear, mouth, or nose can be an indication of chest or head injury. Place the person in a semi-sitting position with the head leaning toward the injured side to facilitate the blood to drain and call for help. Internal bleeding is characterized by tenderness, pain, swelling, and discoloration of the urine, stool, vomit, and sputum. Don't move the person if internal injuries are suspect until help has arrived.

WHEN TO SEE YOUR M.D.

Seek medical attention for the following wounds:

- Are so wide a butterfly bandage can't hold them together.
- Are very deep.
- Affect a finger or joint.
- Are due to a broken bone or human or animal bite.
- Are due to a broken artery.
- Have caused the loss of function of a body part.
- Have a high risk of tetanus.
- Can't be well cleaned but need to be.

If the object that caused the wound is still imbedded in it, attempting to remove it could increase bleeding. Cover the wound gently so that the object will not be forced in deeper and seek medical attention.

HERBS THAT STOP BLEEDING

The herb yarrow, a potent astringent, can seal up a wound so quickly that dirt could still be trapped in it, so you'll need to clean if first with a good antiseptic soap. Use yarrow topically because it has an astringent or tightening effect.

GOOD TO KNOW!

Spider webs contain a coagulating substance that can be applied to cuts. Just make sure there is no spider in the web and that the web looks clean!

Thrifty Cures!

Apply slices of raw potato or cucumber on the area to cool inflammation and reduce pain and swelling. If you have them in your garden, you can collect some plantain leaves, shred them up with a bit of water, and apply them over the closed eye as a poultice.

Just grab a handful of the fresh plant's leaves. Chop it up a bit and press into the wound to stop minor bleeding.

Nettles are a good herb to give people prone to excessive bleeding as they contain vitamin K, which aids in blood clotting. Take 2 to 4 capsules (internally) daily if needed.

An excellent Chinese patent medicine to stop bleeding is Yunnan Pai Yao (made from tienchi ginseng, which has strong blood-clotting properties). Take either topically and/or internally as directed on the packaging. Avoid internal use during pregnancy as its safety has not been studied for use during that time.

Drawing Out Splinters

It's easy to get a splinter. As a first step, use tweezers sterilized with a bit of alcohol to remove the splinter. If the splinter is deeply imbedded, freeze the area with ice first to help anesthetize the area and try using a sterilized needle. Once the splinter is out, wash with soap and water and then apply an antiseptic solution such as echinacea tincture, tea tree or lavender

Thrifty Cures

Apply cayenne powder on the wound to encourage it to stop bleeding (note that this does sting). Just sprinkle some on a bleeding wound and apply pressure. Avoid contact with the eyes or mouth, which could burn. You can also take cayenne pepper powder internally in cases of bleeding. Take 1 teaspoon (2 g) in 1 cup (235 ml) of water.

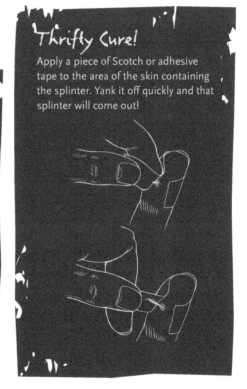

Thrifty Cure!

Apply a piece of Scotch or adhesive tape to the area of the skin containing the splinter. Yank it off quickly and that splinter will come out!

Cures from Grandma's Kitchen

Draw splinters out by taping a slice of raw onion to the area. (Onions pull objects to the surface of the skin.) Apply overnight and use a band-aid to keep in place. In the morning, the splinter should come out.

HOMEOPATHIC HELP FOR SPLINTERS

Homeopathic Ledum can help a stubborn splinter rise to the surface. Other homeopathic remedies include Silicea to help expel a foreign object. Hepar sulph is used when the area is sore and tender to the touch and helps it come to the surface. Take 3 or 4 pellets under the tongue three times daily for a few days until the splinter is removed.

Soothing and Healing Sprains

Sprains can happen during athletic activities, but they can also happen just by stepping off a curb and landing with your foot in the wrong direction. Sprains result when a ligament (the tissues connected to the bones near a joint) is stretched beyond its normal range of motion. There is likely to be pain, swelling, and discoloration. What's most important is to take action right away.

NATURAL CURES FOR SPRAINS

In addition to the arnica tincture compress mentioned in the "Good to Know" sidebar on page 79, other topical poultices or compresses can be made of apple cider vinegar, tofu, comfrey, plantain, clay, cabbage, onion, grated raw potato, tea tree essential oil, turmeric, burdock leaf, or ginger tea. You can also mix apple cider vinegar with sea salt and gently apply it to the area. Cool any teas well before applying. Use enough to cover the area well. (For directions on how to make a poultice or compress, see page 18 and 19.)

BEST FOODS AND SUPPLEMENTS FOR SPRAINS

Eat foods rich in the photochemical anthocyanadin, such as blackberries, blueberries, cherries, and raspberries, to strengthen blood vessels and muscles.

Take a daily supplement of calcium (1,000 mg)/magnesium (500 mg) supplement to keep muscles supple. Vitamin E (400 IU) and potassium (99 mg) supplements can also be taken. Taking bromelain in 100 milligram doses 3 times daily can help reduce pain and swelling.

Turmeric is another herbal ally to reduce inflammation. Take one or two capsules three times daily. Take 1,000 mg of vitamin C with bioflavonoids every 2 hours to reduce inflammation.

HOMEOPATHIC HELP FOR SPRAINS

Homeopathic Arnica and arnica oil can be applied topically. Homeopathic Byronia is used when the injury is hot, red, and swollen, when pain is worse from movement, and when the injury needs to be held tightly.

℞ WHEN TO SEE YOUR M.D.
Get medical attention if the splinter is large, deep, made of broken glass, if the object is embedded near an artery or the eye, or if the area becomes swollen, red, and bleeds.

℞ WHEN TO SEE YOUR M.D.
If pain and swelling do not diminish after 2 or 3 days, consult a medical professional to be sure the bone is not broken. If you are in doubt as to whether you have a sprain or a fracture, treat the injury as a broken bone and seek medical attention.

Homeopathic Ledum is for sprains that are purple and puffy, when the injury feels cold, yet when cold compresses bring relief. Homeopathic Rhus tox is for sprains that feel better with movement, especially when the ligament is damaged, worse when initially moved, but better after repeated motion. Homeopathic Ruta graveolens is for old sprains that are worse from being still and better with movement.

Soothing Scars

Your skin gets plenty of wear and tear. Fortunately, skin has an amazing ability to heal and regenerate. In general, there are three stages of skin healing. In the first stage, a scab forms and is often accompanied by tenderness, swelling, and redness. During the next stage, new skin forms underneath the scab as the body produces collagen and reforms what constitutes the intercellular matrix. The last stage is where the inner and outer layers of skin rebuild. As time passes, the scab decreases, redness

GOOD TO KNOW!
In case of injury such as a sprain, remember the acronym RICE, which stands for Rest, Ice, Compression, and Elevation. Rest means you'll need to lie down to prevent further trauma to the area. Avoid using the injured area and immobilize it by using a sling or splint. Ice helps to constrict blood vessels, which will minimize bleeding and swelling. Fill a plastic bag with some ice and secure it before applying to the injured area. You may want to be prepared by wetting a washcloth and keeping it in a secured plastic bag in the freezer so you have it ready for emergencies. When the area begins to feel numb from the cold, remove the cold compress until the numbness subsides and reapply. This can be repeated routinely for at least six to twelve hours following the injury.

Make a compress by adding 10 drops of lavender oil to a pint (475 ml) of cold water, mixing, soaking a washcloth or face towel with the solution, and applying to the injured area. Next, elevate the injured area above the body if possible such as propping an injured foot onto a pillow. Keep the afflicted area above heart level. After a couple of days, pain and swelling should be relieved. At that time, alternating hot and cold compresses can further speed up healing but avoid heat until at least a couple days after the injury.

Cures from Grandma's Kitchen

Make a liniment for sprains by adding 1 tablespoon (5 g) cayenne pepper and ½ teaspoon (475 ml) oil of birch to a pint of apple cider vinegar. Apply topically to the injured area, cover with a cloth if desired, then elevate and rest.

and inflammation are reduced, and the skin hopefully returns to normal. Many scars can be prevented. Here's how.

NATURAL CURES THAT HEAL SKIN

If you have a wound attempting to heal, you'll want to allow the skin to breathe as much as possible to prevent scarring. If a bandage must be used, make sure it is breathable or use gauze with tape only at the sides of the wound. Remove any coverings at night if possible. Keep the damaged area clean but don't overclean.

A small amount of aloe vera gel can be applied for its biogenic (new skin growth) stimulating properties. Research published in the *Journal of the American Podiatric Medical Association* in 1989 showed that aloe vera speeds wound healing.

After the wound has healed somewhat, to promote further healing, apply salves that contain skin-softening avocado oil, calendula flowers, castor oil, cocoa butter, comfrey, honey, plantain, shea butter, and vitamin E. These are all allies to treat and prevent scars.

ESSENTIAL OILS THAT HEAL SKIN

Good essential oils that help heal and prevent scars include frankincense, geranium, lavender, and neroli. Natural food stores carry salves that carry various combinations of these remedies. Keep using these after the scab has gone. Scars can take from several months to two years to heal.

Scars are best treated when they are newer, but calendula and castor oil and plantain have even helped old scars. AHA (alpha-hydroxy acids) peels or laser resurfacing can help reduce any scar that is persistent. Talk to a licensed esthetician about these procedures.

VITAMINS AND FOODS THAT HEAL SKIN

Vitamin E (400 IU) taken both internally and topically is a favorite remedy for preventing scars. Taking zinc (25 mg to promote wound healing), vitamin C (1,000 mg daily for collagen production), and bromelain (500 mg three times daily to reduce inflammation) internally may also help prevent and treat scar formation.

If there is a potential for a scar, consume foods rich in beta-carotene, vitamin C, and vitamin E, all of which support collagen production. Especially good are apples, apricots, cucumbers, millet, rice, rye, apricots, and sea veggies. Vegetable juices of diluted carrot, celery, endive, lemon, and pineapple are also beneficial.

Healing Faster from Surgery and Accidents

Not only does your trusted physician say surgery is in your best interest, you've had two second opinions. Or perhaps you have been incapacitated by an accident and are in need of long-term rest. Remember that often our problems in life can be transformed

Skip This!

Avoid using heavy pore-clogging creams on any wound. They will prevent the wounded area from getting adequate oxygen. Nix synthetic fragrances or harsh cleansers as well. Avoid getting lots of sun with a wound that has the potential for scarring as it can render the scar more permanent. Picking at scabs can cause scarring that might not have occurred otherwise.

into opportunities! Here are some ideas that promote healing so that you can come through the ordeal like a champion.

BEFORE SURGERY

Read about the procedure so you know what to expect. Discuss your fears and feelings with your doctor, family, and spiritual counselor. Get your personal affairs in order, including naming someone to have power of attorney in case it is needed. Let your doctor know about any herbs, drugs, or supplements you are currently taking at least 1 week before surgery. Consider making a donation of your own blood, so that if blood is needed, a safe, perfect-for-you type is available.

Do your best to be in good health before surgery. Cut out or minimize the use of health-robbing substances such as cigarettes, coffee, alcohol, and junk food. Lose or gain weight reasonably if appropriate. If you feel yourself getting nervous as surgery draws near or in dealing with the aftermath of an accident, Rescue Remedy can be an excellent ally.

DURING SURGERY

Music during the operation as well as during any recovery phase can reduce anxiety and blot out noise pollution that could be detrimental. Taking an mp3 to the hospital will assure that you hear what you need and want to hear.

HERBS THAT HELP YOUR BODY HEAL

The following herbs can be taken as tea, tincture, or capsules and can be used three times daily following surgery:

- Chinese ginseng and Eleuthero help the body acclimate to stress.
- Nettles are high in iron and minerals that aid in blood building if the patient has lost blood.
- Ginger can help allay some of the residual nausea from anesthesia.

- Turmeric helps reduce inflammation and reduce pain.
- Gotu kola promotes wound healing. Research shows that the triterpenoids in Gotu kola help prevent scar formation after surgery.
- Aloe vera also speeds wound healing time and stimulates new cell growth.
- Using astragalus, echinacea, and reishi mushrooms can help you be more resistant to infection.

VITAMINS AND SUPPLEMENTS FOR HEALING

Vitamin A (10,000 IU) works as an antioxidant and promotes the repair of epithelial tissue. Beta-carotene (10,000 IU), which is converted into beta-carotene in the body, has the same properties. Both help prevent post-surgical infections and normalize white blood cell counts.

Vitamin C (1,000 mg) helps promote wound healing and is needed for the syntheses of collagen. Zinc (915 mg) promotes tissue repair and improved immune function. These vitamins, including vitamin E (400 IU), are all helpful for one recovering from an accident.

Bromelain (250 to 500 mg) taken three times daily can reduce post surgical and traumatic swelling, inflammation, and pain. Calcium (1,000 mg) and magnesium (500 mg) can promote bone healing.

Consider daily doses of the above supplements following surgery and for at least a month afterwards.

BEST FOODS FOLLOWING SURGERY

After surgery or an accident, you may need to follow certain dietary guidelines for important reasons. Depending on your dietary guidelines, the following simple and nourishing foods will help aid in your recovery:

- Unsweetened applesauce is high in pectin, which helps to normalize bowel function.
- Miso soup and yogurt help replenish your system with friendly intestinal flora.

- Pureed vegetables and soups are a simple way of getting a variety of nutrients without having to consume many different dishes if you have a decreased appetite.
- Seaweeds help prevent the body from absorbing radiation from x-rays.
- Winter squashes and yams are filling and nutrient rich.
- Bioflavonoid-rich foods such as blueberries and rose hips have capillary strengthening abilities.
- A congee, which is a watery nourishing porridge that is easy to digest, can be prepared by cooking one part rice with seven parts water.
- Chi and blood tonics like ginseng root and dong quai are invigorating and can help you regain your energy.

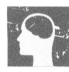

GOOD TO KNOW!
After surgery, you can take vitamin E (400 IU) both internally and externally to help reduce scarring. You can also use it topically after sutures have been removed. If you have been given lots of drugs or anesthesia, use alterative herbs (which can help detoxify the body of drug residue) such as alfalfa leaf, burdock root, raw dandelion root, nettles, and red clover blossom. They can be taken as teas three times daily. If you have been on antibiotics, take probiotic capsules three times daily to prevent fungal overgrowth. You can also take homeopathic Arnica before and after surgery to reduce swelling and trauma. Put four pellets under the tongue three times daily.

If the hospital staff tries to give you chemical green electrolyte beverages, if you can, take an alternative from the health food store without dyes and artificial flavors. When friends come to visit, ask them to bring a fresh vegetable juice of carrot, beet, and celery, which can be diluted and enjoyed. Enjoy homemade meals and other healing gifts your friends know how to provide.

SOOTHING PRACTICES AFTER SURGERY

Would having your own colorful sheets brighten your spirits more than antiseptic white ones? Bring them. You may also prefer to have your own comfortable and familiar pajamas from home with you instead of hospital garb.

Allow healing sunlight and adequate fresh air into the room. Cleanliness and brightness will help inspire health and good cheer.

CDs with beautiful healing music (such as Bach, Mozart, and Vivaldi) and an aromatherapy diffuser that is electric (candles are a fire hazard) can lift your spirits during a hospital stay. The smell of lavender essential oil is both uplifting and antiseptic.

Consider bringing an easel so you can display a piece of beautiful inspirational art with you to have in your hospital room. This will do a lot more for your psyche than white walls

GOOD TO KNOW!
A salve made of comfrey, calendula, and vitamin E can be used to heal bedsores should they occur. Apply topically using enough to cover the affected area.

or generic hospital art! Bring oxygen-giving green plants into the recovery room. Invite a stuffed animal to share your bed.

Read some of the books you've always wanted to. Spend some time studying. Maybe there's a subject you've always been interested in but never had the time to pursue? This may be the only time in your life you decide to read about a period of history or art that interest you. Check out books on tape if you are not up to reading.

Remember and enjoy the art of drawing and coloring. Learn to play some games.

Visualize placing your healing and consciousness into the parts of your body that need it. Send healing light and colors to all parts of your being. Take time to pray and give thanks for the things that are right in life.

This may be a good time to keep a journal. Tell the story of your life, illness, or your accident. Do it again in two weeks and see how it might be different. Or write the story of how you want your future to look. You can also use a journal to learn more about the meaning of dreams. Write poetry and short stories.

Sleep as much as you can. Use this time for healing, to regenerate and renew so that you emerge with new strength and vitality. Use this time to do anything that soothes you and promotes your healing.

When it is time to get back on your feet, do it gradually with care and moderation. Take care and revel in the taking time out for your own healing process!

Skip This!

There are many herbs to avoid before surgery, including the following:

- Ephedra: Can elevate blood pressure.
- Feverfew: Can increase bleeding.
- Garlic: Can decrease blood platelet aggregation.
- Ginkgo: Can decrease blood platelet aggregation.
- Ginseng: Can increase bleeding in some people.
- Goldenseal: Might increase blood pressure.
- Kava: May increase the effects of some antiseizure medications.
- Licorice: May aggravate electrolyte imbalance and increase blood pressure.
- Valerian: Can increase the effects of some anesthesia or antiseizure medications.

Also a week before surgery, avoid aspirin, Motrin, Advil (anti-inflammatory nonsteroidal drugs), vitamin E, COQ10, selenium, ginger, white willow bark, hawthorn, and turmeric (okay in food) as they all have blood-thinning properties.

Emotions that are unexpected and sometimes irrational are likely to occur and can be part of the healing process. Screaming into a pillow for no more than ten minutes can be releasing and therapeutic if you feel a need for it during the recovery process.

Treating Poison Exposure

A skull and crossbones on a container in a B movie means poison. But you can become poisoned from household cleaners, plants, and substances in the air like carbon monoxide. Kids can take poisonous substances out of a trash container or get access to such substances when visiting people who do not have childproof homes. Using poisonous volatile substances in a poorly ventilated area can cause them to be inhaled and absorbed through the body. Symptoms of poisoning include dizziness, nausea, headache, impaired speech, visual disturbances, chest pains, convulsions, and even paralysis..

NATURAL REMEDIES TO THE RESCUE

Dilute poisons by drinking lots of water or milk (which has some fat content to buffer caustic substances ingested). However, drink slowly enough to avoid vomiting if vomiting is contraindicated, such as after consumption of corrosive substances such as ammonia, bleach, and detergents. If there are burns around the lips, this can be an indication that the substance ingested was indeed corrosive. A universal antidote for poisoning is:

2   parts burnt toast
     (charcoal to adsorb toxins)
1   part strong black tea (tannic acid
     to offset alkaline)
1   part Milk of Magnesia (alkaline
     to offset acids)

Just using charcoal by itself is good to pass the poison out of the body.

Homeopathic remedies for poisoning include the following:

- Homeopathic Arsenicum: Can help when there is intense vomiting with restlessness and anxiety.
- Nux vomica: For poisoning that results in nausea that persists.
- Veratrum album: For serious vomiting with a cold sweat on the forehead.

Vomiting is often recommended for noncorrosive substances such as toxic plants and most drugs. If Poison Control suggests vomiting, give syrup of ipecac with lots of water. The standard dose is 1 tablespoon (15 ml) for children and 2 tablespoons (28 ml) for adults followed by 1 or 2 cups (235 to 475 ml) of water. Repeat in 20 minutes if vomiting doesn't occur. Sticking a finger or spoon in the back of the throat can also induce vomiting.

WHEN TO SEE YOUR M.D.
Call your local poison control center if poisoning has occurred. Have the poison container in your hand when you call. Be prepared to give the approximate weight and age of the person poisoned. Try to find out if they have vomited. If there is a sample of vomited material, scoop it into a container along with the poison container for analysis. If the poisoned victim is unconscious, make sure they are breathing, that their air passages are clear (place them in a position that allows for ventilation and be sure their air passages are not blocked by vomit or mucus), loosen their clothing, and get them to a hospital.

After vomiting, give the person 1 to 2 table-spoons (14 to 18 g) activated charcoal in a glass of water to adsorb remaining poisons. Since charcoal can adsorb even the syrup of ipecac, do not administer charcoal until after vomiting has occurred.

FOR CHEMICAL POISONING THROUGH THE SKIN

If the poisoning is from a dry chemical, first brush away as much as possible with a soft brush or duster. Be careful to protect your hands. Next, remove contaminated clothing and rinse the body off. If the poisoning is from a wet chemical, rinse repeatedly with plenty of water for about 10 minutes. If needed, seek medical assistance.

FOR POISON THROUGH INHALATION

Carbon monoxide is colorless, odorless, and hard to detect. Stoves and all forms of fire are potential causes of carbon monoxide poisoning. Get the victim into fresh air and encourage them to breathe deeply and evenly as you call for medical attention. Loosen tight clothing. Maintain an open airway and perform artificial respiration or CPR if needed and you are qualified. After exposure to carbon monoxide, consuming some sort of stimulant like coffee or black tea can be helpful.

KEEP IN MIND

Household chemicals and medicines should be stored out of sight and reach of children, preferably in a locked cabinet. Avoid storing chemicals and medicines on the same shelves as food. Make sure everything is properly labeled and do not transfer poisonous substances into unmarked bottles, cups, or glasses.

Never take medications in the dark without turning on the lights, and always read labels before using.

Avoid taking medicines in front of small children who will want to imitate you. Drugs that are colorful or sugar coated are especially tempting to them.

Never leave poisonous substances open "just for a minute." Most poisoning fatalities occur in children between the ages of one and three.

Soothing Crushed Fingers

Ouch! Slamming your finger in the car door is truly painful. First, be sure the finger isn't broken by bending it in different directions. If you can't bend your finger, seek medical attention.

If your finger is merely bruised, think CPR-Cold, Pressure, and Raise it. Soak the finger in ice water immediately until the cold feels painful (usually not more than 30 seconds). Then raise and squeeze the finger, and repeat the cold, pressure and raise technique up to a few dozen times. These remedies can also help.

Skip This!

Never give food or liquid to an unconscious person. Do not induce vomiting unless directed by poison control and never in an unconscious person. Never induce vomiting in cases of ingestion of strong acids, strong alkalis, and petroleum products. They can be inhaled on their way up the esophagus and absorbed into the lungs.

NATURAL REMEDIES THAT REDUCE SWELLING

Apply a plantain poultice, Saint-John's-wort oil, or herbal salve, using enough to cover the injured area, to reduce swelling. (See page 19 for directions on making a poultice.) Take 3 or 4 homeopathic Arnica pellets internally under the tongue and apply arnica salve topically to move fibrin, a blood protein that forms at the site of injury and causes swelling.

NATURAL REMEDIES THAT RESTORE FEELING

Homeopathic Hypericum is good for injuries where there are lots of nerves as it has a restorative effect on the nerves. Rescue Remedy also has a restorative effect. Take 2 drops under the tongue or in a glass of water. Another quick fix is to squeeze the fingers (or toes) of the opposite uninjured hand (or foot) firmly to cause nerve pain to travel down a less painful pathway.

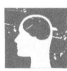 **GOOD TO KNOW!**
If you feel you may faint from heat, try rubbing an ice cube or a cold-water compress on your wrists. Lie down in a cool place and drink liquids. If you are feeling faint after long periods of standing, try rocking gently from the balls of your feet to the heels.

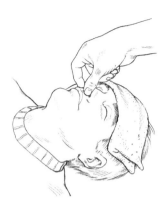

Recovering from Fainting

Fainting is a brief loss of consciousness usually caused by a decrease in blood supply to the brain. If you feel you may be about to faint, lie down (preferably) or bend over with your head at knee level. Even better, lie down with your feet and torso elevated, with your head lower than your heart. If you are attending to someone who has already passed out and is lying down, leave them lying but elevate their feet 8 to 12 inches (20.3 to 30.5 cm) and try to position their head below heart level, turning it to the side. Loosen tight clothing.

Cures from Grandma's Kitchen

Use a simple grated onion poultice on damaged fingers or toes to reduce pain and inflammation. Use enough to cover the area and leave on for 10 to 20 minutes.

You can also pinch the fleshy part between the upper lip and nose using a slightly upward pressure, which is an important acupressure point known as GV 26 that increases alertness. Applying cold moist towels to the neck and face can help as well. Do not give anyone who is unconscious anything to eat or drink, but when they are conscious, sips of cool water are fine. Be sure to allow access to fresh air, which may be blocked by looming crowds. Here's what else can help bring that someone around.

NATURAL REMEDIES FOR FAINTING

Simply smelling the essential oils of lavender, peppermint, or rosemary can help prevent fainting or bring someone out of fainting. Smelling a strong raw onion can also be helpful. The nasal cavities are in close proximity to the brain, and smelling something with a strong aroma sends a different message to the brain. A few drops of Rescue Remedy can be placed behind their ears or onto their lips or wrists. If they are revived, two drops of Rescue Remedy can be taken in water or directly under the tongue.

Cooling Off Heat Stroke and Heat Exhaustion

If you've been exercising in high temps, working in the hot sun, or even tanning yourself too long, you can suffer from heat stroke, which is the overheating of the body due to fluid depletion Heat exhaustion is more serious and the result of the loss of minerals and the body's heat regulation system stops functioning. Symptoms of both heatstroke and heat exhaustion can include disorientation, headache, rapid heartbeat, nausea, dizziness, high body temperature, red, hot, dry skin, thirst, and strong rapid pulse. Victims may become unconscious. With heat exhaustion, the victim's skin will be normal temperature, but with heat stroke, a high temperature will be present and the person may become disoriented and unable to notice their predicament.

Before using any natural remedies, get the person out of the sun and remove or loosen their clothing. Lie them down and slightly elevate their head. Use a hand towel and sponge their bare skin with cool water and fan them vigorously with anything available.

WHEN TO SEE YOUR M.D.
Most people recover from fainting within a few minutes, but encourage them to remain calm and still for a few minutes after they recover. Get emergency medical help if the person does not become conscious within 5 minutes, if there is a serious health condition involved, or if the person is elderly. Place them in the recovery position and check their breathing and heart periodically. If you faint without knowing why, consult a competent health professional.

GOOD TO KNOW!
Vitamin C can help prevent heatstroke or heat exhaustion. Siberian ginseng in capsules, tincture, or tea can also help people acclimate to changes in climate.

ESSENTIAL OILS FOR HEAT STROKE OR EXHAUSTION

To help cool a person with heat stroke/exhaustion, make cool compresses by soaking washcloths in a sink full of cool water to which 10 drops of essential oil of cooling lavender or peppermint have been added. Compresses can be applied to the forehead, over the wrists, and around the neck to help cool body temperature. Alternatively, make a spritzer by filling an 8-ounce (235 ml) spray bottle with spring water, 2 teaspoons (10 ml) of witch hazel, and 10 drops of lavender and 10 drops of peppermint essential oils. Spritz over the person's face (with glasses removed, eyes and mouth closed), neck, and upper chest for a cooling and reviving gentle blast.

BEST FOOD AND BEVERAGES FOR HEAT STROKE OR EXHAUSTION

Make an electrolyte beverage by adding $1/4$ teaspoon each of baking soda and sea salt to 8 ounces (235 ml) of water. A bit of fruit juice can be added to improve the flavor. Watermelon juice is also helpful in cases of heatstroke. Hibiscus flowers, lemon balm, strawberry leaf, and peppermint tea all make cooling beverages, especially when chilled. Squeeze lemon or

WHEN TO SEE YOUR M.D.
Heatstroke can be fatal. Should the victim of heatstroke become unconscious, place them in the recovery position and seek medical attention immediately.

lime into water for a cooling effect. Give sips of fluid every 10 minutes. However, give fluids cautiously as one suffering from heatstroke can be more likely to choke.

Both cucumbers and watermelon are very cooling to eat. Many victims of heatstroke are deficient in potassium, so if you feel you may be at risk, be sure to include potassium-rich foods in your diet, such as bananas, cantaloupe, and potatoes. During hot weather, eat lighter fare like salads, yogurt, smoothies, melons, and green leafy vegetables.

Skip This!

Drink lots more fluids but avoid alcoholic beverages and stimulants such as coffee, which can be further heat the body and are diuretic, causing the body to lose more important minerals.

Skip This!

Immersion in very cold water is vasoconstrictive and can result in death or brain damage by preventing the heat from escaping. But after initial cooling takes place, one can slowly get into tepid water feet first, parts at a time. Ice packs can also be placed under the armpits, behind the neck, on the wrists and forehead, and over the groin.

To prevent heatstroke or heat exhaustion, take a nap during the hot part of the day when you are likely to feel low in energy. Avoid strenuous exercise during midday and instead exercise early. Go for a walk after sunset. Have sex later in the evening when the weather has cooled rather than during the heat of the day.

Wear lighter cotton or hemp clothing. Use a hat with a brim and make sure your arms and legs are covered with light-colored clothing. In the morning of hot days, apply coconut or sunflower oil to the body before bathing to help you feel cooler. Slow down your activities.

In cases of heat cramps (symptoms include dizziness, shallow breathing, nausea, and muscle cramps), get into the shade and drink water to which a pinch of salt has been added to 1 pint (475 ml) of fluid. Since most heat cramps occur in the legs, elevate them and apply firm pressure on cramped muscles.

Avoiding Hypothermia

Exposure to cold, wind, and rain can bring on hypothermia, as can exhaustion, lack of clothing, food, or shelter, and not being prepared. Mild hypothermia can occur when the body temperature drops to 95°F (35°C). The brain is one of the first organs affected, so it's not surprising that the first symptoms of hypothermia include confusion. Symptoms of later stages of hypothermia include slurred speech, stumbling, irrational behavior (such as sudden bursts of energy followed by fatigue), blurry vision, abdominal pains, and unconsciousness. The elderly, very young, and very thin are most prone to hypothermia. Anyone pulled from cold water can be assumed to be suffering from hypothermia. Here's how to warm up fast.

R WHEN TO SEE YOUR M.D.
If you have severe hypothermia, you should go to a hospital as soon as possible.

Skip This!

Cigarettes are vasoconstricting and will reduce blood flow. Avoid contact with cold metallic objects as well as cold foods, water, and wind. Avoid wearing rings and metal jewelry, which can impair circulation. Avoid a hot bath before going into cold weather, as the blood vessels will dilate on the skin's surface. Avoid over-washing, which can strip the body of its natural oils.

Unless it is to get the victim out of the cold, avoid moving them. Avoid rubbing or massaging them and put them into a warm not hot bath. Putting them into a hot bath can send cold blood to the heart and cause ventricular fibrillation.

BEST FOODS FOR AVOIDING HYPOTHERMIA

First, seek shelter from the cold and wind, preferably indoors. If outside, build a fire. Next, get into dry clothes, one garment at a time. Drink sweet hot drinks such as spiced apple cider, ginger tea, or warm soups. Sprinkle a bit of cayenne pepper between your shoe and socks to keep your feet warm.

When the weather is very cold, to stay warm longer outdoors, eat more warming foods—such as anchovies, buckwheat, butter, oatmeal, parsnips, and soups—rather than salad. Use more cayenne, garlic, and ginger as warming condiments. Teas of angelica, cinnamon, ginger, fenugreek, nettles, and roasted dandelion root help you stay warm longer as well.

PRACTICES TO AVOID HYPOTHERMIA

You can also place warmth (warm hand, warm rocks, hot water bottle) in areas where blood is close to the skin (at the stomach, armpits, small of the back, back of the neck, wrists, and between the thighs). This can then transport heat throughout the body. Don't put warmth on the legs or arms, which will draw blood away from the torso. Scrunch your face and then relax and exercise your hands by shaking them or clenching then releasing to keep circulation moving.

Huddle together. Take turns putting different people in the middle, which is the warmest position. Toes and feet can be warmed by placing them on the belly of a friend. Keep an eye on each other. If one succumbs to hyperthermia, others in the group may follow. If the condition is severe, get naked in a sleeping bag or warm bed with the victim of hypothermia. Skin to skin is the most warming.

Sleeping with your clothes on inside the sleeping bag will ensure warmth. Wear a waterproof hat and remove it every once in a while if your head gets hot. Have appropriate waterproof gear. Mittens are warmer than gloves. An extra pair of socks can be used as mittens. Tight clothing will impair circulation.

If clothes are damp, spread them between the bag liner and sleeping bag or beneath the sleeping bag and sleep on top of them. If clothes are dry, roll them up and use as a pillow inside the sleeping bag so they will be warm in the morning. Replace wet clothing with dry whenever possible.

Skip This!

If you plan on spending a long time out in the cold, to avoid hyperthermia, don't drink too many liquids as this can make you colder.

Thrifty Cure!

Stuff your clothes with dry grass, moss, leaves, or rumpled newspaper to provide your body with warmth. Avoid depending on lightweight space blankets as your only way to get warm as they will keep moisture from evaporating and end up making you colder if used for long periods. Waterproof outer clothing can be life saving.

Should you fall into water and quickly get out, rolling immediately in fluffy snow will blot up much of the moisture. Should your boots get wet, stepping into a snow bank will absorb some of the water perhaps to the extent of keeping it from wetting the feet.

Stopping Nosebleed

A nosebleed can result from a trauma to the nose or when the nasal passages are dried out and blood vessels or capillaries rupture. Blood-thinning medications (including aspirin and anti-inflammatory drugs), allergies, nose picking, hypertension, blood disorders, and even smoking or alcohol abuse can make one more likely to have nosebleeds.

Most nosebleeds don't last longer than 15 minutes. As a first step, it can be helpful to blow vigorously one time to discharge any blood clot that is keeping the blood vessels open. Loosen any clothing around the neck. Lie down with head and shoulders elevated and mouth open. Lying down flat will cause you to swallow blood (which may cause stomach upset).

Pinch the soft part of the nostril closed by pressing with the thumb and index finger below the cartilage for at least 10 minutes and then slowly release. Open your mouth to avoid choking on blood. If bleeding is still occurring, keep closing your nose. Breathing through your nose will help dry up the blood, but it may be easier to breathe through your mouth.

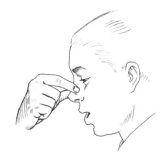

 WHEN TO SEE YOUR M.D.
Seek medical attention in the following situations:

- Blood flows from both nostrils.
- The nosebleed occurs after a head injury.
- Bleeding lasts for longer than 30 minutes despite applications of cold and pressure.
- Bleeding is from a severe blow that causes dizziness and nausea.
- The nose looks crooked and could be broken or fractured.
- The patient is elderly, has high blood pressure, or is using blood-thinning drugs.
- You are having recurrent nosebleeds for no apparent reason.

Senior citizens, especially those with hardening of the arteries, should give home remedies a try for 10 minutes and then seek medical attention if still needed.

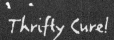

Thrifty Cure!
Placing a clean plantain leaf, a dime, a copper penny, or even a piece of brown paper bag (or tightly rolled strip on undyed, unscented tissue) under the upper lip (acupuncture point GV 26) will stimulate a point that controls circulation and will help stop the bleeding.

Try not to swallow a lot of blood. Take it easy and rest for at least 30 minutes after your nose stops bleeding. Avoid vigorous exercise for a day or two afterward so that the nose doesn't start bleeding again. Here's what else you can do.

NATURAL REMEDIES FOR NOSEBLEED

When dealing with an acute situation, apply a cold water or vinegar compress of 2 teaspoons (10 ml) apple cider vinegar and 1 cup (235 ml) of cool water to the base of the neck and to the top of the nose to help constrict blood vessels. You can also drink 2 teaspoons (10 ml) apple cider vinegar mixed with 1 cup (235 ml) of water for its astringent effect. Do this daily if bothered by frequent episodes of nosebleeds.

If nosebleeds occur frequently, eat more green leafy vegetables, which are high in vitamin K and promote blood-clotting ability. Consider taking a supplement of vitamin C (1,000 mg) with bioflavonoids (500 mg) and three doses daily of nettles, shepherd's purse, or yarrow in tea, tincture, or capsule form to strengthen the capillaries and promote healthy blood clotting.

If the nose is bleeding due to excessive dryness, apply a bit of herbal salve inside the nose at the area of bleeding. Use a humidifier to moisten the air and drink more water.

Thrifty Cure!

Placing a clean plantain leaf, a dime, a copper penny, or even a piece of brown paper bag (or tightly rolled strip on undyed, unscented tissue) under the upper lip (acupuncture point GV 26) will stimulate a point that controls circulation and will help stop the bleeding.

CHAPTER 5

NATURAL REMEDIES FOR COMMON AILMENTS

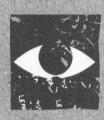

How to care for all the parts of our being that serve us so well is worth learning about. Here are some techniques from around the planet that can help heal.

Treating Eye Ailments

The precious gift of sight, which brings light and color into our lives, is worth all the attention we can focus toward achieving and maintaining healthy vision. Our eyes are long-range preceptors. All organs give the purest part of their energy to the eyes, helping to create their alertness and brightness. Our eyes are much like a camera. The lenses at the front of the eye collect and focus light rays. The colored iris works as an aperture. The retina is compared to film, which captures the image. Tears are fluids that help to wash the lens with lysozyme, a powerful germ killer. Crying can actually be a therapeutic way to clean and heal the eyes! Keep in mind that eye problems are usually a long time in the making and consistency is needed to allow natural remedies to demonstrate their full benefits. Let's get started!

HERBS FOR SHARPENED EYE SIGHT

During World War II, Air Force pilots were given bilberry jelly, which is actually a type of blueberry, to improve their night vision. Bilberry extract is even available in capsule form these days. Take as directed on the bottle daily.

Also helpful are goji berries. These sweet, reddish dried berries are considered helpful for blurred and poor vision. I like to use goji berries like raisins, mixed into cereal or added to trail mix. Consume $^1/_8$ cup (15 g) daily.

The herb eyebright has a long history of use in treating eye disorders. The French often refer to this herb as "casses lunettes," which means "break your glasses." Ancient peoples found this herb slightly resembles an eye and used it for poor sight. Eyebright has a cool, acrid, slightly bitter taste that stimulates liver function, thus improving blood supply to the eye. Eyebright

Cures from Grandma's Kitchen

Herbal eyewashes have long been used to strengthen the eyes and improve vision. To make an herbal eyewash, pour 1 cup (235 ml) of boiling water over 1 heaping teaspoon (5 g) of herb such as cornflower, eyebright, and or fennel seed. Allow to steep for 15 minutes. Strain well (through a clean coffee filter) and wait until the tea is lukewarm to use. Make fresh each day to avoid introducing any bacteria into the eyes. Herbs that can be used as eyewashes include chamomile, cornflower, eyebright, fennel seed, and violet leaves.

can be taken internally in tea, capsule, or extract form using a dose of either 2 to 3 times daily. Many have also found that using the strained tea as an eyewash helps to reduce eye inflammation.

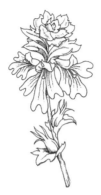

Other herbs that benefit the eyes when included in teas and tinctures (one dose taken three times daily) include the following:

- Barberry root, which contains the alkaloid berberine, long used for eye infections and redness.
- Calendula flowers, which can be used in a compress or as drops and are anti-inflammatory and a circulatory stimulant.
- Ginkgo, which improves circulation to the retina, tones capillaries, and increases visual acuity.
- Nettle and schizandra berries, which improve vision.
- Parsley leaf, which is great for eyestrain.
- Antiseptic and nutritive violet leaves, which can be used as a compress or in an eyewash for sore eyes.

VITAMINS FOR HEALTHY EYES

Vitamin A is often referred to as "the eye vitamin" because it helps to strengthen the mucus membranes of the eyes. It is manufac-

tured in the liver from carotene. The rod cells in our eyes contain a substance known as visual purple or rhodopsin. If the body is deficient in vitamin A, the cells' ability to make visual purple is impaired, and night blindness, dry eyes, and loss of color vision may result. People who work in bright lights, sunlight, or snow, who face car headlights, or who have to see in the dark may benefit from this nutrient.

Beta-carotene is present in orange-colored foods, which gets converted into vitamin A in the body. Beta-carotene can also help prevent dry eyes and reduce the risk of macular degeneration. 10,000 IU daily of either can be used.

Vitamin B1 deficiency may lead to dimness of sight. Riboflavin, also known as Vitamin B2, is also essential. It is thought that light enters the eyes through a screen of riboflavin before reaching the visual purple. A deficiency in riboflavin can manifest in extreme light sensitivity (photophobia) or in bloodshot eyes that burn, itch, and water frequently. People deficient in B2 may rub their eyes a lot.

The lenses of our eyes contain more vitamin C than any other body part, except some endocrine glands. Vitamins C and E may both help prevent cataract formation by preventing oxidative damage. In cases of cataracts, vitamin C is usually deficient.

The omega 3 fatty acids can be used for dry eyes, macular degeneration, glaucoma, and diabetic retinopathy. The omega 6s are anti-inflammatory and enhance lubrication of the eyes. Pycnogenol (100 to 200 mg daily) which is found in pine bark and grape seeds, elevates, elevates glutathione levels and can benefit cataracts, glaucoma, and macular degeneration. DHA (docosahexaenoic acid) nourishes the eyes and brain to delay bone degenerative rod loss in the eyes (350 IU 2 times daily).

BEST FOODS FOR THE EYES

Besides eating a wholesome diet, foods that are known to be particularly beneficial to the eyes include colorful antioxidant-rich blueberries, raspberries, raw sunflower seeds, black beans, black sesame seeds, beets, carrots, celery, green leafy vegetables (especially kale, dandelion greens, spinach, and watercress), leeks, sweet potatoes, barley, dates, mulberries, goji berries, and raisins.

According to research in the *Journal of Nutrition*, the antioxidants lutein and zeaxanthin found in dark green leafy veggies like kale, spinach, collard and turnip greens, and broccoli all help protect your eyes from UV light, which can cause cataracts. Aim for nine servings of fruits and vegetables a day for optimal ocular health.

Spirulina is also beneficial as it is rich in beta-carotene and can be added to smoothies. Use chervil, cilantro, paprika, and parsley frequently as they improve blood flow to the eyes. Garnish your meals with fresh dandelion, calendula, or marigold petals which are rich in lutein.

You can also make a tasty beverage in your blender that is rich in many nutrients for visual health. Good juices to mix are cholorophyll- and beta-carotene-rich beet, carrot, celery, endive, parsley, and spinach. Drinking several cups of barley water daily moistens the liver, which governs the eyes and moistens them.

BEST EXERCISES FOR THE EYES

Eyes should get exercise just like any other part of the body. Attached to our eyeballs are six little muscles that can be tonified. Eye exercises can also increase circulation to the eye area.

When reading or focusing for long periods, squeeze your eyes shut for a few seconds to increase blood flow to the area. If you spend your days looking at close objects, every half hour, take a break and gaze off into the distance. It truly is worth the time to improve circulation and strengthen the muscles attached to the eyes to keep them in working order.

You can also use the following exercise to improve your vision:

1. Keeping your head still, look up and down 7 times. Close your eyes and rest 10 seconds.
2. Look from one side to the other 7 times. Close and rest 10 seconds.
3. Look diagonally from one direction to the other 7 times. Close and rest 10 seconds.
4. Look diagonally from the opposite direction to the other 7 times. Close and rest for 10 seconds.
5. Roll your eyes in an upper half circle and back 7 times. Close and rest for 10 seconds.
6. Roll your eyes in a lower half circle and back 7 times. Close and rest 10 seconds.
8. Place the backs of both hands over closed eyes and rest for a full minute.

Another simple way to exercise your eyes is to hold a finger or pen 10 or 12 inches (25.4 or 30.5) away from your face, focus on the tip, and then look off into the distance. Turn your head from side to side as if saying no emphatically. Repeat several times.

ACUPRESSURE FOR EYE HEALTH

Acupressure on the feet can benefit the eyes, especially if you pay special attention to the bottom of the second and third toes. If your eyes need some extra help, you may want to massage the correlating reflex points at the base of the bottoms of the second and third toes in a firm circular motion. Deep massage at the base of the neck may help to relieve tension that impairs vision.

KEEP IN MIND

If you spend your days in front of computers, keep the lighting in the room low with screen brightness three to four times that of the room. Consider using full-spectrum lighting in the home and workplace. Natural light improves visual acuity and helps prevent eyestrain.

Minimize glare by keeping monitors away from light sources such as windows. Consider using an antiglare screen. Make sure characters on the screen stand out sharply. Have the screen positioned 14 to 20 inches (35.6 to 50.8 cm) away from eyes just below eye level. The colors of display characters on a computer that are easiest on the eyes are amber and green. Fifteen minutes out of every hour, try to do some non-computer sort of work.

When it is safe and can be done without strain, try to spend a few minutes each day without anything covering your eyes (glasses, sunglasses, or contact lenses). Close your eyes and allow the sunlight to rest upon your closed eyelids for 3 to 5 minutes. Another beneficial eye strengthening technique is called "sunning." It is done by standing or sitting with closed eyes (though no glasses or contacts). Then move your head slowly from the left to the right, allowing the sun's rays to gently cross over closed eyes. This is best done outside, preferably when surrounded by the calm, cooling, healing green colors of nature. An ancient folk remedy to benefit the eyes is to gaze at the cooling rays of the moon!

NATURAL REMEDIES FOR PUFFY EYES

Your eyes can get puffy from crying, but puffiness can also be a sign of a food allergy, sinus problems, weak kidneys, sulfites in wine, alcohol consumption, excess sugar or fat consumption, and exhaustion. If your eyes are red, itchy, burning, and begging for attention, give them some genuine nurturing rather than using synthetic eye drops, which provide only temporary relief and can lead to more irritation later.

Apply cooling and anti-inflammatory slices of raw peeled potato (red ones are best, according to traditional folklore), apple, cucumber, melon, or tofu over each eye.

To make an eyewash for puffy eyes, bring 1 cup (235 ml) of distilled water to a boil and remove from heat. Add 1 heaping teaspoon (5 g) of herb such as cornflower, eyebright, and or fennel seed and allow to steep while covered for 15 minutes. Strain through a coffee filter. When the tea is cool, place into a clean eyecup and gently apply and bathe the eyes several times daily. Make fresh daily and refrigerate any unused portion to avoid introducing any bacteria into the eye. If you do use an eyewash or eyedrops, close your eyes for a couple of minutes to retain the benefits of the remedy.

EXERCISES FOR PUFFY EYES

An exercise for puffy eyes is to squeeze both eyes shut tight. Looking inwards, draw the lids inward toward the nose without using your hands, just the muscles in the corners of the eyes. Keep the eyes relaxed and then move the eyelids outward. Hold for three seconds. Repeat seven times. This exercise works quickly. Start by doing it every night for ten nights and then reduce the frequency to three times a week.

KEEP IN MIND

Sleep on your back, as sleeping on your side causes creases in your face, leading to permanent lines. Using two pillows to elevate your head keeps fluids from pooling around the eyes. Puffy eyes could also be related to allergies to the bedding, such as a down pillow or comforter.

Beware of heavily chlorinated pools or swimming in unclean water, which can cause eye infections or irritations. Wear watertight goggles if necessary.

NATURAL REMEDIES FOR CATARACTS

Cataracts are a degenerative condition that result in visual cloudiness or opacity in the lenses of the eyes. Cataracts develop from the slow deterioration of the lens's protein, often caused by oxidation, and can cause gradual vision loss. (Follow the guidelines given on page 97 for eye foods, exercises, and herbs.)

NATURAL REMEDIES FOR CONJUNCTIVITIS

The conjunctiva is a thin protective tissue over the sclera (white) of the eye. When it is inflamed, it is commonly known as pinkeye. Causes can include allergies, overexposure to the elements, viewing overly bright objects (such as electric welding) with the naked eye, bacteria, virus, "burn out" (adrenal exhaustion), as well as foreign objects such as dust and pollution. Conjunctivitis is highly contagious and can be spread through washcloths, towels, and fingers, so keep them clean and separate from others. Here's what else can help.

Eating cooling cucumbers and mung beans is also helpful if you have conjunctivitis. Take cooling anti-inflammatory herbs, such as burdock, chickweed, Echinacea, and red clover blossom, in tea, tincture, or capsule form three times daily. A probiotic supplement taken three times daily between meals helps inhibit unfriendly microorganisms that may be contributing factors in the infection.

Skip This!

Cheap sunglasses filter only some rays and may allow harmful rays to penetrate. The best sunglasses are gray, green, then brown in that order.

Thrifty Cure!

Splash cold water over your eyes several times a day to improve circulation. Ahhh!

Cures from Grandma's Kitchen

To make a compress to reduce puffiness in the under-eye area, make a tea of chamomile, cornflower, elderflower, eyebright, marshmallow root, peppermint, and/or black tea, strain, and chill. Soak a small clean cloth in the chilled brew and lie down and relax with the compress over your eyes. Black tea bags, which have been used to make tea, can be set aside to cool and applied later. Also helpful for sore eyes is to soak cotton balls in cool milk and apply over closed eyes.

NATURAL REMEDIES FOR FOREIGN OBJECTS IN THE EYES

Got something in your eye? The first step is to blink frequently to induce the eyes to tear and wash the object out. If that doesn't work, try these tips.

You can flush the foreign body out with 2 drops Saint John's Wort tincture in 8 ounces (235 ml) plain water or simply 2 drops of warm olive oil directly to wash out the particle. One drop of fresh lemon juice in 1 ounce (28 ml) of warm water used to rinse the eye is soothing and helps remove the particle.

You can also blow your nose vigorously while closing the nostril on the opposite of the affected eye to dislodge the foreign object. If this is unsuccessful, gently flood the eye with water using a gentle spray kitchen sink nozzle or fill a clean sink with water, place your face in it, and while holding your eye open, move your head from side to side while the water flows over the eye.

GOOD TO KNOW!
Be sure you aren't using an eye cream you are allergic to. Eye creams are designed to be richer and thicker than other moisturizers as the area around the eyes lacks oil glands. If the puffiness disappears as the day wears on, fluid retention may be the cause, which is ultimately a kidney concern.

Try pulling the upper eyelid out and down over the lower lid, which can help dislodge pesky particles. If you are helping someone else dislodge a particle from their eye, have them look up and down and left and right as you examine their eye. If the particle is visible, use a clean handkerchief to remove it. Do not use cotton or tissue as they have fibers that can come loose in the eye.

NATURAL REMEDIES FOR GLAUCOMA

Glaucoma is a degenerative disease in which the pressure inside the eye is too high (referred to as intraocular pressure). Glaucoma results from an imbalance between the production and outflow of the aqueous humor. Symptoms of glaucoma include morning eye pain, blurry vision, halos around light, peripheral vision loss, and inability to adjust to a dark room. There are usually no symptoms until damage has been done to the eyes.

A folk remedy for both cataracts and glaucoma is to make a juice out of the aboveground portion (including the flower) of greater celandine. Apply the juice to the outer eyelids daily. Do not apply directly to the eye. Refrigerate any unused portion, which will keep fresh for up to six days. You can also follow the tips for cataracts.

WHEN TO SEE YOUR M.D.
Consult with a competent, preferably holistic-oriented optometrist or ophthalmologist for problems such as seeing colored rings around lights, blurred or double vision, seeing imaginary spots, lines, or flashes of light, and burning, watery, or itchy eyes for a proper diagnosis.

NATURAL REMEDIES FOR MACULAR DEGENERATION

Macular degeneration is a retinal disorder that can block central vision and is one of the leading causes of blindness in the elderly. There is a dry form of the disease, which can cause blurry vision, and a wet form caused by abnormal blood vessel growth behind the retina, causing the retina to separate from the eye. The dry form of macular degeneration can develop into the wet form. Smokers, postmenopausal women, and those with light-colored eyes seem to be at highest risk. Overuse of aspirin can be a causative factor in macular degeneration, as can excessive sun exposure. Follow the same guidelines regarding food, herbs, and supplements for vision health and cataracts.

GOOD TO KNOW!
Safety glasses can help prevent eye accidents. Look for glasses with shatterproof lenses and use them for hazardous carpentry, art projects, sports, and cleaning.

NATURAL REMEDIES FOR STYES

A stye is an infection of the eyelid oil gland or hair follicle, sometimes caused by Staphylococcus. The eyelid lining may have a pimple and can become red, sensitive to light, burn, sting, and produce discharge. Styes can occur when a person's eyes are tired and they have been rubbing their eyes excessively.

To promote drainage, apply a hot compress using antiseptic herbs such as barberry, calendula, elderflower, eyebright, goldenseal, parsley leaf, and raspberry leaf for 15 minutes up to four times daily using a fresh clean washcloth each time. You can also apply aloe vera juice to the outside of the closed eye several times daily for its soothing antimicrobial effect. Black tea bags can be used as a compress as they contain antibacterial and astringent agents. Alternatively, you can use a charcoal poultice over the closed eye to help draw out the infection. Drinking alterative (blood purifying) teas like burdock, echinacea, and red clover three times a day will also help prevent and treat styes.

Skip This!

If you have a stye, avoid dairy food and foods that contain gluten as they are likely to cause excess phlegm.

Cures from Grandma's Kitchen

To help with cataracts, make an eyewash from chamomile, eyebright, and fennel and apply 3 drops with an eye dropper 3 times daily. You can also put one drop of pure honey or two drops of castor oil in the eyes nightly before bed. You can also put 1 drop of pure coconut juice into the eyes daily. (See page 20 for directions on making an eyewash.)

℞ WHEN TO SEE YOUR M.D.
If the eye has been penetrated, get emergency care immediately. Cover the eye loosely and get someone to take you to an urgent care facility. Also seek medical attention in the following situations:

- You are unable to remove the object.
- The object is made of glass or metal.
- The person will not stay still for the eye to be examined.
- The object can't be located.
- The object appears to be embedded.
- The object is on the pupil or iris.

After the object has been removed, seek medical attention if there is swelling in the eye or sharp or even mild pain 24 hours later. Also seek medical attention if there is light sensitivity, visual disturbances, the eye is unable to stay open, or it still feels as if something is in the eye.

Treating Ear Ailments

Our ears tune us in to the sounds of the world. They enable us to listen to the voices of our loved ones, the melodies of music, and the orchestra of our natural (and unnatural) environment. Because our sense of hearing is so precious, it is well worth protecting this vital sense.

NOTE: For earache, see "Natural Remedies for Baby and Child Care."

Thrifty Cure!

For babies, a few drops of mother's milk, which is high in antibodies, can be applied directly to the eyes 3 times daily.

Skip This!

Avoid hot spicy food, coffee, and alcohol. According to Asian medicine, the health of the eyes is governed by the liver. Anything that dries or irritates the liver also affects the eyes.

Skip This!

Avoid rubbing the eyes or using any instrument to remove a foreign object.

Cures from Grandma's Kitchen

Use an herbal eyewash, especially of chamomile, eyebright, goldenseal, or barberry, for conjunctivitis. (See page 20 for directions on making a soothing antimicrobial eyewash.)

NATURAL REMEDIES FOR TINNITUS

The word tinnitus comes from Latin roots, meaning "tinkle like a bell." For this annoyance, it is important to determine the cause and attend to the source of the problem. Ear ringing is sometimes caused by excess consumption of coffee, alcohol, or aspirin, medication, catarrh, smoking, trauma, exposure to loud noise, arteriosclerosis, and allergies. If only one ear is affected, it is more likely to be the left ear.

Ginkgo biloba taken orally (a dose daily of tea, tincture, or capsule) can help diminish the sounds of tinnitus by improving nerve signal transmission as well as increasing the brain's utilization of oxygen. Other herbs that help diminish the sounds of tinnitus include elder flowers (opening to the channels, including Eustachian tubes), oregano (which moves blockage), black cohosh (which is antispasmodic), violet leaves (which have been used since ancient times to open the ears), and chamomile (which calms inflamed nerves). Look for combinations of some of these herbs at natural food or herbal stores and take a dose three times a day as a tea, tincture, or capsule.

Niacin supplementation may also help by improving circulation to the ears and moving blockages. Try 50 mg three times daily. (Note that this will make you feel hot, red, and prickly for up to 10 minutes as it improves circulation.) Drink some water and rest or take with a meal.

NATURAL REMEDIES FOR AIRPLANE EARS

Also known as barotitis, this complaint occurs when a plane ascends or descends and the surrounding air pressure changes and causes vacuum pressure to form in the middle ear, causing pain. Simple remedies include swallowing, yawning, and chewing gum. (Look for chewing gum at a natural food store; otherwise, you might be stuck with artificial sugary stuff from the airport.) Infants can be nursed (most comforting) or given a bottle or pacifier during takeoff and landing to remedy airplane ears. You'll find more information about treating baby's earache in the section on "Natural Remedies for Baby and Child Care."

NATURAL REMEDIES FOR SWIMMERS' EAR

Swimming exposes the ears to a number of possible problem-causing bacteria and fungi. To prevent swimmers' ear, shake the head somewhat vigorously or jump up and down with the head tilted to one side after being in water. If necessary, you can make a simple solution to put in the ears after swimming by adding 1 teaspoon (5 ml) of white vinegar to 4 tablespoons (60 ml) of freshly boiled water (allow to cool before using). After swimming, put 2 drops of the mixture in each ear up to three times daily. Store in the refrigerator.

 GOOD TO KNOW!
Should you accidentally get a foreign object in your ear or disobey your mother and put beans in your ears, remember that an imbedded object is best removed by a doctor, who will have the tools to do so without puncturing the delicate membrane of the ears.

NATURAL REMEDIES FOR A BUG IN THE EAR

To remove a bug from your ear, turn your ear toward the sun, as many bugs are attracted to the light. If it's nighttime, darken the room and shine a flashlight in the ear to draw the pest out. If this does not work, pour 1 teaspoon (5 ml) of warm olive oil in the ear and let it sit with the ear turned upward for 1 to 2 minutes. The last resort is to gently fill the ear with warm water. These last two remedies drown the bug and get it to float to the top.

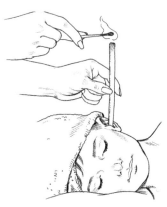

NATURAL REMEDIES FOR EARWAX

The purpose of earwax is to lubricate and protect the ears. It is also considered antiseptic. An excess of this substance (called ceruminosis) may be due to over-consumption of fats and sugars in the diet. Putting cotton swabs in the ears can also push dirt and wax further into the ears, causing wax buildup.

To safely remove earwax, add several drops of mullein flower oil into the ears every night for a week. You can also use special earwax candles (find them in your health food store) based on a tradition used be ancient Egyptians and Native Americans. These uniquely designed hollow candles are placed in a person's ear one at a time while the person is lying down, a towel protecting his or her hair and face. An assisting person holds the candle and lights the top. When it burns down and feels warm to the person holding it, the candle is plunged into a nearby glass of water.

If you examine the candle, the bottom portion will be filled with one to several inches of wax (and also some ash from the candle). I have found these candles beneficial in improving hearing and relieving blockages such as airplane ears and even in some cases of earaches.

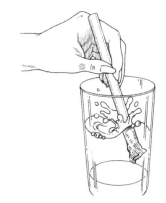

NATURAL REMEDIES FOR HEARING LOSS

More than 12 million people in the U.S. are deaf, and the number is increasing. Hearing loss can be aggravated by genetic tendencies. Pinched nerves in the neck or upper spinal column can impair hearing. Accumulations of fat and mucous in the inner ear can also impair hearing, thus it may be helpful to eliminate foods like fatty meats and dairy products.

The auditory nerve vibrates in response to sound, and if it is coated, it can lose its sensitivity. The cochlea contains a fluid that transmits sound vibration. Should this fluid become overly thick and sticky due to dietary imbalances, sound transmission may also be impaired. An eardrum that is overly loose (often due to excess use of sugary, cold foods and drugs) will not be able to conduct sound well. The food most likely to contribute to ear congestion is ice cream—dairy, cold, and sugary. Massaging a few drops of cajeput oil in front and behind the ears helps to improve hearing by increasing circulation. Applying a ginger compress over the ears and kidney area helps to break up accumulations of fat and mucous.

The herb ginkgo has also been shown to be beneficial in improving hearing loss, especially when due to nerve deafness. Ginkgo leaves increase cerebral and peripheral blood flow and improve nerve transmission. This herb may be taken in tea, extract, or capsule form 2 to 3 times daily.

In Oriental medicine, the ears are said to correlate to the kidneys. The kidneys are often treated with acupuncture or moxibustion to help improve the ears. It is interesting that the ears and kidneys are similarly shaped. You can practice acupressure by tapping the ears firmly with two fingertips with the top portion of the ear gently folded over the ear opening, of the other hand 50 to 100 times every day. Also gently tap the sides of the head above the ears.

GOOD TO KNOW!
Foods that have a long tradition of being considered beneficial to the ears based on their antioxidant properties include colorful fresh fruits and berries (especially blueberries and blue elderberries); adzuki; kidney and black beans; green leafy vegetables like kale, collards, and mustard greens; dark yellow vegetables such as pumpkin, acorn, and butternut squashes; garlic; and onions. I am very fond of eating wild violet leaves in salads for strengthening the ears. An antioxidant vitamin is also helpful in protecting our hearing. A vitamin D deficiency can contribute to hearing loss of the higher frequencies. Taking a supplement of 1,000 IU daily may be helpful.

GOOD TO KNOW!
Yoga postures that improve various ear disorders include the Palm Pose, the Lion, the Wheel, the Plow, the Shoulder Stand and the Neck Pose.

Treating Foot Ailments

We need our feet to get from A to B, so it's important to do everything we can to keep them in shape. Follow these tips for your tootsies, and you'll walk with ease.

NATURAL REMEDIES FOR ATHLETE'S FOOT

You don't have to be an athlete to suffer the itching irritation of athlete's foot. Those who frequent public pools, gyms, and shower rooms, who sweat a lot, or wear tight nonbreathable shoes are the most likely to develop this problem. Athlete's foot is seven times more prevalent in men than women and is more common where conditions are hot and humid. Prolonged exposure to moisture, nail injuries, and cuticle damage can all lead to fungal infections. With all foot conditions, it's important to take care of little problems in the feet so that they don't become big problems.

Create an antifungal foot powder by mixing $1/4$ cup (55 g) baking soda with 10 drops each of essential oils of tea tree, geranium, and lavender. Combine ingredients and store in a glass jar. Liberally apply to affected areas. You can also try soaking your feet in 3 quarts (2.8 L) of warm water to which 1 cup (235 ml) of apple cider vinegar has been added. Dry the feet well, especially between each toe, and apply some tea tree oil, an excellent anti-fungal agent, to the affected area.

GOOD TO KNOW!
Avoid sharing pedicure tools like nail clippers. Wear rubber sandals when showering in public places.

KEEP IN MIND

As much as possible, air your feet out in the sun for short periods of time. Wear natural fiber socks that are changed often and shoes made of natural materials that allow your feet to breathe, rather than synthetic materials. Alternate the shoes that you wear so that shoes have the opportunity to air out. Many health professionals feel that athletes' foot can also be a symptom of yeast overgrowth in the body. Keep in mind that sugar, fruit juice, alcohol, and yeasted breads may all be foods contributing to yeast overgrowth in the body.

NATURAL REMEDIES FOR BUNIONS

Bunions are bony bumps, often on the sides of the toes. Although they can be hereditary, tight shoes can cause this otherwise painless ailment to be irritated. As a first step, you can cushion the area with a foam pad when wearing shoes.

Exercise can also help with bunions. Loop a big rubber band around the big toe and then pull the toe away from the smaller toes, holding each pull five seconds. Repeat ten times. Also practice spreading the toes.

Castor oil can also be applied to bunions twice daily to penetrate the skin deeply and help move congested hardened tissue.

NATURAL REMEDIES FOR CALLUSES AND CORNS

A callus refers to hardened skin, often on the ball or foot heel, caused by the way we walk or foot pressure on shoes at odd angles. A corn occurs when the skin over the toe forms a hard protective coating, usually due to pressure. As a start, insert insoles into your shoes to cushion the area.

 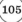

Corns can be softened by soaking the feet in warm salt water for 10 minutes and then using a pumice stone before applying castor oil twice a day to the afflicted area. Apple cider vinegar can also be applied directly to corns and calluses twice daily to increase circulation to them, thus helping them break up.

NATURAL REMEDIES FOR SORE FEET

Do your feet feel sore and tired? After being on your feet all day, it feels delightful to soak your feet in a basin of warm water to which 7 or 8 drops of pure essential sage, rosemary, or lavender oil has been added. Also consider wearing insoles in the shoes and supportive house shoes (rather than outdoor shoes that track in dirt and pollution) rather than walking barefoot on hard surfaces.

You can find foot massage tools at any natural food stores. A foot massage feels heavenly! You can give one to yourself or show the one you love just how pleasurable this can be. Then you can trade!

NATURAL REMEDIES FOR FOOT ODOR

If your nose runs and your feet smell, you are built upside down! Foot odor can often be improved by taking 3 capsules of chlorophyll daily, which acts as a natural deodorizer. You can also put sage leaves in your shoes for weeter-smelling feet. And remember to choose natural fiber footwear so that your skin can breathe.

R̺ WHEN TO SEE YOUR M.D.
If you have "burning soles," it may indicate diabetes or other health conditions, including nerve damage, fungal infection, or excess alcohol consumption.

Cures from Grandma's Kitchen

The following are great treatments for athlete's foot.

ANTIFUNGAL FOOT SOAK
1 gallon (3.5 L) comfortable hot water
¼ cup (60 ml) apple cider vinegar
5 drops tea tree oil
5 drops lavender oil

Soak for 20 minutes once or twice daily.

NATURAL REMEDIES FOR INGROWN TOENAILS

An ingrown toenail usually occurs on the big toe. To prevent this ailment, be sure to cut the toes nails straight across rather than in a sloping fashion.

To treat an ingrown toenail, soak the foot in hot water and apply a healing herbal salve to help reduce inflammation. You can also secure a juicy slice of lemon to the affected area with a Band-Aid before going to bed, and in the morning the nail should be soft enough to be eased away from the skin and trimmed. Do your best to keep the skin away from the nail by taping some athletic tape and gently pulling the skin away from the toe.

If the problem is chronic, a misshapen toenail may be the problem. Consult with a podiatrist.

GOOD TO KNOW!

Be sure to choose shoes that fit well and don't cause unnecessary pressure. Avoid buying shoes in the morning, as the feet expand during the day and what fits perfectly at 10 am might seem too tight by 6 pm. If you walk to work or a ways to the subway or bus, consider wearing sneakers and then changing into other shoes during work.

Cures from Grandma's Kitchen

Poultices that can be applied to bunions include grated lemon peel or chopped onion soaked in apple cider vinegar held in place overnight by a bandage, allowing the circulatory-stimulating properties of the poultices to move stuck energy and help break down the bunion.

A folk remedy for corns is to tape the inside of a fresh lemon peel to the area overnight for several nights in a row. Garlic oil can also be applied to calluses twice daily.

GOOD TO KNOW!

For tired, aching feet, simply prepare the herbs below as you would for drinking tea, strain, cool slightly, and then pour into a bucket and soak your sore feet:

HERB	BENEFITS
• Chamomile	For sore, swollen feet
• Lavender	Refreshes tired feet
• Marjoram	For tired, achy feet
• Peppermint	Stimulates tired feet
• Thyme	For fungal infections, also refreshes tired feet

GOOD TO KNOW!

To deodorize your feet simply prepare the herbs below as you would for drinking tea, strain, cool slightly, and then pour into a bucket and soak your feet:

HERB	BENEFITS
• Horsetail	Reduces perspiration
• Lovage	Strong natural deodorant
• Rosemary	Naturally deodorizing
• Sage	Antiperspirant, deodorizing

GOOD TO KNOW!

For healthy feet, keep these tips in mind:

- Spend some time with your feet elevated by lying on a slant board or spending a few minutes a day in the shoulder stand yoga posture.
- Sit with your legs outstretched in front of you and rotate your feet in circles a dozen times in each direction to keep your ankles flexible.
- Whenever possible and safe, spend time barefoot to tone your feet. When trying on shoes, wriggle your toes to make sure they are roomy enough.

Helping Hypothyroidism

The thyroid is a butterfly-shaped gland on either side of the windpipe directly below the Adam's apple. The thyroid gland has many functions, including governing metabolism and aiding in digestion, mental processes, sex drive, muscle and cardiac activity, and bone repair.

When your thyroid gland is underperforming, it's called hypothyroidism. Symptoms of hypothyroidism include fatigue, brain fog, moodiness or depression, weight gain, constipation, dry skin and hair, headaches, low libido, high cholesterol, poor short-term memory, anxiety or panic attacks, poor sleep, flu-like symptoms, hoarseness, hypersensitivity, and fluid retention. Heredity, viral infection, fluoridated water, and some medications can all affect the thyroid adversely. Here's how to boost your thyroid function.

NATURAL SUPPORT FOR HYPOTHYROIDISM

Nature provides herbs that can naturally boost thyroid health. Nettle seed is a natural thyroid tonic, being both nourishing and providing trace minerals needed by the thyroid. Look for it in tincture form and take a dropperful three times daily. You can also gather it wild and dry the seeds to sprinkle on food.

Irish moss, a seaweed, moistens dry skin and soothes swollen glands. It is a nutritive and moistening tonic for the body. It can be found in capsules and taken as directed, usually three times daily.

A deficiency of vitamin A can reduce the thyroid's ability to assimilate iodine and contribute to goiter. In cases of hypothyroidism, it's better to take a vitamin A (10,000 IU) supplement rather than its precursor, beta-carotene, which becomes vitamin A in the body. An iodine supplement, which is usually derived from kelp, should also be taken as sea vegetables contain the minerals needed for all endocrine functions. You can also look for combination remedies in natural food stores that contain herbs and vitamins to support the thyroid.

ESSENTIAL OILS FOR HYPOTHYROIDISM

Essential oils are powerful fragrances that are able to improve circulation to parts of the body that need attention. Massage Saint-John's-wort oil in the area of the thyroid gland several times each day to invigorate it by increasing its circulation to function more optimally. You can boost the thyroid's effectiveness by adding 5 drops of essential oils of frankincense, geranium, or catnip to 1 teaspoon (5 ml) olive oil or coconut oil. The ideal massage technique is to grasp the front of the throat at the gland level using all fingers and move the area up and down.

BEST FOODS FOR HYPOTHYROIDISM

If iodine is deficient, the thyroid gland tends to swell, and blood vessels get hardened. The Japanese, known for their diet high in iodine seafoods and sea vegetables, such as dulse, kelp, and hiziki, rarely have goiter associated with hypothyroidism. The sea vegetables, constantly bathed in the rich brine of the ocean, have a softening and cleansing effect. Do your best to consume at least 1 gram daily. It is simple to sprinkle kelp or dulse on dishes.

Apricots, parsley, Swiss chard, tahini, and watercress are considered beneficial foods for thyroid health. Include some in your regular regimen. Coconut oil is made primarily of medium-chain fatty acids, which increase metabolism and promote weight loss. Coconut oil can also raise basal body temperatures while increasing metabolism, benefiting those with low thyroid function.

Harmonizing Hyperthyroidism

Hyperthyroidism means your body is producing too much thyroid hormone. This can result in heart palpitations, hot sensations, sweating, weight loss, chest pain, and muscle weakness. A goiter can also form around the necklace line of the neck due to poor thyroid function.

NATURAL CURES FOR HYPERTHYROIDISM

Motherwort herb calms heart palpitations, hot flashes, anxiety, skin hypersensitivity, and thyroid enlargement. Mullein leaf is also used for hyperthyroidism and reduces glandular inflammation. Take each in tea or capsule form three times a day.

A supplement of essential fatty acids three times daily may help decrease excessive thyroid hormones. The amino acid L-tyrosine (500 mg 2 times daily) is a precursor to the thyroid hormones, meaning it becomes transformed into thyroxin and triodthyronine. The thyroid gland has a high need for vitamin B1, especially when overactivity is the problem. Niacin, or vitamin B3, is needed for smooth functioning of all the endocrine glands. B6 improves iodine assimilation. Taking a vitamin B complex (50 mg) once daily should help nourish both hypo- and hyperthyroid conditions.

Balancing Hypoglycemia

If you get jittery when you haven't eaten in awhile, you may have hypoglycemia. Many people think of hypoglycemia as the opposite of diabetes, but this is not true. With diabetes, there is a deficiency of insulin; in hypoglycemia, excess insulin is produced. If this process continues, the pancreas may become exhausted, lose its ability to produce insulin, and diabetes may occur.

Some of the symptoms of hypoglycemia include allergies, appetite fluctuation (such as ravenous hunger to no appetite, feeling hungry after a meal), depression, dizziness, fatigue, food cravings, headaches, hyperactivity, inability to concentrate, and waking up exhausted after a full night's sleep. Consulting with a qualified health professional to get a glucose tolerance test should help give you a clearer idea of what you are dealing with. In order to treat hypoglycemia, the pancreas needs to be re-educated and the adrenal glands strengthened. These natural cures can help.

Skip This!

Foods that inhibit thyroid function include millet, peanuts, and soybeans. Eating large amounts of foods in the Brassicaceae family, such as broccoli, cabbage, cauliflower, kale, rutabaga, turnips, and Brussels sprouts, inhibits the uptake of iodine, a necessary nutrient. However, consuming plenty of mineral-rich sea vegetables makes this concern less. The thyroid gland becomes damaged by excessive consumption of caffeine, sugar, and refined carbohydrates, all of which stimulate pituitary activity and damage its ability to produce the necessary hormones that activate thyroid function. Fluoridated water can also inhibit thyroid function.

SUPPLEMENTS TO BALANCE BLOOD SUGAR

If you have hypoglycemia, important nutrients include B complex (50 to 100 mg), magnesium (500 mg), and zinc (15 mg), all given in daily doses. Research published in the medical journal, *Metabolism* (1987) has also shown that taking 200 mcg of chromium (as chromium chloride) twice daily for three months improves hypoglycemia symptoms. If any of these are deficient it can make one more predisposed to hypoglycemia. As a bonus, chromium reduces the craving for sugar.

 GOOD TO KNOW!
A simple test called the Barnes Basal Temperature Test checks thyroid function. Refrain from drinking alcohol that night. Before bed, shake down a thermometer and place it by your bed. In the morning, put the thermometer firmly in the armpit and rest for 10 minutes. A normal resting reading will be 97.8°F. (37°C). Repeat the next day. If it is lower than that, you may have an underactive thyroid. Women should do this after their menses is complete, as temperature levels will fluctuate more during this time.

BEST FOODS TO BALANCE BLOOD SUGAR

Folklore for improving hypoglycemia is to eat small frequent meals. It is also important to consume complex carbohydrates such as potato, sweet potato, pumpkin, and winter squash rather than refined grains. Avocados help to suppress excess insulin production. Also enjoy lots of cooked high-fiber vegetables, such as asparagus, cabbage, cauliflower, corn, green leafy vegetables, kohlrabi, and string beans, which nourish the pancreas and increase the fluids in the body. Snap beans are very alkaline (note: the green beans are more nutritious than the yellow ones). They are rich in beta-carotene, B complex, calcium, and potassium. Sea vegetables improve the entire glandular system.

It is important to have some protein at every meal. Whole grains such as barley, wild rice, buckwheat, millet, quinoa, black beans, and tahini are good protein sources. Almonds and hazelnuts also make good protein-rich snacks. High-protein super foods include spirulina, blue-green algae, and chlorella. Nutritional yeast, rich in protein, chromium, and B vitamins, is a blessing for hypoglycemics, helping to keep blood sugar levels stable.

Moderate amounts of fresh fruit that is not excessively sweet, such as tart apples, papaya, and strawberries, may be enjoyed. If a sweetener is desired, consider stevia, which stabilizes blood sugar levels in hypoglycemic people. On occasion, moderate amounts of barley malt or brown rice syrup can also be used as sweeteners.

BEST BEHAVIORS TO BALANCE BLOOD SUGAR

Learn to manage your stress. You'll find benefits in yoga, meditation, relaxation tapes, or stress management programs. Erratic blood sugar levels can contribute to erratic moods. Find multiple ways to get grounded.

Pay attention to underlying cravings for sweetness and gratification in life.

Look at any unexpressed feelings that leave one bitter, overburdened, and hopeless, which are said to correspond to blood sugar problems.

Skip This!

Eliminating refined sugars and grains (such as white rice, white bread, and other white flour products) is essential. Refined grains are too rapidly absorbed. Fruit juices as well as sweet vegetable (carrot and beet) juices should not be consumed; they are too sweet, lack the fiber of whole food, and tend to overstimulate the pancreas. Dried fruit, dates, grapes, artificial sweeteners, and honey are also too concentrated if you are hypoglycemic. Heavily salted foods can cause insulin overreactions.

GOOD TO KNOW!

A diet that is rich in sweets and lacking in fiber sets us up for the blood sugar blues. When blood sugar levels elevate too fast due to glucose overload, the pancreas "panics" and over-secretes insulin, which then causes the blood sugar level to drop very low. At this point, we are likely to crave another sweet fix and begin the cycle over again. As this is repeated, the pancreas becomes hypersensitive. Overusing stimulants also contributes to hypoglycemia, as this raises blood sugar levels by over-stimulating the adrenal glands. This causes a flight or fight reaction, causing insulin to be released. After years of this process, the adrenal glands become exhausted and unable to function properly. Heredity can also be a factor in hypoglycemia. Allergies can also cause stress on the body and can be exhausting to the adrenal glands.

WHEN TO SEE YOUR M.D.

Hypoglycemia should not be taken lightly. If it persists, it weakens the body and can be a factor in many other disorders. So pay attention when your body speaks. Walk in balance!

CHAPTER 6

NATURAL REMEDIES FOR WOMEN'S SPECIAL CONCERNS

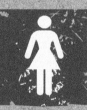

This section covers natural remedies for conditions that affect women. You'll learn how to use food, herbs, vitamins, minerals, and other natural therapies to help you center yourself and feel more balanced. Women are often the ones who give care to others. Here are some simple yet effective ways to give back to ourselves.

Regulating Appetite: Anorexia and Bulimia

If you are anorexic or bulimic, your food intake is out of balance. Anorexia nervosa is chronic undereating and obsession with thinness and a fear of weight gain. Bulimia nervosa is a repeated cycle of eating excessively, called binging, and then purging, either by vomiting or through the abuse of laxatives.

Both anorexia and bulimia are more likely to occur in women (about 90 percent), but they do occasionally occur in men. Practicing prayer, meditation, guided visualization, and yoga can all help you become more serene and stable.

So can these practices.

HEALING HERBS FOR ANOREXIA AND BULIMIA

Herbs that can be used in connection with anorexia and bulimia are listed below. Since many of them fit into the category of a digestive bitter, they are best used in capsule or tincture form, taken three times daily 10 minutes before a meal.

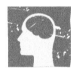

GOOD TO KNOW!

If you are anorexic or bulimic, it's important to correct any underlying health problem (such as low thyroid or biochemical imbalance). It can also help to get counseling by a professional trained in eating disorders.

Cures from Grandma's Kitchen

To soothe the digestive tract, try my Slippery Elm Gruel. Just mix a spoonful of slippery elm powder with a pinch of cinnamon powder and drink in a cup of hot water. Slippery elm provides a soothing protective coating on an irritated digestive tract, reduces inflammation, and is very nourishing and easy to digest.

HERB	BENEFITS
Ashwaghanda	Builds stamina and calms stress
Centaury	Stimulates and normalizes appetite; improves digestion; used for anorexia
Chamomile	Restores an exhausted nervous system; improves digestion
Gentian	Stimulates and normalizes appetite
Ginger	Eases nausea and indigestion
Hops	Helps you to gain weight; used for anorexia, anxiety, indigestion, and irritable bowel
Licorice	Soothes a digestive tract irritated from bulimic vomiting
Marshmallow Root	Soothes a digestive irritated tract from bulimic vomiting
Oatstraw	For debility associated with appetite loss; eases anxiety and mild depression
Peppermint	Relieves indigestion, irritable bowel, and stomachache
Saint-John's-wort	Inhibits serotonin breakdown while enhancing its efficiency; used for anxiety and depression

You can also look for a product in your health food store called a "digestive bitter combination," which stimulates digestive secretions and improves appetite.

VITAMINS THAT IMPROVE APPETITE AND WELL-BEING

Research published in the medical journal *Lancet* in 1985 showed that anorexics are deficient in zinc. If you can't taste a solution of zinc sulfate or if it tastes just like water, you may need this nutrient—50 mg of zinc sulfate taken three times daily with meals can help improve your sense of smell and taste.

If you are anorexic, you can also benefit from supplementing with essential fatty acids, according to a study in the *American Journal of Clinical Nutrition* (1985). Essential fatty acids in fish oil can also help ease depression and stabilize the emotional body by feeding the brain. Take 1 teaspoon (5 ml) of fish oil daily. Taking 500 mg of the amino acid l-tyrosine one to three times daily can reduce depression.

For bulimics, taking 10,000 IU of a beta-carotene supplement daily can help heal mucus membranes irritated from lack of nourishment as well as vomiting and laxative use.

BEST FOODS FOR ANOREXIA AND BULIMIA

Eat foods that calm the spirit, nourish the stomach and spleen, and tonify the heart, such as barley, rice, well-cooked beans, organic chicken, corn, pumpkins, sweet potatoes, and winter squash. Watery-cooked grains with some vegetables cooked into them are ideal.

Thrifty Cures!

Stimulate your appetite by adding cilantro, cinnamon, garlic, and ginger to your food.

Include raw juices and fruits like persimmons and ripe pineapple, which are rich in enzymes that help digestion and reduce inflammation. Consume soothing foods like soaked chia seeds and mashed avocado (which contains the enzyme lipase, which aids in the digestion of fats). Add these foods in gradually to your diet, a little at a time.

Keep a daily food journal to observe mood patterns and what foods are binge triggers and to promote awareness.

Overcoming Infertility

Fertilization occurs only when an egg cell (ovum) fuses with a sperm cell. Women reach peak fertility in their early 20s. It diminishes from the mid-30s in women and about 10 years later for men. After 30, one in four women will have some difficulty conceiving. It is estimated that one sixth of all married couples are infertile. Infertility can be due to any combination of factors, including blockage due to scar tissue, fibroids, or endometriosis. Hormonal imbalances can also be a factor.

Some ulcer medications as well as many other drugs lower sperm count and so can heat from hot baths, tight underwear, jock straps, tight jeans, long bike rides, and even hot car seats. If nerve damage occurs in men due to diabetes, it can cause ejaculated semen to back up into the bladder. Erectile dysfunction or premature ejaculation can make it difficult to conceive. Even sitting for extended periods of time can lower sperm count!

Many women whose mothers took the drug DES (diethylstilbestrol) have experienced fertility problems and reproductive disorders. Irregular menses or lack of menses can make it difficult to predict when or if ovulation is occurring. No matter whether the problem is more with the woman or the man, both should work together for the best results.

Knowing when ovulation occurs and having sex close to that time will greatly increase your chances of conceiving. Chart your temperature to determine when ovulation occurs using special thermometers or kits from a pharmacy. Take your temperature every morning before

Skip This!

Eliminate caffeine, which can aggravate feelings of anxiety and depression and increase the desire to binge eat. Some people with eating disorders may actually have food intolerances such as to gluten, which when consumed can cause damage to the intestinal lining. This makes food abusers more likely to choose foods that require little digestion, such as sugar, white flour products, and alcohol, which are best avoided. Yeast overgrowth, also known as candida, can also be a contributing factor in eating disorders. Sugar feeds unfriendly yeast microorganisms, making them proliferate and you miserable. You can learn more about beating sugar addiction in the book *Beat Sugar Addiction Now!* (Fairwinds Press 2010).

doing anything. On the day of ovulation, your temperature will rise 0.4 to 1°F (-17.5 to -17.2°). Chart your menstrual cycle too. Notice when your cervical mucous is stringy, like an egg white, when held between two fingers; this is another sign of fertility. Fertile mucous is stretchy and doesn't soak into toilet paper. Infertile mucus is pappy and breaks apart easily. Learn to read your body to improve your timing. Here are some other ways to increase your chances of getting pregnant.

BEST HERBS FOR FERTILITY

Ashwaganda root is a male reproductive herb that increases sperm count. Asparagus root is an ovarian tonic that supports estrogen activity. It's also an aphrodisiac. False Unicorn Root is an alkaline uterine and ovarian tonic. One of my teachers said, "It's the next best thing to sperm for getting you pregnant!" Take in tea, tincture, or capsule form three times daily.

Ginseng nourishes the entire female reproductive system and can also help correct erectile dysfunction and low sperm count. Women should stop using if they become pregnant. Licorice root encourages normal ovulation. It contains phytosterols that provide the raw material for hormonal production.

Oat straw helps relieve exhaustion and stress, nourishes the nerves, and makes tactile sensations more pleasurable. It's also an aphrodisiac. Raspberry leaf helps regulate hormones. Red clover blossom is very alkaline, nutritive, and phytoestrogenic. Vitex berry affects the pituitary gland and stimulates ovulation. Vitex can also be used the first trimester of pregnancy to maintain the corpus luteum in women with a history of miscarriage before the twelfth week. Take a dose of herbal tea, tincture, or capsules three times daily.

GOOD TO KNOW!
Lubricants can slow down sperm motility. Even saliva, which contains the enzyme amylase, may have an inhibitory factor. Egg white at room temperature is one of the only things that can be used as a lubricant that won't adversely affect conception. However, if one of the partners is allergic to eggs, this is best avoided. Remember, foreplay is the best way to stimulate the body's natural lubrication.

Skip This!

Female smokers have a 40 percent higher rate of infertility than nonsmokers. Male smokers show a 33 percent rate of reduced sperm motility. Even electromagnetic energy from microwaves, electric blankets, waterbeds, computers without protective screens, x-rays, pollution, and toxins can affect fertility. Stress can also affect your ability to conceive. It can interfere with both sperm production and the female reproductive cycle. Avoid toxic cleaning products, heavy metals, and chemicals. Drink pure water. Love the weeds, learn to eat them, and stop using herbicides!

BEST SUPPLEMENTS FOR FERTILITY

Vitamin E (400 IU daily) helps prevent sterility in men and women and also prevents miscarriage. A deficiency in vitamin E can contribute to sluggish sperm. According to in vitro studies, taking a vitamin E (400 IU daily) supplement enhances the ability of sperm to penetrate an egg. Taking 200 mcg of selenium also improves the activity of vitamin E.

Zinc is found in the outer layers of sperm, in seminal fluid, and in vaginal lubrication. It is essential for the growth and maturity of the gonads and can help to increase the number and motility of sperm. Men with azoospermia (absence of living sperm) and oligoosperma (low sperm count) have both benefitted from zinc supplementation. Taking 15 mg daily improves testosterone production.

Taking 500 mg of L-arginine three times daily is essential for sperm formation and to promote normal sperm count and motility. Note, however, that arginine may aggravate existing herpes conditions and should be used only after other nutritional approaches have been tried.

BEST FOODS FOR FERTILITY

Foods beneficial for fertility are also good for health and sexuality. Buy organic. Raw sunflower, black sesame seeds, chia seeds, and pumpkin are rich in potent zinc and vitamin E. Almonds, pine nuts, and walnuts are also great as they provide vitamin E and zinc.

Whole grains such as wild rice and quinoa contain beneficial complex carbohydrates. Oatmeal and barley help build sexual fluids. Other fertility fruits include seed-rich elderberries, figs, goji berries, pomegranates, and raspberries. Seeds contain the germ of life. Indeed, if you were to plant some of them they would grow into plants themselves! Use them liberally.

Carrots, yams, and winter squash are also good foods for fertility. Consider drinking vegetable juices made from beet, carrot, and spinach three times a week. Since juices are sweet, dilute them with 50 percent water. Miso, unpasteurized tamari, sea weeds, and Celtic salt are rich in trace minerals and therefore beneficial condiments when used in small amounts, particularly for low sperm count.

Avoid margarine, shortening, and hydrogenated oils as these can contribute to blockages.

Cures from Grandma's Kitchen

If you are trying to conceive, make this shake. It's great for both of you in providing protein and essential fatty acids!

1 1/2 cups (355 ml) fresh raw almond milk
1 tablespoon (15 g) raw tahini
1 tablespoon (20 g) raw honey
1 tablespoon (4 g) raw pumpkin seed
2 ripe bananas

Mix ingredients together well. Share the mixture and make a toast to each other and to new life.

ESSENTIAL OILS FOR FERTILITY

Essential oils that can be used to increase fertility in massage, bathing, and inhalations include angelica, anise, basil, Clary sage, cumin, fennel, geranium, jasmine, lemon balm, neroli, and rose. Note, however, that these are not suggested during pregnancy as they have not been studied for safety during that time.

KEEP IN MIND

The best position for conception is the missionary position. If the woman can put her feet on her partner's shoulders, this is enhancing. Other beneficial positions include rear entry and lying on your sides. The positions least likely to promote conception are those that involve sitting, standing, or woman on top. It is not imperative for a woman to have an orgasm for conception to occur, yet she should be

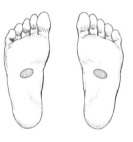

GOOD TO KNOW!
Try Reflexology
The kidney point is a reflexology point located at the center of the ball on each foot that connects through the meridians to the kidneys. It is beneficial to stimulate the foot reflex point in a circular motion for three minutes a day to increase fertility. Also work on the area of the Achilles heel, which correlates to reproductive organ points on both men and women.

stimulated enough to produce vaginal mucous. When the man ejaculates, he should go deep and stop thrusting.

After union, the woman should lie on her back with her knees elevated to her chest (urinate before sex so you won't need to urinate right after) for at least 20 minutes. Use a pillow or two to elevate your hips. The very adept yogini can stand on her head after intercourse during her fertile period. (If you're not adept at yoga, don't try it!) A shoulder stand can help too. Most importantly, keep in your hearts and minds the love and good feelings you have for one another and trust the process of life.

Preventing Miscarriage

About one in ten pregnancies end in miscarriage. Environmental pollutants, drugs, stress, overexposure to radiation, fibroid tumors, infection, structural abnormalities, and nutritional deficiencies can all be contributing factors to miscarriage. Miscarriage is sometimes nature's way of letting go of a being that may be less than perfect. It is only during the first stage, referred to as threatened miscarriage, that one can prevent the end of the pregnancy. Bleeding, spotting, and cramping are all symptoms. When the blood becomes heavy and bright red, it is considered too late to prevent. These natural remedies may be able to help, but of course it's wise to consult your doctor or midwife as well.

Black haw is a powerful uterine sedative, strengthens a weak cervix, and has helped many women continue a threatened pregnancy. Women who have had repeated miscarriages may want to take a dropperful in a bit of water 3 times daily to prevent problems before they begin. If you can't find black haw, cramp bark, a close relative, can be used in the same way. Keep using these daily until the threat of miscarriage has passed.

Another herb to prevent miscarriage is wild yam, which is an antispasmodic. It can be used in tea, tincture, or capsule form; one dose is taken three times daily.

Foods to consume that strengthen the reproductive system and have high nutritional profiles, and can help prevent miscarriage according to folkloric traditions, include black beans, millet, quinoa, wild rice, and winter squash.

Low thyroid function can also be a factor in miscarriage. Consider eating more sea vegetables or taking a kelp supplement.

Easing Morning Sickness

Morning sickness is kind of a misnomer because this condition can last all day long when you are expecting. Causes can include low blood sugar and the increased protein requirements of the developing fetus, the liver not being able to break down the extra hormones, stress, certain aromas, and diet.

But nausea during pregnancy may be a positive sign. It causes us to pay attention to ourselves. Research shows that women who have nausea early in their pregnancies may have a lower risk of miscarriage, perhaps because hormonal levels are high. And here's more good news. For many, morning sickness disappears by the end of the first trimester of pregnancy. Here's what to do until it passes.

Note: It is always wise to let your midwife or doctor know before taking any herbs or supplements while you are pregnant.

BEST HERBS FOR MORNING SICKNESS

For thousands of years, women around the world have relied on healing botanicals to help with morning sickness. Herbs such as peppermint leaf, anise seed, red raspberry leaf, and ginger root have all been helpful in relieving morning sickness. They are all available as tea and capsules, and ginger is also available in honey-sweetened sodas, candies, and syrups. If you choose to use candied ginger, rinse the sugar off before you eat it.

BEST NUTRIENTS FOR MORNING SICKNESS

Vitamin B6, in doses of 25-50 mg, can really help reduce nausea. But before adding, B6, note how much is already in your prenatal vitamin formula. Take no more than 150 mg as a total daily dose unless recommended by your physician or midwife.

Low levels of magnesium have been found to be a contributing factor in morning sickness. Green leafy vegetables and almonds are good sources of this nutrient.

GOOD TO KNOW!
Homeopathic remedies to consider for threatened miscarriage include Apis mellifica, which helps calm premature labor and stinging ovarian pains. Arnica montana can prevent miscarriage brought on by physical trauma such as falling.

BEST FOODS AND BEVERAGES FOR MORNING SICKNESS

Morning sickness is often worse when the stomach is empty and blood sugar level lowest. Small, frequent, bland complex carbohydrate meals throughout the day may be beneficial. Have a high-protein snack such as raw almonds before bed. If carbohydrates are all you can tolerate, see how you feel about sweet potato, chia seed porridge, or flax crackers. If nausea is worse at certain times of the day, eating something half an hour beforehand may help. You can also suck on frozen honey lemonade popsicles or chew a natural peppermint or spearmint gum to ease the nausea.

Drink between meals rather than with meals. Sip 2 teaspoons of apple cider vinegar (10 ml) and honey (13 g) in a cup (235 ml) of warm water. If you do experience vomiting, be sure to consume adequate fluids to prevent dehydration, preferably in small sips between meals which is easier to keep down.

HELPFUL HOMEOPATHICS FOR MORNING SICKNESS

Homeopathic remedies that help morning sickness include Ipecac, Nux vomica, Phosphorus, and Sepia. Talk to a homeopath about which remedy would best suit you.

℞ WHEN TO SEE YOUR M.D. Get professional attention if you lose weight (more than a couple of pounds [0.9 kg]), become dehydrated and do not urinate, or can't keep anything down (including water, tea, or juice small occasional sips are best tolerated) for over four to six hours.

OTHER NATURAL REMEDIES FOR MORNING SICKNESS

Take up to seven deep inhalations of essential oil of lemon or peppermint to calm nausea.

Use Sea Bands that gently press on acupressure points known as Pericardium 6 on the inside of the wrist to help alleviate morning sickness, available in health food stores.

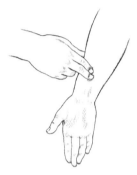

Place a cool lavender-scented compress on your forehead and a warm vinegar compress over your rib cage to ease morning sickness. Lie totally still with the eyes closed for best effect.

Get out into fresh air and take a walk every day.

Find pleasant diversions such as reading uplifting books and doing gentle exercise. My daughter Rainbeau has an amazing yoga DVD called *Zen Mama* (www.rainbeaumars. com) that may help.

Try to maintain a positive attitude about this time in your life. A healthy baby makes it all worthwhile!

Soothing Stretch Marks

Stretch marks are a common aftermath of pregnancy. It's important to lubricate your body daily to help prevent them. This is especially important the last three months of pregnancy so your skin will be supple and stretch during delivery. You'll want to apply this Pregnant Belly Butter to the perineal area, belly, hips, thighs, and breasts, which are all areas where stretch marks can occur. Here's how to make it:

Pregnant Belly Butter

2 cups (475 ml) olive oil or coconut oil

½ ounce (15 g) calendula flowers

½ ounce (15 g) comfrey leaves

1 tablespoon (15 ml) vitamin E oil

5 drops essential oil of lavender

In a dry, clean glass jar, place the crushed herbs and oil. Allow to steep for two weeks. Strain through a clean dry cotton cloth while squeezing the oil out of the herbs. Discard the herbs. Stir in the vitamin E and lavender oil. Bottle. Apply to areas prone to stretching at least twice daily.

Bettering Breastfeeding

Mother's milk is the perfect temperature, requires no preparation, is easy to digest, is free of bacterial contamination, is available at no extra cost, creates bonding and emotional security, promotes facial and muscular development and, best of all, is totally fresh! The benefits of breast-feeding are enormous. Babies that are breastfed are less likely to suffer from allergies, colic, diarrhea, ear infections, eczema, and infections. Breast milk helps protect babies from microbes including bacteria, fungi, and viruses and from disorders such as celiac disease and Crohn's disease. Breast milk also seems to contribute to higher IQs, perhaps because it is higher in essential fatty acids omega 3, 6, and DHA (docosahexaenoic acid). Here's how to boost production.

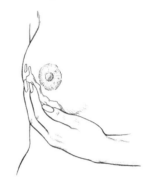

HERBS THAT BOOST MILK PRODUCTION

Galactagogue is the word for herbs that encourage milk production. It comes from the word galax, meaning "milk," and is from the same root as the Milky Way Galaxy. Galactagogue herbs that increase lactation include the following:

- Alfalfa leaf
- Anise seed
- Blessed thistle
- Caraway seeds
- Dandelion leaf
- Dill seed
- Fennel seed
- Fenugreek
- Goat's rue
- Hops
- Nettles
- Oatstraw
- Red clover

Marshmallow root helps to increase the fat content of breast milk and thus aids weight gain in the baby. Vitex causes the pituitary gland to produce more prolactin, which governs lactation.

You can find all of these in your health food store. Drink three to four cups daily or look for teas or capsules already prepared at natural food stores such as Nursing Mothers Tea by Traditional Medicinals or Nursing Support by Yogi Teas.

Hops, another herb, promotes lactation in mothers who are stressed and anxious. Good dark beers that are rich in hops can help relax a new mother and increase milk production. Nonalcoholic beers are available that provide the same benefits. One nightly should be enough.

Essential oils such as anise and fennel can enhance milk production too. Add 10 drops to 1 ounce (28 ml) of coconut oil in a small jar and massage a teaspoonful into the breasts using gentle circular motions daily. Rinse the breasts off before nursing.

BEST FOODS FOR BREASTFEEDING

Good nutrition is as important when you are breastfeeding as it was during your pregnancy. To support healthy milk production, choose plenty of calcium-rich foods like almonds, apricots, asparagus, barley, string beans, beets, carrots, green leafy vegetables such as beet and dandelion greens, kale, parsley, watercress, peas, pecans, sesame and sunflower seeds, oatmeal, brown rice, sea vegetables, sweet potatoes, and winter squash. Do your best to eat at least three servings of a selection of these foods daily.

When you are nursing, it's common to get depleted of essential fatty acids, especially the omega-3 fatty acids. A deficiency can result in postnatal depression and developmental deficiencies in your baby. Flax and chia seeds, a good source of essential fatty acids, also increase milk supply. Sprinkle freshly ground flax seeds (get them at your health food store) on cereal and yogurt. Soak chia seeds overnight and eat as an omega 3 source.

GOOD TO KNOW!
It is best to wean a child slowly to make the transition easier for mother and child. The World Health Organization suggests nursing for at least two years. As a child nurses less, less milk will be produced. The milk becomes saltier and thicker. To decrease milk production, drink a cup (235 ml) of sage tea up to eight times daily and drink less of other fluids.

Thrifty Cures

Check and see if you already have any of these galactagogue herbs on your spice shelf such as anise, dill, fennel, and caraway. It's simple to make a tea from them by steeping 1 heaping teaspoon (5 g) of the crushed herb (use a mortar and pestle or blender) in 1 cup (235 ml) of hot water for 10 minutes.

Nursing mothers need to drink plenty of fluids, at least half a gallon (3.8 L) a day. Good choices include barley water, green smoothies, and carrot juice (diluted with at least 50 percent water).

NATURAL REMEDIES THAT EASE BREAST TENDERNESS

If your breasts aren't emptied, it is easy for them to become painfully engorged. As a first step, you'll want to increase lactation. It can also be soothing to alternate hot and cold compresses, simply by soaking a cloth in hot or cold water briefly and then wringing it out and applying the hot compress until it cools down and then the cool compress until it warms up (about 5 minutes each). Cover the wet compress with a dry towel to hold in either the heat or cold longer. Cover the chest after doing compresses to prevent getting a chill.

Soothe sore nipples by applying a salve of calendula and comfrey available at natural food stores. Aloe vera gel can be used but it must be rinsed off before nursing. You can even apply some of your own breast milk, which has anti-bacterial properties and lubricating oils.

KEEP IN MIND

To promote healthy lactation, it is important to have a good "latch on." Elevate your baby to the level of your nipple and encourage him to latch on to the areola rather than the nipple. Start each nursing time with a different breast and vary positions so that the areola doesn't get too much intense pressure. Have your baby do all of her sucking when breastfeeding. Frequent use of pacifiers can reduce nursing time, and many of them are made of polyvinyl chloride, bisphenol, and pthlates.

Be calm when you are nursing. Relax and nurture the relationship and focus on the nursing experience rather than nurse while cleaning house or watching TV.

Soothing Mastitis

Mastitis is a breast infection that is more likely to occur in mothers who are overdoing things and tired. Does this sound like you? Plugged ducts from the mother not drinking enough fluids or the baby not nursing long enough to empty the breasts can all contribute. As a first step, slow down and rest more. Next use these helpful suggestions.

HERBS THAT REDUCE SWELLING

To reduce engorgement, it's a good idea to take cleavers herb and dandelion leaf in tea or tincture form to cleanse the lymphatics. Take a dose of the Thrifty Cure below every two hours. You can also use a dropperful of echinacea tincture orally every two hours to combat infection and boost white blood cell count. Also take 500 mg of vitamin C every three hours. If you have a fever, drink a hot

Thrifty Cures!

Add 2 teaspoons (10 ml) each apple cider vinegar and honey (13 g) to 1 cup (235 ml) of hot water and sip every hour until the infection has passed to reduce infection and inflammation. Eat plenty of celery and cucumbers (or juice) to cool the inflammation from the inside.

infusion of elderflower, which is diaphoretic and will help eliminate toxins through sweat. Essential oils that can be used in compresses, massage oils, or in a bath for sore swollen breasts include fennel, geranium, lavender, and rose. (See page 23 for aromatherapy guidelines.)

OTHER NATURAL METHODS TO RELIEVE SWELLING

Look no further than your fridge to relieve swelling. A poultice of grated raw potato can be applied directly to the breast to help relieve pain and blockage. Remove after about 20 minutes and repeat with a fresh potato several times during the day.

Cabbage leaf compresses reduce swelling of the breast caused by breast infection. Cabbage has both antibiotic and anti-irritant properties. It contains sinigrin (allylisothiocya-nate) rapine, mustard oil, magnesium, and sulphur. This mixture of ingredients helps decrease tissue congestion by dilating (opening) local capillaries (small blood vessels), improving the blood flow in the area.

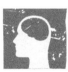

GOOD TO KNOW!
Nursing the baby on the side where infection occurs will not pass infection on to the baby and can help drain the breasts. Though it will be painful, it can help. If the condition is too painful or an abscess occurs near the nipple, nurse on the other side for a day while you actively treat the infected side with compresses and salves.

To make a cabbage leaf compress, rinse common green cabbage leaves and cut a hole for the nipple. Right before applying, crush the veins of the cabbage leaves with a rolling pin (or roll a glass bottle over the leaves) to break open the veins. Apply the cabbage leaves directly on the breast. Usually one or two leaves per breast works well. Make sure to cover all inflamed or engorged tissue with a cotton bra (synthetic fibers can trap sweat, contributing to a moist environment that encourages infection) and a clean T-shirt.

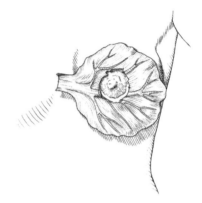

In 1 to 2 hours, when the cabbage leaves have wilted, remove the leaves and reapply fresh leaves. Repeat 4 to 6 times for a total of 8 hours. Use the cabbage leaves only until the engorgement subsides. Prolonged use of cabbage leaves on the breast can reduce milk supply according to folklore.

℞ WHEN TO SEE YOUR M.D.
Any fever that occurs in the mother within the first few weeks of birthing should be reported to your health care practitioner to determine whether a uterine infection, also known as childbed fever, could be occurring. This is a serious condition that needs to be treated.

Easing Menstruation Woes

Women, like the moon, are always going through changes. In fact, the word menstruation comes from the Latin mensis, meaning "month," which is derived from the word for moon. Menstrual time can be a time of healing, rest, and regeneration. Many women experience this as a time of increased awareness.

The process of menstruation occurs between the brain, hormonal levels, and female reproductive system. The pituitary gland releases follicle stimulating hormones (FSH), which signal the ovaries to secrete estrogen into the blood in the middle or follicular phase of the cycle. This signals a blood supply to build up in the uterus. An egg is released into the uterus. Progesterone is secreted, while lutenizing hormone (LH) flows into the blood from the brain and causes more blood to supply the uterus in preparation for a baby. This is the luteal or last phase of the cycle. When bleeding begins, the body prepares for a new cycle by releasing FSH from the pituitary, which causes the next egg to begin maturing within the ovary.

When menstrual bleeding occurs at irregular intervals or outside the duration of normal menses, it is called metrorrhagia. Menses that are delayed 8 or 9 days longer than a 28-day cycle could be due to a cyst, late ovulation, or lack of ovulation (anovulation). Here's how to fix menstrual difficulties in a natural way.

GOOD TO KNOW!

If you exercise regularly, you're less likely to have menstrual difficulties. Exercise improves circulation and liver function and stimulates endorphin production. It also can help relieve emotional problems related to physical disharmonies by detoxifying the body, causing perspiration, and helping to regulate fluids. Brisk walking and swimming are two helpful forms of exercise for menstrual difficulties.

GOOD TO KNOW!

If you get cramps, try using pads rather than tampons. The blood is trying to flow out and anything that is keeping it inside will cause the body to cramp more to expel what it is trying to get rid of.

GOOD TO KNOW!

If you have premenstrual syndrome (PMS), it can feel like you are on edge and out of sorts. Symptoms include breast swelling, mood swings, sweet cravings, depression, crying spells, irritability, anger, and agitation. Being more accident-prone or absent-minded are also common symptoms. Besides using the herbs mentioned here, find ways to nurture yourself during your "moon" time. Take an aromatherapy bath. Drink warming herbal teas. Get a massage for tense parts of your body. Play relaxation tapes. Practice deep breathing. Take a long walk. Take a day off around the first day of your menses for self nurturing.

Excessively early or late menses can be due to a chi deficiency, or general lack of energy. Menses that come early may be due to an insufficiency of progesterone. If menses occuring early is due to lack of ovulation, estrogen may be deficient.

MENSTRUAL HERBS

Some of the herbs that help PMS and menstrual difficulties work by inhibiting prostaglandins that have inflammatory actions. Plants with phytosterols can help keep hormonal levels from plunging. Herbal therapy can improve circulation, build the blood, improve liver function, and be diuretic. Herbs that can help regulate the cycle include vitex, dandelion root, and raspberry leaf. If the menses is always coming too early, avoid dong quai but use sage and rose hip teas. For delayed menses, raspberry leaf may be used. Here is some information about these herbs and others:

HERB	BENEFITS
Alfalfa leaf	Improves anemia and fatigue with its rich mineral content and its phytosterols help nourish estrogen receptors
Crampbark	An antispasmodic; calms cramps and emotional upheaval
Ginger root	Improves circulation, helping amenorrhea (lack of menses), dysmenorrhea (painful periods), and nausea
Nettle herb	Prevents anemia and helps control excessive bleeding (thanks to vitamin K); is a circulatory stimulant, diuretic, hemostatic, nutritive, and thyroid tonic
Raspberry leaf	Contains calcium, magnesium, and iron as well as phytosterols, helping amenorrhea, anemia, dysmenorrhea, and menorrhagia; is also a hormonal regulator
Red clover	Builds the blood and resolves blood clots; is anti-inflammatory, antispasmodic, diuretic, nutritive, and phytoestrogenic
Vitex berry	Helps regulate too heavy and frequent periods; for amenorrhea, breast tenderness, dysmenorrhea, metrorrhagia and PMS; also helps menstruation-related acne and headaches

SUPPORTIVE MENSTRUAL SUPPLEMENTS

Taking 50 mg of B complex daily supports the liver.

Taking 400 IU of vitamin E daily can help ease breast tenderness. Bioflavonoids inhibit estrogen by competing with its receptor sites and they also strengthen the capillaries.

ESSENTIAL OILS DURING MENSTRUATION

Essential oils that bring comfort to both body and mind during menses include basil, chamomile, Clary sage, fennel, geranium, hyssop, jasmine, juniper berries, lavender, marjoram, myrrh, neroli, peppermint, rose, and rosemary. These can be used as inhalations, in the bath, or diluted for massage once daily. (See Aromatherapy on page 23 for more ideas.)

BEST FOODS DURING MENSTRUATION

Green leafy vegetables and seaweeds help build the blood and prevent deficiencies. Seaweeds also can help regulate erratic menstrual cycles by providing missing minerals and nourishing thyroid function. Carrots also help regulate the cycle. Cruciferous vegetables such as broccoli, cabbage, and cauliflower can also keep estrogen levels normal by helping the liver do a better job in breaking down hormones no longer needed.

Soy products such as tofu, tempeh, and miso are good sources of phytoestrogens, which can help reduce the body's production of its own estrogen. These are best consumed as fermented foods such as miso and tempeh, making them easier to digest and less allergenic.

Eating a high-fiber diet and using acidophilus as a supplement can help normalize estrogen levels.

Cutting down on salt will help prevent water retention and bloating. Eat foods that are naturally diuretic such as artichokes, asparagus, watercress, and watermelon (including the seeds). Drinking more water helps the body to excrete sodium and excess fluids. Add the juice of half a lemon to a cup of water at least once a day to improve liver function.

NATURAL REMEDIES FOR MENSTRUAL CRAMPS

Dysmenorrhea is derived from the Greek word meaning "difficult menstrual flow." After ovulation, the uterine lining prepares itself for a fertilized egg, and arteries become enlarged. If fertilization doesn't occur, the uterine membranes start to die off and the lining is shed during the menstrual blood flow. The arteries may spasm as the lining dies off. The cramping usually ceases as menstrual blood helps to clean out the area. Constipation can cause pressure on the uterus and contribute to cramping. If the spine is out of alignment, pinched nerves can cause cramping. This can be remedied by yoga, bodywork, and/or chiropractic adjustments.

Black cohosh, chamomile, cinnamon, cramp bark, ginger, peppermint, raspberry leaf, and yarrow are all antispasmodic, relaxing cramps and spasms. Take them in tea, tincture, or capsule form up to three times daily when needed.

℞ WHEN TO SEE YOUR M.D.
If cramps become suddenly worse or change locations, get a proper diagnosis.

Eat a high-fiber diet to prevent constipation, which creates pressure in the digestive region. Include omega 3 and omega 6 fatty acids such as fish oils, chia, and flax seed, which can nourish brain function. Green leafy veggies such as kale and collards can also help reduce cravings, breast tenderness, and PMS weight gain by improving liver function, where hormones get broken down. One meal a day should be green leafy vegetables.

For painful menses, essential oils that can be used in massage, bathing, and inhalations include anise, carrot seed, Clary sage, jasmine, and rose.

KEEP IN MIND

Women who practice deep diaphragmatic breathing are less likely to get cramps.

It is a good idea to wear loose clothing during your period. Cramming yourself into tight jeans and belts will make you more likely to suffer from cramps.

Do leg lifts and you'll ease menstrual cramps by moving stuck energy in the pelvic cavity.

Do acupressure on the Achilles tendon to relieve menstrual cramps. Acupuncture has helped many women open channels of blockage in their bodies.

Stay warm during menstrual cramping times. Avoid cold drinks and icy foods, which can cause muscle contractions. Keep the kidneys warm so the rest of the body doesn't get chilled.

Thrifty Cures!

Try these thrift cures to relieve cramps:

- Castor oil compresses are messy but worth the effort for cramping. (For directions on how to make a compress, see page 18).
- Salt packs retain heat well and can easily be reused. Warm some salt in a dry pan and pour the salt into a cotton pillowcase. Secure well and apply the salt pack to the sacrum, at the base of the spine.
- A hot water bottle is a great folk remedy to place on a sore womb or painful lower back.

℞ WHEN TO SEE YOUR M.D. In cases of extreme menstrual difficulties, get a checkup to rule out conditions such as fibroids, endometriosis, cysts, or cancer. See your doctor if you have any concerns.

NATURAL REMEDIES TO STOP EXCESSIVE BLEEDING

Menorrhagia is excessive bleeding. See your gynecologist to have an exam and rule out a cyst, tumor, or a complication in pregnancy. Then try these natural remedies for relief.

Herbs that can decrease the flow of blood due to their natural astringency (usually from their natural tannins) include cinnamon bark, ladies mantle, nettles, raspberry leaf, shepherd's purse, uva ursi, and yarrow. Use any of them or in combination in tea, tincture, or capsule form three three to five times daily as needed.

Taking 1,000 mg vitamin C with 500 mg bioflavonoids daily can help strengthen capillaries and therefore reduce bleeding.

GOOD TO KNOW!

Include plenty of blood-building foods such as beets and dark green leafy vegetables to compensate for blood loss. Cold-water fish such as salmon, herring, sardines, and mackerel as well as essential fatty acids from chia, flax seed, evening primrose, or black currant seed oil can help normalize hormones. Seaweed nourishes the thyroid gland, which helps to regulate all the cycles of the body, including the menstrual cycle, and replenishes minerals lost through bleeding.

NATURAL REMEDIES FOR LACK OF MENSES

In women who are past puberty, not pregnant, lactating, or in menopause, a lack of menstruation is called amenorrhea. An imbalance in hormones, infertility, tumors, nutritional deficiency, glandular problems, weight imbalances, environmental toxicity, stress, certain medications, and less than 18 percent bodyfat can all be factors. First, schedule a thorough physical to determine the cause. In addition, try these natural cures.

Herbs that can help amenorrhea by building the blood and improving circulation to the pelvis include angelica, basil, blue cohosh, burdock root, cinnamon bark, licorice root, nettles, and raspberry leaf. Take them in tea or capsule form 2 to 3 times a day. Take a good multi-vitamin and mineral that contains vitamin B complex too, along with 400 mg of vitamin E.

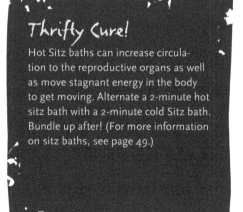

Thrifty Cure!

Hot Sitz baths can increase circulation to the reproductive organs as well as move stagnant energy in the body to get moving. Alternate a 2-minute hot sitz bath with a 2-minute cold Sitz bath. Bundle up after! (For more information on sitz baths, see page 49.)

Blood-building foods include beans, beets, blueberries, green leafy vegetables, parsley, raspberries, and nettles. Increase foods rich in iron (to build blood) and take an essential fatty acid supplement. Also nourishing for women who have amenorrhea are sea vegetables, brown rice, wild rice, quinoa, oats, fish, eggs, and organic dairy products.

For menses that are scanty, always late, or nonexistent, essential oils to use topically include Clary sage, fennel, lavender, and rosemary. Combine 1 tablespoon (28 ml) of olive oil or coconut oil scented with about 5 drops essential oil total. Massage beginning in your lower right abdominal area, using clockwise circles, and move up toward your ribcage, laterally across your navel to your left lower ribcage area, and down to your lower left abdominal region.

Handling Menopause

Menopause is more than the normal cycle of life in which menstrual cycles cease. It's a rite of passage that can be empowering, freeing us from monthly periods and the need for contraception. It can also be a catalyst for positive change, a chance to start over in midlife.

Menopause can be natural, premature (occurring before age 40), or surgically induced. It may occur quickly or take several years. Smoking cigarettes, illness, and genetic tendencies can bring menopause on earlier. Here's how to handle it gracefully:

HERBS FOR MENOPAUSE

Plants are sometimes referred to as being phytoestrogenic or phytoprogesteronic. This means that the plants have molecular structures similar to hormone molecules. The molecules of these plants can occupy the receptor sites in the body that would normally be taken up by hormones. Therefore, plants can in some cases can both increase and decrease hormonal levels in the body. Some herbs can

Skip This!

Sugar raises glucose levels, which then crashes, leaving us on an emotional roller coaster. Keep blood sugar levels stable by eating smaller, more frequent meals. Alcohol consumption can contribute to fatigue and headaches, so avoid drinking excessive alcohol as well. Eat less animal fat to keep estrogen and prostaglandin levels lower. Remember too that many commercially raised farm animals are fed estrogen-type drugs to promote earlier maturity, weight gain, and higher yields of milk and eggs. This can definitely raise our own levels of estrogen unfavorably, so be careful with your consumption of these foods.

even provide the raw material so that the body can produce its own hormones. Herbs to help menopause include the following:

- **ALFALFA** can raise or lower estrogen levels by providing the raw material to create estrogen or by binding to estrogen receptor sites and decreasing its production. (Avoid using this if menstrual bleeding is excessive.)
- **BLACK COHOSH** contains phytoestrogens, which bind to estrogen receptor sites. Because it's a muscle relaxant and a sedative, it helps improve edema, hot flashes, heart palpitations, depression, and headaches. A study reported in the *International Journal of Cancer* in 2007 showed that Remifemin, a specific formulation of black cohosh, also lowers the risk of breast cancer by up to 60 percent!
- **MOTHERWORT** is a bitter member of the Mint family. It cools and lessens frequency of hot flashes, emotional upheaval, heart palpitations, and night sweats, and also calms uterine pain associated with stress. It nourishes vaginal walls and decreases vaginal dryness.
- **NETTLES** as a food, tea, or juice is rich in minerals, tonifying the bones and muscles. Nettles also break down fat and build the blood. Their vitamin K content can curb excessive bleeding.
- **RASPBERRY LEAF** is rich in calcium, magnesium, and iron and aids in regulating menses and reducing hot flashes.
- **RED CLOVER BLOSSOM** contains phytoestrogens including diadzein and genestein as well as the estrogenic isoflavones biochanin and formononet, helping to calm hot flashes and night sweats.

Look for these herbs in your unsprayed fields and gardens. Learning to include them as teas and tonics three times daily is easy! (See page 13 for how-to instructions.)

SUPPLEMENTS FOR MENOPAUSE

Vitamins that can help a woman through changes include vitamin A or beta-carotene (10,000 IU of either daily) to nourish mucus membranes. Hot flashes can deplete B vitamins. Taking 50 mg of a B complex daily will boost your energy, strengthen the kidneys, and reduce nervousness. Vitamin E (400 IU daily) can reduce hot flashes, balance mood swings, and prevent vaginal dryness.

Vitamin C with bioflavonoids support immunity, nourish the adrenal glands, and are needed for collagen production so that skin remains elastic. They can ease some of the problems of heavy and irregular bleeding, relieve hot flashes, and increase vaginal lubrication. Take 500 mg twice a day. Calcium (1,000 mg) and magnesium (500 mg) are important for bone health and promote calmness and good sleep.

Skip This!

Minimize your intake of alcohol, sugar, caffeine, carbonated beverages, fried foods, and high-fat products as excessive consumption can worsen hot flashes.

If menstrual bleeding is excessive, an iron supplement can help prevent anemia. Evening primrose oil aids estrogen production and can decrease menstrual flooding. A fish oil supplement can help keep the skin moist. Of course, you can also focus on eating foods rich in these nutrients, like leafy greens.

ESSENTIAL OILS FOR MENOPAUSE

Essential oils of basil, geranium, grapefruit, lavender, lemon, and peppermint help relieve hot flashes and can be used as inhalations, in the bath, or in massage on a once daily basis (see Aromatherapy on page 23 for other ideas). Clary sage and cypress can help counteract vaginal atrophy. Use Clary sage to scent some olive oil and apply it to vaginal tissue. Clary sage can also help irregular menses and lift depressed spirits when diluted and applied to the skin. Oils that have estrogenic activity include Clary sage, sage, anise, fennel, angelica, coriander, cypress, and niaouli.

BEST FOODS FOR MENOPAUSE

Eat foods that build blood and strengthen the liver, such as barley, beets, beet greens, black beans, black sesame seeds, deep sea fish, green leafy vegetables, jujube dates, goji berries, millet, mulberries, mung beans, pomegranates, string beans, sweet potatoes, walnuts, and wild rice. Seaweed is mineral rich and helps promote vaginal elasticity.

SOOTHING PRACTICES FOR MENOPAUSE

Personality changes may occur with menopause. Take more time to yourself. Many women have spent their lives pleasing others, often not taking care of themselves in the process. A personal retreat can be wonderful and soul enriching. Take a class or learn about what has always been a passion you had to put off.

Stretching helps maintain flexibility. Kegel exercises help keep reproductive organs in good tone.

Simplify your life. Let go of activities that get in the way of keeping yourself in good spirits and health. Menopause can also be a good time to clean your karma. Are there people in your life to whom you owe an apology, a letter, perhaps flowers? Are there people who you need to confront to clear the energy—a parent or an old lover? This may be a good time to record your life story on paper. Complete any unfinished business. Enjoy this time of changes and growing wisdom.

Skip This!
Avoid washing with drying soaps as these may further dry the vaginal tissues.

GOOD TO KNOW!

Hot flashes feature warmth that is intense and often accompanied by heart palpitations, anxiety, faintness, flushing, headache, and night sweats. The average hot flash lasts about three minutes, but anything between half a minute and an hour can occur. It may be helpful to keep a record of what is going on and under what conditions hot flashes occur.

When hot flashes occur, ride the wave. Wear cool clothes and dress in layers so you can dress and undress as need be. Use a fan to cool yourself. Try pinching the fleshy area between the nose and upper lip to cool off.

Drink lots of cool beverages. Consume cooling foods like cucumbers, celery, melons, lemon, and fresh chickweed salad, which are considered refrigerants, literally cooling the body. Make your own dressing with extra virgin olive oil, as commercially heated oils congest the liver, causing it to become overheated and thus result in hot flashes. Avoid hot and spicy foods. If hot drinks bring on hot flashes, drink your teas at room temperature.

Spritz your chest, neck, and face (with glasses off and eyes and mouth closed) with water scented with essential oils such as cooling peppermint or lavender when you feel the heat come on. Avoid oil-type massages if you are suffering from hot flashes. Instead get shiatsu or other bodywork that is done without heavy oils, as oil massage is heating to the body.

A hydrotherapy technique for hot flashes is to walk or stand in a tub filled with 6 inches of cold water. (You can also add 3 drops of essential oil of peppermint or some lemon peels from your last salad dressing project.) Then dry your feet, put on your shoes, and go for a short walk.

Herbs to use as tea or tincture three times daily to curb hot flashes are motherwort and sage, both of which are astringent.

Finally, express your feelings in a healthy way. Bottled up emotions can cause you to heat up and blow your top!

Alleviating Vaginal Dryness

During menopause, vaginal secretions decrease because there is less estrogen to nourish mucus membranes. What's the good news? One of the best ways to prevent drying and atrophy of the vagina is to keep having orgasms! Sexual activity can stimulate vaginal secretions and blood flow. Make sure to engage in plenty of delicious foreplay to get your love juices flowing. Other natural cures can also help. Here's how.

To make a suppository for vaginal dryness, melt 1 ounce (28 g) of cocoa butter and add the following powdered herbs:

- 1 tablespoon (14 g) dong quai
- 1 tablespoon (14 g) licorice root
- 1 tablespoon (14 g) wild yam
- 1 tablespoon (14 g) marshmallow root or slippery elm bark powder
- 2 tablespoons (30 ml) vitamin E oil

This can also be scented with a couple of drops of pure essential rose oil. Pour into a glass baking dish and cut into suppository size pieces. Store in the refrigerator in a covered container. Insert one vaginally before bed.

Yeast overgrowth can be a contributing factor in vaginal dryness. It can be curbed by a probiotic capsule that is vaginally inserted to help produce lubrication.

Many creams containing wild yam are available in health food stores that can be used topically as a vaginal lubricant. Cotton swabs lubricated with sesame oil can be inserted vaginally overnight to improve dryness. You can also take vitamin E oil from a pricked vitamin E capsule and apply it to vaginal tissues. Use a 400 IU capsule daily. Be aware that latex condoms can be broken down by oils.

Takinge a sitz bath with emollient herbs such as comfrey or marshmallow root can also be a comfort. Black cohosh can help build vaginal mucus membranes, when taken as a tincture or capsule three times daily.

An omega 3 fatty acid capsule helps lubricate the body from within.

KEEP IN MIND

Remember your Kegel exercises, which strengthen the pubococcygeus muscles, building tone and elasticity in the pelvic region.

R WHEN TO SEE YOUR M.D.

If a rash or ulceration appears on the skin, it may indicate a more serious condition than surface varicose veins and should be checked by a competent health professional. Varicosities around the ankles are more inclined to rupture and bleed. Should this happen, apply pressure and seek medical attention.

Cures from Grandma's Kitchen

Apply apple cider vinegar to varicose veins and drink 2 teaspoons (10 ml) of apple cider vinegar in warm water three times daily to strengthen the venous system. You can also apply a cabbage leaf or cottage cheese poultice or apple cider vinegar compress overnight. (For more information on how to make a compress or poultice, see page 18 and 19.)

Vanishing Varicose Veins

Varicose veins are veins in the lower legs that are distended, widened, and in some cases twisted. Normally, blood flows into the veins after it has deposited its nutrients into the capillaries and returns to the heart so it can be reoxygenated. But when the valves in the legs that help move blood upward aren't working properly, blood can pool in the legs, causing pressure and bulging varicose veins. You usually find varicose veins on the sides of the legs, the upper parts of the calves, and the inner thighs. Varicose veins may also appear around the anus and are called hemorrhoids.

Symptoms of varicose veins include cramping, dull aching pain, heavy feeling in the legs, swollen ankles, itching, and tingling and burning sensations in the skin of the legs. Women are about four times more likely to be affected than men (which is why we cover them in this chapter on women's special concerns). Obesity, heredity, pregnancy, and age put one greater risk. When the veins are near the surface, they are more of a cosmetic problem than a health threat. However, a blockage of deeper veins can lead to thrombophlebitis, pulmonary embolism, stroke, and myocardial infarction. Here's what you can do to help.

NATURAL REMEDIES TO EASE VARICOSE VEINS

For ulcerations, apply a soothing salve or poultice of calendula, chickweed, comfrey, or liquid chlorophyll (available in bottles from natural food stores). To ease the pain or discomfort of varicose veins, apply a moist warm compress of mullein, sage, and white oak bark yarrow tea, all of which are astringent and tonifying. (For more information on how to make a compress or poultice, see pages 18 and 19.)

Bilberry helps to improve the strength of capillaries. Take one 80 to 160 mg capsule of 25 percent anthocyanosides three times a day. Butcher's broom also helps improve the strength of capillaries and it contains a compound called ruscogenin that reduces swelling. Research published in the medical journal, *Drugs Under Experimental and Clinical Research* showed that taking butcher's broom eased the symptoms of varicose veins such as pain, leg cramps, itching, and swelling. Take 150 mg three times a day.

GOOD TO KNOW!
Doctors have a nebulous catchall phrase, chronic venous insufficiency or CVI, to describe vein circulation problems. All this means is that a person's vein circulation system is failing, and blood is backing up either in the tissues or veins. Symptoms of CVI include nighttime leg swelling, leg pain, and cramping.

GOOD TO GROW!
Put an aloe vera plant in your windowsill and use the gel to relieve varicose vein itching!

Studies done in Europe found that horse chestnut helped to increase blood flow up and out of the legs, strengthen connective tissue, tighten up veins, decrease redness and swelling, and relieve painful leg conditions caused by poor circulation. One of its compounds, aescin, has been found to close the small pores in the walls of the veins, making them less permeable. This strengthens the vein walls and reduces leakage of fluid into the surrounding tissues. Take horse chestnut capsules containing 50 to 300 mg of aescin two to three times a day or 1 to 5 drops of horse chestnut tincture three times a day. Improvement should be within six weeks.

Avoid horse chestnut if you have liver or kidney disease or if you are pregnant or breastfeeding. You can find products in natural food stores that contain capsules of combinations of these herbs, which can be used three times daily.

A quart (946 ml) of nettle and/or horsetail tea daily is rich in silica, which helps build strong connective tissue.

You can apply a witch hazel compress as an astringent twice a day to the veins.

Supplement with daily doses of 1,000 mg vitamin C and 500 mg bioflavonoids to help strengthen the capillaries. Vitamin E helps the blood utilize oxygen better and prevents blood clots so 400 IU a day supplement is recommended.

A supplement of 500 mg omega-3s three times daily can also help prevent blood platelet aggregation and keep vessels more flexible. Take two tablets of 6x calcium fluoride, mornings and evenings, to impropve elasticity of blood vessel walls.

FOODS TO IMPROVE VEIN HEALTH

Eat more ginger, garlic, and onions as these foods help break down the fibrin surrounding the varicose veins. Add them to every dish you eat if you can!

Varicose veins are rare in parts of the world where a high-fiber diet is common. When fiber is lacking, one is likely to be constipated and tend to strain during bowel elimination, putting pressure on the veins. So it's important to eat more vegetables (especially dark leafy greens, beets, cabbage, okra, and sea vegetables) and salads. Use purslane raw as a salad green as it is a rich source of omega-3s. Also add small amounts of cayenne pepper to food to improve circulation.

Thrifty Cures!

At night, alternate hot and cold foot baths to alleviate varicose veins. Begin with hot water and end with cold.

Skip This!

Avoid deep massage atop a varicose vein as loosening a blood clot may be dangerous. However, gently applying some arnica oil to the area can gradually help disperse congestion. Do this only on unbroken skin.

Eat fruits high in bioflavonoids, such as berries and cherries. Whole grains beneficial to the circulatory system include barley, buckwheat, and oats. Also good to strengthen the vascular system are fish, especially bass, cod, flounder, hake (whiting), halibut, mackerel, salmon, snapper, trout, tuna, whitefish, and yellow perch. Consider using fiber supplementation such as flax seed (best if freshly ground before use), chia seed, or psyllium seed (take 1 teaspoon [2 g] in a bit of water three times daily).

Eat a relatively low-fat diet to avoid creating viscous blood. Cut down on red meat, high-fat dairy products, fried foods, and baked goods laden with fats. Nix margarine or hydrogenated oils. Be sure to drink plenty of fluids.

KEEP IN MIND

The following are some additional ways you can avoid or heal varicose veins:

- If you stand for long periods of time or do lots of heavy lifting, pressure in the veins increases. Instead, move around, walk, or bike ride. Do deep knee bends and a short walk when taking a break instead of drinking another cup of coffee. This helps pooled blood move back into the circulatory system.
- Regular exercise helps strengthen muscle tone and improve circulation. Brisk walking, roller-skating, aerobic dancing, swimming, cross-country skiing, and biking are all excellent activities for one prone to varicose veins.
- Wriggle the toes and flex and rotate the feet. Raise up on the toes and slowly sink to the heels. You can also practice isometric exercises by tightening the muscles and then relaxing. The old high school gym exercise "bicycling," where you lie on your back, elevate the hips and legs, and make a bike pedaling motion, is also excellent.
- Avoid long periods of sitting, especially with your legs crossed. If you must cross your legs, do so at the ankles, not the knees. Elevate your legs when sitting if possible. If you have a desk job, adjust your chair so that there is not a lot of pressure on the backs of your thighs. Sit on the floor with your legs stretched in front of you whenever possible (like when watching an occasional movie on TV).
- Raise the foot of your bed by four inches (10.2 cm). Before jumping out of bed in the morning and applying sudden pressure on your legs, stay in bed a few minutes and stretch and flex your legs and feet before getting up.
- Whenever possible during the day, elevate your legs. Use a slant board to elevate the feet above the heart. If you are into yoga, the shoulder stand or head stand is a great way to ease varicose veins.
- Use color therapy to ease varicose veins. Focus on lemon yellow, which helps to dissolve clots, and turquoise, which is a blood-purifying agent.
- According to those that study psychoneuroimmunology, standing in a situation which one hates, feeling overworked, overburdened, and not being able to stand up for oneself can be contributing psychological factors to varicose veins. Do your best to improve these situations.

- Do your best to avoid walking on paved surfaces and choose more natural uneven places to promenade so that you use a wider variety of muscles.
- Clothing that is too tight, including shoes or boots, will restrict circulation and may cause varicose veins by not allowing the blood to properly flow through your body. Snug-fitting girdles, pantyhose, and belts, tight socks, and shoes—especially high-heels—cut off circulation, thus forcing blood to seek alternative routes or causing pressure on the veins. Support hose, on the other hand, help promote circulation. Make sure they are the kind that is tighter at the ankles, gradually decreasing in pressure as they get higher up the leg. If you can't find a good over-the-counter brand, they can be medically prescribed.

Stopping Yeast Infections

Candida is a yeast (scientifically, a single-celled fungi known as *Candida albicans*) that grows on the surface and mucous membranes of most living organisms, including people, animals, grasses, drinks, and food. Pregnancy can increase yeast overgrowth as the vagina becomes less acidic and as more sugar gets stored in the vaginal walls. Some women experience candidiasis during PMS.

Use of antibiotics can also cause yeast to overgrow. That's because antibiotics kill both good and bad bacteria. When good bacteria aren't present in the gut in sufficient amounts, yeast will proliferate. Symptoms of a yeast over-growth include acne, allergies, asthma, bad breath, bloating, chronic fatigue, craving sweets, depression, diaper rash, diarrhea, and emotional swings. Frequent sinus and bladder infections also indicate a yeast overgrowth. Here's what you can do to keep yeast in check.

NATURAL CURES FOR CANDIDA

Interestingly, probiotics and candida have similar binding sites in the intestines. The more acidophilus is present in the intestines, the fewer sites for candida to flourish. As a first step, take a probiotic capsule four times daily for at least three months.

Soaking in the bathtub with 1/2 cup (60 ml) apple cider vinegar or sea salt (or use both) will help give relief from candida itchiness and clear up the condition. While you want to avoid using douches too much as this can wash away friendly vaginal flora, a good douche can be done by combining 1 tablespoon (15 ml) of apple cider vinegar to a pint (475 ml) of water twice daily. Other possible douches include 1 teaspoon (5 g) of acidophilus in 1 quart (945 ml) of water or 1 teaspoon (6 g) salt and 1 teaspoon (5 ml) 3 percent hydrogen peroxide to 1 quart (950 ml) of water. This should be done just for a few days during an acute condition.

Skip This!

Sugar feeds yeast and needs to be avoided. Minimize high-carbohydrate foods, such as peas, potatoes, winter squashes, and lima beans. Use stevia, a natural sweetener, instead of sugar. Other key foods to leave out of the diet until the yeast is under control include breads (which contain yeast), fruit juices, coffee, alcohol, peanuts, and mushrooms, all of which contain yeasts.

Afterwards, insert some plain cultured yogurt (chock full of acidophilus) vaginally using a diaphragm jelly applicator or soaking a natural fiber tampon before inserting. Wear a cotton sanitary pad to avoid having yogurt dripping down your clothes.

You can also insert a "00" size capsule filled with boric acid (don't ingest) or two capsules of probiotic. Look for probiotics containing the *bifidus* and *bulgaricus* strains. Just make sure you are using capsules that dissolve and not some enteric coated capsules that won't break down as easily. Insert the capsules high into the vagina for five to seven nights in a row.

Note that if you are pregnant, avoid putting anything into the vagina, including a douche, without consulting your health professional.

It's also very effective to use a garlic clove vaginal suppository. Simply peel the paper off a single clove of garlic, and without breaking the skin of the garlic, gently insert it vaginally before bed. In the morning, remove it. Some women are frightened that they may never find the clove again. Although this is highly unlikely, you can put the clove into a piece of cheesecloth and tie it securely with some dental floss, leaving a string of floss hanging out far enough to aid retrieval of the garlic-filled cloth the next day. Squatting while bearing down will also expel the clove. Be sure not to cut the clove or it can be irritating to delicate tissues.

After having a bowel movement or urinating, it can be helpful to wipe the perineal area well and squirt onto the area some antifungal herbal teas such as calendula, echinacea, garlic, myrrh, rosemary, thyme, or yarrow. (For directions on how to make tea, see page 13.) Keep a week's supply in the refrigerator and take out one day's supply and leave it in the bathroom so it will be at room temperature. What isn't used in a day's time should be discarded.

TREATING THRUSH

Thrush is a fungal condition caused by the yeast organisms Candida and Monila. Monila normally exists in the vagina but is a problem when it overgrows. A white cottage cheese like discharge may occur in the vagina along with itchiness, soreness, and burning. It can also affect the perineum area. Follow the same suggestions as treating candida.

MORE NATURAL CURES TO FIGHT YEAST

You can use a therapeutic bath to inhibit yeast. Just add 1 cup (235 ml) of apple cider vinegar or a pound of salt (455 g) or seven drops of tea tree oil to a clean bathtub. Tea tree oil is antiseptic, germicidal, and antifungal. It can even be used topically on yeasty areas of the skin such as athlete's feet or jock itch. It is one of the few essential oils that can be applied "neat," meaning straight and undiluted.

Other essential oils that can be used in bathing, massage, or inhalations that inhibit candida are allspice, chamomile, cinnamon, cloves, eucalyptus, geranium, lavender, patchouli, and rosemary. Add seven drops of your choice after filling the bath. The body's cleansing process can also be aided with colon cleansers and saunas.

When bathing, use coconut-based soaps. Lubricants that contain glycerin are sweet and can feed yeast overgrowth. Diaphragms and tampons can keep yeasts inside the vagina, encouraging an environment for their proliferation.

BEST FOODS TO STAY YEAST-FREE

Start each day with a pint (475 ml) of warm water to which the juice of a fresh lemon has been added to help the body's natural process of detoxification. The sour flavor stimulates liver and bowel cleansing.

Yeast flourishes on gluten-rich grains such as wheat, rye, and barley, so eat these foods in moderation, if at all. Millet, buckwheat, amaranth, quinoa, and wild rice are better grains to use. Lots of fiber is important as a slow-moving bowel becomes more alkaline, an environment that candida thrives on.

The best vegetables are low in carbohydrates, such as asparagus, beet greens, collards, kale, celery, cucumber, lettuce, broccoli, cauliflower, onions, radish, and spinach. Eating dandelion greens, nettles juiced, and chickweed as wild foods can be helpful in curbing yeast overgrowth.

Green foods are rich in chlorophyll, which promotes healthy intestinal flora and cools this damp heat condition. You can also top a salad with an olive oil dressing to stop the proliferation of yeast. It contains oleic acid, which inhibits candida growth. Coconut oil contains caprylic acid, another antifungal agent.

When cooking, use warming culinary herbs such as black pepper, cayenne, cinnamon, cloves, curry powder, garlic, ginger, oregano, and turmeric, all of which help dry damp conditions and inhibit yeasts. Seaweeds contain beneficial yeasts that outnumber the undesirable yeasts. Before modern drugs were available to treat yeast, iodine, found in seaweeds, was the drug of choice in treating yeast!

Contrary to what you may have heard, using some fermented foods helps to defeat candida. Rather than killing the candida, outnumber it! So do use some fermented food products such as yogurt, unpasteurized sauerkraut, unpasteurized apple cider vinegar, and miso.

KEEP IN MIND

Damp, muggy weather can often worsen candidiasis symptoms. While you can't do anything about that, it is important to eliminate dampness in the home. Mold can grow in damp basements and in carpeting. Sprinkle Borax as an antimold agent in damp areas. Get rid of piles of damp clothing and old newspapers that can harbor mold. Severe mold may necessitate replacing old carpets with wood flooring.

Leaky gas stoves can also pollute our internal environment. Have your stove checked and fixed or replace with electric if needed. Do your best to eliminate airborne chemicals in the home.

Use only white unscented toilet paper as it exposes you and the environment to less irritating chemicals. Avoid pantyhose, synthetic fabrics, tight-fitting clothes, and sleeping in underwear. Change out of wet clothes as soon as possible. When privacy is available, a five-minute air and sunlight bath of affected areas can clear up yeasts quickly. And of course wipe from front to back.

Stick with the program. Candida is resilient and many give up too soon or don't realize how easy it is to sabotage progress by cheating. There are some health practitioners that blame everything on candida and some that barely recognize its existence. It's important to find a holistic doctor who will work with you to get well. Get a culture of unusual discharge to determine what is the cause.

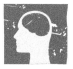

GOOD TO KNOW!
When beginning a yeast control program, it is not unusual to feel temporarily worse. Proteins from dead yeast can cause a histamine reaction, resulting in irritating symptoms like anxiety and fatigue. But taking a high dose of powdered vitamin C (1,000 milligrams) once a day will help clear the symptoms. Taking 300 mcg of biotin, a part of the vitamin B complex, daily helps prevent candida from transforming from a yeast vacuole into a fungal mycelia, which contributes to more yeast formation.

Caprylic acid, made from coconut and palm kernel, has been used as a natural antifungal agent since the 1940s. It can be taken orally to inhibit yeast. Pau d'arco tea can also help yeast die off. Take one to two capsules or three cups of tea daily.

Skip This!
Avoid vitamin formulas that use yeast as a base.

CHAPTER 7

NATURAL REMEDIES FOR BABY AND CHILD CARE

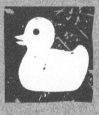

**Babies respond well to the gentleness of natural remedies.
Here is how to treat little ones safely and effectively.
When in doubt, always see your pediatrician.**

Children's Dosing Info

When offering your child herbal remedies, it's easier for kids to take an herb as a tincture than to swallow pills or drink tea. To figure out a dosage for children, follow one of two rules:

1. Cowling's Rule: Take the child's age at his or her next birthday and divide by 24. The resulting fraction is the amount of the adult dosage the child can have. For example, a five-year-old will be six at his next birthday. The number 6 divided by 24 equals $1/4$; this child should have $1/4$ of the adult dosage.
2. Clark's Rule: Divide the child's weight by 150. The resulting fraction is the amount of the adult dosage the child can have. For example, for a 50-pound (23 kg) child, 50 divided by 150 equals $1/3$; this child can have $1/3$ of the adult dosage. Look for products specially made for children such as Wishgarden Herbs and and dose according to their directions.

Calming Colic

Colic can be stressful both for you and your baby. The most common symptom of colic is when babies draw their knees up to their stomach and furrow their forehead. Colic happens when trapped gas causes spasms in the still-developing digestive system. Tension in the home environment can also be a contributing factor. It is also possible that the baby is sensitive to something the nursing mom is ingesting (see sidebar, page 146). These tips can provide much-needed relief.

HERBS FOR COLICKY BABIES

Herbs to treat colic can be taken by the nursing mother. Ideally, the nursing mother will drink a cup of the tea or take capsules 3 times daily. These herbs can also be taken in tablespoon doses in bottles by infants older than three months of age.

Cures from Grandma's Kitchen

Make your own teething solution with 5 drops each of essential oil of cloves and anise diluted in 2 tablespoons (18 ml) olive oil. Rub a small amount on the afflicted area up to four times daily.

The following herbs are gentle and help ease digestion by increasing circulation to the digestive tract due to their presence of essential oils:

- Anise seed
- Catnip herb
- Chamomile blossom
- Cumin seed
- Dill seed
- Fennel seed
- Lemon balm
- Peppermint herb
- Spearmint herb

Nursing mothers can also take a magnesium supplement (500 mg daily), which helps prevent the spasms of colic in your baby by relaxing the muscles.

SOOTHING PRACTICES FOR COLICKY BABIES

Massage the baby's abdomen gently in a circular clockwise motion (up on the baby's right, across and down on the left; the directions the intestines move food through) with 1 ounce (28 ml) of olive oil scented with 5 drops of anise, chamomile, fennel, ginger, or peppermint oil.

You can also give your baby a warm bath in which you add three to five drops of one of these essential oils or several cups of herbal tea such as catnip or chamomile.

You can also soothe your baby by applying a warm (not hot) compress of ginger or peppermint tea over the baby's abdomen. Cover with a dry towel to hold the warmth in. (See page 18 on how to make a compress.) You can also wrap a warm (not too hot) hot water bottle in a towel and apply it next to the baby's belly to provide relief.

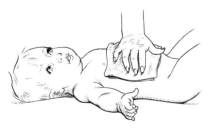

It helps to carry a colicky baby with his or her belly against your shoulder. Rocking and car rides can also be soothing. Be sure and keep the baby's feet warm, which helps them feel more relaxed and secure, thus calmer!

Exercise can also help a colicky baby. Gently take the baby's legs and pretend it is pedaling a bicycle by pressing the legs to the baby's stomach and then out and down. Lay the baby across your knees and gently rub his or her back.

Feed babies who suffer from colic small frequent meals rather than large ones to minimize gas. Be in a relaxed state when feeding the baby as babies pick up on your stress and tension. Keep the baby's head above the feet when feeding, which allows burps to be released more easily.

After you've tried everything, it might just be time to drink a cup of relaxing tea yourself!

GOOD TO KNOW!

For some babies, sensitivity to cow's milk that the mother is consuming can cause infant colic. So try switching to goat's milk, which is much easier to digest than cow's milk. Adding 1 tablespoon (28 ml) of liquid acidophilus per 8 ounces (235 ml) of milk can also help digestion. Learn to make nut milks. (For more information on raw food preparations, read my book, *Rawsome!*)

Moisturizing Cradle Cap

Cradle cap is a type of infantile seborrheic dermatitis caused by overactive sebaceous glands or in some cases by a yeast called Pityrosporum ovale. It is not caused by poor hygiene. Babies may have flaking of the skin and redness on the scalp and head and also under the arms and groin area. It is not itchy, contagious, or painful and tends to bother the parents more than the child. It usually begins between two weeks and three months of age and can last until the toddler stage. These natural remedies can help.

Skip This!

Signs that might indicate that the baby is allergic to something the mother is eating include red cheeks, constipation, frequent ear infections, dark circles under the eyes, spitting up frequently, gas, and sweating while nursing. Foods to avoid because they can cause colic include wheat, corn, beans, sugar, chocolate, nuts, and curries. Foods that are likely to give the mother gas such as cabbage, broccoli, cauliflower, kale (all in the Brassicaceae or Mustard family), as well as beans, garlic, and onions, all high in gaseous sulfur, are also likely to aggravate colic in infants. Cucumbers, green peppers, tomatoes, fried foods, eggs, alcohol, peanuts, and caffeine are all also notorious contributors.

HERBAL AID FOR CRADLE CAP

At night, rub the baby's scalp with 1 teaspoon (15 ml) of olive oil or coconut oil scented with 3 drops of lavender or rosemary essential oil. You'll also want to avoid using harsh soaps and shampoos on the baby. Instead, wash the baby's scalp with a tepid tea of burdock root, chamomile, chickweed, meadowsweet, or violet leaf. Leave the tea on the scalp and when it is dry, apply some cocoa butter on the scalp to soften the crusts. Use a fine-tooth comb to loosen the afflicted spots.

SUPPLEMENTS FOR CRADLE CAP

When you are nursing, add two omega-3 capsules and burdock root tea to your daily diet to respectively help in fat metabolism as well as in controlling any fungus, as both poor fat metabolism and yeast overgrowth can be causes for cradle cap.

Skip This!

If your child has diaper rash, avoid rubber or plastic pants as well as disposable diapers. They keep the skin from breathing and create a damp moist environment where rashes proliferate.

Thrifty Cures!

Make a cloth bag and fill it with oatmeal. Use the oatmeal that exudes from it to wash your baby's scalp.

Soothing Diaper Rash

Diaper rash can be painful. Ask any baby! It can occur when either the mother's or baby's diet is overly acidic. It may indicate that tomatoes, citrus products, sweets, and even fruits are being over consumed. To heal diaper rash, as a first step, keep the baby's bottom diaper-free as much as possible, ideally exposed to sunlight, and change the diapers more often. These remedies can also help ease baby's sore bottom!

You can apply plain yogurt to your baby's bottom to help clear up a persistent diaper rash. Also consider giving your baby an internal probiotic supplement that is formulated for infants. (Nursing mothers may also want to use an adult acidophilus supplement.) Acidophilus, a type of probiotic, is a friendly bacteria that naturally occurs in yogurt. Since many diaper rash conditions can be due to yeast overgrowth, this is outnumbered by the probiotics.

You can also apply calendula salve to your baby's bottom. Find it at your health food store.

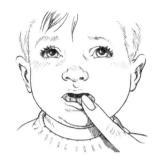

Soothing Teething Pain

Teething is a time that may leave both parent and child sleepless and slightly frazzled. Here's how to soothe your baby.

If you are a nursing mom, try drinking catnip and chamomile tea. Both herbs are quite calming. You can also soak a washcloth in the cooled tea and allow your baby to chew on the cloth.

Unsulfured dried apple rings make handy teething food. One of their virtues is that you can put the fruit ring around a couple of the baby's fingers, thus prolonging the amount of time before the object falls to the floor. Several types of natural teething cookies are also available.

Look for natural teething solutions to apply topically to the gums at your natural foods store. Many have also found homeopathic teething tablets effective in bringing relief.

> ### Thrifty Cures!
> If you launder your own cloth diapers, add ¼ cup (60 ml) apple cider vinegar to the final rinse water. This will make them softer for your baby's skin.

 GOOD TO KNOW! Anytime you allow a baby to chew on anything, be present, in case he should choke!

Fighting Ear Infections

Babies and young children often have earaches. Earaches are classified as either Otitis externa, which is an infection and inflammation of the external ear, or Otitis media, which pertains to the middle ear. In the latter, excess fluid and mucous impair drainage through the Eustachian tubes. Symptoms of ear infections include pain, throbbing, discharge, and/or a feeling of fullness. Infants too young to talk may cry shrilly, pull and rub their ears, and have low-grade fever and/or diarrhea.

One of the causes of earaches is an allergy to cow's milk and other dairy products. Other common allergens include wheat, eggs, corn, soy, citrus, peanuts and peanut butter, and tomatoes. A food sensitivity may cause an increase in mucous production and even swelling, thus creating blockage and pressure. For those with extreme sensitivities, even a tiny amount of the offending food may be a catalyst to an ear infection. For breastfed babies, the mother may need to be scrupulous in her avoidance of the offending substance, as it would be passed on to the baby through her milk. Here's how to get natural relief from ear infections.

NATURAL REMEDIES FOR EAR INFECTIONS

To help the body fight an ear infection, use the very effective herb echinacea (Echinacea purpurea, E. angustifolia). This herb has large polysaccharide molecules, which the body perceives as a bacteria, thus white blood cell production becomes activated, making the immune system stronger. One simple way to administer echinacea to a baby is in an extract or tincture form. Dosages on the bottle will usually be for an adult unless you purchase a product dosed for kids such as Wishgarden

GOOD TO KNOW!
Bottle-fed babies have more frequent ear infections than those who are nursed. Not only is there more exposure to possible allergenic substances, but the baby given a bottle has to suck harder, which creates more negative pressure in the Eustachian tubes. Breastfeeding or bottle-feeding while the baby is lying in a prone position may also contribute to more frequent ear infections as milk or fluid can drain into the ears. It is best to hold the child slightly more upright. Teething infants are often prone to ear infections, especially when molars are coming in, as this may cause swelling in the maxilla bone plate.

Cures from Grandma's Kitchen

Make your own teething solution with 5 drops each of essential oil of cloves and anise diluted in 2 tablespoons olive oil. Rub a small amount on the afflicted area up to four times daily.

Herbs. Look for kid-friendly tinctures made with vegetable glycerin rather than alcohol. They can be placed directly in the child's mouth or added to tea, juice, cup, or bottle.

MASSAGE TO SOOTHE EAR INFECTIONS

When an ear infection is present, gently massage behind the ear, around the outer ear and ear opening, and pull slightly on the earlobes, massaging gently down the neck to encourage lymphatic drainage. Rubbing the temples helps increase blood flow to the area as well as to move toxins. Using a drop or two of essential oil of lavender makes this antiseptic as well.

Stimulate the reflex points to the ears by pressing deeply for about 20 seconds in a circular motion at the base of and between the fourth and fifth toes. These points may be tender yet often provide relief.

Massaging children with two drops essential oil of lavender will help to relieve congestion and alleviate pain. Massage behind the ear, down toward the neck. Keep away from the eyes and mouth.

BEST FOODS FOR EAR INFECTIONS

For children old enough for food, give plenty of warm fluids (tea and soups) or lemon in water or 2 teaspoons each of apple cider vinegar (10 ml) and raw honey (13 g) in 1 cup (235 ml) of water to help thin mucus secretions. (Note: Do not give honey to babies under a year old because of the slight danger of botulism spores.) Goat's milk is more easily tolerated, and its high fluorine content actually helps to improve lymphatic drainage.

GOOD TO GROW!
I often make my own ear drops in the summer by gathering the fresh picked golden blossoms of mullein, layering them in a clean glass jar with slices of garlic, and covering the mixture with olive oil. Cover the mixture with a piece of cheesecloth secured around the jar with a rubber band. This allows excess moisture to evaporate while keeping dust and debris out. In two weeks, strain and rebottle the liquid portion into amber-colored dropper bottles. These can be stored in the refrigerator for up to two years.

Thrifty Cures!

A simple way to treat an ear infection is to position the ear so that the sun's rays are directly warming the painful region. Keep doing for up to a minute for a child or three minutes for an adult at a time, repeating if needed. It doesn't cost a thing!

Skip This!

Avoid congesting foods (dairy and wheat are common culprits) if you are nursing a baby with an ear infection.

REMEDIES FOR OLDER KIDS AND ADULTS

The remedies on page 148 work for older kids and adults. Here are a few more that older kids and adults can try:

- Deliberate yawning may also help to open blockages in the ear.
- For those familiar with yoga, the simple lion pose also helps to open the ears.
- During the night, it is best to elevate the head slightly to promote better drainage of the ears. (In the case of children, do this only if the child is old enough to sleep with a pillow.)
- When you are having a treatment done to your ears, breathe deeply and visualize sending healing energy to your ears. A painful ear is an ear calling for attention!

℞ WHEN TO SEE YOUR M.D. If an earache persists for more than 48 hours, if the person has a high fever, or if the earache is accompanied by a discharge of blood or green or yellow pus, it is time to consult with a health professional.

- If anger and turmoil fill your household, it makes sense to create more harmony so you will feel less compelled to "tune out" the negativity by perhaps psychologically blocking the ears. Louise Hay suggests that the person with the earaches, if old enough, frequently repeat the affirmation "Harmony surrounds me. I listen with love to the pleasant and the good. I am a center for love."

Calming Temper Tantrums

Temper tantrums can be a common occurrence if you have a little one. It's a lot easier to stop a tantrum that's just starting than one in high gear. These tips can also help you soothe your agitated child.

WHAT TO DO FIRST

If your child is yelling and screaming, ask him to come to you instead of asking him to stop screaming. It can help to change environments, which will remove the child from the source of the temper tantrum. When your child stops crying (if necessary give a 5 minute time-out), talk about the frustration the child has experi-

Thrifty Cures!

To treat the ears even more directly, I have had excellent results using herbal and oil drops, found in health food stores, usually made with garlic, mullein flowers, and olive oil. Before application, place the closed bottle in a glass of hot water to gently warm the oil for a few minutes, as cold oil does not relax the ear canal.

Have the person with the earache lie down on their stomach with the painful ear facing upward, while putting 2 or 3 drops of oil in the ear. Pull down gently on the earlobe to facilitate the oil getting into the ear. The oil helps with the pain and to fight infection. It is best to treat both ears, even if only one seems afflicted, as infection may be present though not discernable.

enced. Try to help solve the problem if possible. Teach the child new skills to help avoid temper tantrums such as how to ask appropriately for help and how to signal a parent or teacher that he or she knows they need to go to "time away" to "stop, think," and "make a plan."

Teach the child how to try a more successful way of interacting with a peer or sibling, how to express his or her feelings with words, and how recognize the feelings of others without hitting and screaming. Teach children how to make a request without a temper tantrum and then honor the request.

It can also be helpful to reflect back what they are feeling without any judgment, such as "Maybe you're angry because you can't watch TV." Make it clear that despite her feelings, there are boundaries to her behavior. "Even though you are angry, you must not yell and scream in the store."

The best way to bring these feelings under control is to express your love and concern. Reward children with positive attention rather than negative attention. During situations when they are prone to temper tantrums, catch them when they are being good and say such things as, "Nice job sharing with your friend."

NATURAL REMEDIES FOR TEMPER TANTRUMS

Homeopathic Chamomila (6C) is used for children who are irritable and difficult to please, as well as for those with a low pain threshold. (It is also well known for its soothing effect on infant colic and teething.) Do your best to get 2 or 3 pellets into their mouth, which will quickly dissolve.

Chamomile is a gentle relaxant that tones the nervous system for those prone to temper tantrums. It helps restore an exhausted nervous system and relaxes muscles. Chamomile before bed also helps prevent nightmares. It can be given as a tea, $^1/_2$ cup (120 ml) 3 times daily.

After an episode, a warm (not hot) bath scented with 5 drops of lavender essential oil also has a calming effect.

OTHER TIPS FOR AVOIDING TEMPER TANTRUMS

The following are some additional tips that may help you avoid temper tantrums in your little one:

1. Give children control over little things whenever possible by giving choices. A little bit of power given to the child can stave off the big power struggles later.
2. Keep off-limit objects out of sight and therefore out of mind.
3. Distract children by redirection to another activity when they tantrum over something they should not do or cannot have. Say, "Let's read a book together."
4. Signal children before you reach the end of an activity so they can get prepared for the transition. Say, "When the timer goes off 5 minutes from now, it will be time to turn off the TV and go to bed."
5. When you are visiting new places or unfamiliar people, explain to the child beforehand what to expect. Tell them you are there to support and protect them and that they are safe no matter what.

GOOD TO KNOW!
If tantrums occur frequently, see if there is any common food that has been consumed: sugar, artificial color, grains, dairy products, peanuts, citrus, or soy. Allergens and food sensitivities can cause inflammation, which may be affecting brain chemistry.

6. Do not ask children to do something when they must do what you ask. Do not ask, "Would you like to eat now?" Say, "It's suppertime now."

7. It's also important to recognize and avoid flash points. Kids are more likely to freak out when they are tired, hungry, or feeling rushed.

KEEP IN MIND

Family tension can be something that kids pick up on and can manifest itself as a tantrum.

℞ WHEN TO SEE YOUR M.D.
In very rare instances, a child who becomes emotionally upset and holds her breath may have a true seizure. Some neurological problems can also cause seizures, so your doctor may want to evaluate your child to make sure she is in good health. If tantrums increase in frequency, intensity, or duration, consult your child's doctor. Also seek medical attention if the child is self-injurious, hurtful to others, depressed, showing signs of low self-esteem, or is overly dependent on a parent or teacher for support. Your pediatrician or family physician can check for hearing or vision problems, chronic illness, or conditions such as Asperger's syndrome, language delays, or a learning disability, which may be contributing to your child's increasing temper tantrums. Your physician can also direct you to a mental health professional who can provide assistance for you and your child.

Eliminating Bedwetting

If your tot is under 6, bedwetting is to be expected and not a cause for concern. After that, it's important to check to see if something is bothering your child. Perhaps it's a new sibling or problems at school (or home). Other causes can include kidney or bladder problems and food allergies. These tips can help your child feel better and more in control.

HERBS FOR BEDWETTING

Certain herbs can help soothe bladder inflammation and promote the strength and integrity of the bladder. These include corn silk, fennel seed, horsetail herb, marshmallow root, and parsley leaf. It's easier for kids to take an herb as a tincture than to swallow pills or drink tea. Follow the children's dosing guidelines in the beginning of this chapter and give the child's dosage three times daily.

OTHER NATURAL REMEDIES FOR BEDWETTING

Give your child 1 tablespoon (20 g) of honey before bed to help the body retain fluid. (Note: Don't give honey to infants under 1 year of age due to the slight possibility of botulism spores.)

Chewing on a cinnamon stick before bed can also be helpful as it has a drying effect. Also limit beverage consumption after 5 pm.

Check at your health food store for homeopathic Hyland's Bedwetting Tablets, which also help deter bedwetting.

℞ WHEN TO SEE YOUR M.D.
If bed-wetting persists, you'll want to see your pediatrician to rule out the possibility of infection.

Due to their rich multi-spectrum mineral content, black beans, miso soup, celery, chia seed, pumpkin seeds, and wild rice help to strengthen the kidney and bladder. Add these to your child's diet on a regular basis.

SOOTHING PRACTICES FOR BEDWETTING

Nighttime can be particularly stressful for little ones. But these tips can help:

- Use acupressure. When putting a child to bed, take their pinkies with your thumbnails and apply pressure on the two lines of each hand for about 30 seconds to affect the meridians. Teach kids how to apply pressure to the acupressure point on the topside between the little finger and ring finger.
- Put a portable potty close to the bed. This will help your child to urinate without having to travel to the toilet in the middle of the night.
- Have your child try sleeping with his or her legs slightly elevated by putting them on a pillow to reduce the gravity force of urinating.
- Teach your child to do Kegel exercises. To practice Kegels, tighten and then release the muscles that control the flow of urine. To find them, tell your child to stop midstream the next time he or she is urinating. Then release. Suggest they do 7 to 21 Kegels sets three times daily.
- Be sure and provide a night light in the bathroom so it's not scary to go to the bathroom.
- A parent can take the child to the bathroom before they retire for the night.

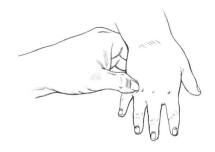

KEEP IN MIND

Scolding kids tends to make them more uptight and more likely to wet the bed. A mother recently told me that she would put on several layers of sheets covered with plastic so she didn't have to completely change the bed in the middle of the night or get overly resentful about having to do laundry so often. Kids older than eight who have to change their own sheets are likely to get more proactive about the situation. Help your kids stay positive too by using an affirmation. "I will wake to go to the bathroom."

Soothing Chicken Pox

Also known as varicella, chicken pox is a common childhood disease that is easily spread by direct contact, through the air, or via contaminated linen. Chicken pox is most common in the winter and spring in temperate climates, yet it occurs year round in tropical climates. At the onset, your child may feel fatigued, have a headache, fever, and cold-like symptoms. An outbreak is most likely from 10 to 21 days after exposure. Lesions appear first like small insect bites and then become blisters,

Cures from Grandma's Kitchen

Using ¹/₂ teaspoon each of apple cider vinegar and raw honey in a glass of warm water to acidify the urine and prevent bacterial growth, which in some cases can contribute to incontinence. Avoid carbonated drinks and orange juice, which can irritate the bladder.

which will eventually form brown crusts. New lesions may appear for 4 or 5 days as the old ones recede. Lesions may even appear in the mouth, vagina, rectum, and urethra. For some kids, the disease is mild, but for those over 10 years old, it's more likely to be severe. Here's how to benefit from natural cures.

NATURAL REMEDIES THAT SOOTHE THE SYMPTOMS

Give your child a 30- to 60-minute hot bath when you first notice the symptoms of chicken pox. Doing so at the outset will help to bring on the pox by being diaphoretic (causing perspiration), thus releasing and eliminating toxins. After that, frequent baths to which 1 pound (455 g) of baking soda or 1 cup (235 ml) of apple cider vinegar has been added will provide comfort and reduce itchiness. Two handfuls of oatmeal (which has soothing qualities) can be securely tied into a washcloth and added to the tub. After a bath, pat the skin dry rather than rubbing it.

Scratching may lead to infection and possible scarring. After bathing, apply calamine lotion or a paste of baking soda mixed with apple cider vinegar made by simply mixing together until it is wet enough to apply and stick to the skin. Aloe vera gel can help cool the inflammation and is also antibacterial and antiviral. To prevent scratching, keep the nails short.

If your child has mouth sores, use saltwater mouth rinses by stirring $1/2$ teaspoon of salt in $1/2$ cup (120 ml) of water, swishing it around in the mouth, then spitting, repeated 3 or 4 times to help dry up the mouth ulcerations. Do this 3 or 4 times daily.

Also offer your child detoxifying herb teas of burdock root, red clover blossoms, cleavers, calendula, and chickweed, all of which help open the body's normal cleansing channels such as the lymph glands, colon, and kidneys. Steep for a few minutes before serving to increase effectiveness. Aim for a cup or two each day.

NATURAL REMEDIES THAT PREVENT SCARRING

Give your child supplements of vitamin C (250 to 500 mg), vitamin E (100 to 200 IU), and beta-carotene (10,000 IU) to promote healing and to prevent scarring as these antioxidants help promote skin regeneration. A study in the medical journal *Free Radical Biology* and Medicine in 2004 showed the protective antioxidant effects of beta-carotene on the skin.

To help speed healing of lesions and prevent scarring on the eyelids, apply a salve made with comfrey and calendula, available at natural food stores. Place carefully on eyelids (not eyes) or any other part of the body needed.

BEST FOODS FOR CHICKEN POX

Keep the diet light and simple, as there may be sores in the mouth that will be stung by salt or acids. Fare such as applesauce, fruit kantens (see sidebar), soups, and fare that is not too spicy, salty, and acidic is best. Avoid citrus fruits as they can also sting the inside of the mouth.

KEEP IN MIND

Change the bed linen daily and clothe your child in light natural fibers that are warm but allow the skin to breathe. Do everything you can to make your child more comfortable. Stories, picture books, uplifting videos, and foot massages can all help your child feel better.

Skip This!

Never give aspirin to children under 19 as this may increase the likeliness of Reye's Syndrome.

WHEN TO SEE YOUR M.D.
Get medical attention for the
following situations:

- Fever lasts more than four days or goes above 102°F (39°C).
- There is a severe cough or breathing difficulty.
- An area of the rash leaks pus or becomes red, warm, swollen, or sore.
- Lesions are on the eyeballs.
- The patient has a severe headache, is unusually drowsy or confused, experiences extreme light sensitivity, has problems walking, is very ill, vomits, and/or has a stiff neck.

Boosting Attention in ADHD

If your child can't sit still or focus, he or she may have attention deficit hyperactivity disorder (ADHD). Approximately 4 percent to 6 percent of children in the United States have ADHD. Many will continue to have ADHD concerns as adults. There are a number of contributing factors to ADHD, which can include environmental toxins such as molds and chemicals,

 GOOD TO KNOW!
Natural food stores carry herbal tinctures that can help ADHD. Look for tinctures that use vegetable glycerin rather than an alcohol base, which can be too strong for a child.

Cures from Grandma's Kitchen

Berries are cooling to a fever, rich in vitamin C, and have antimicrobial properties. Use this recipe to give your child relief from chicken pox.

BERRY KANTEN
2 tablespoons (16 g) agar flakes
1 cup (235 ml) cold water
1 cup (235 ml) boiling water
1 cup (235 ml) unsweetened pineapple juice
½ cup (170 g) honey
1 tablespoon (15 ml) lemon juice
2 cups (145 g) raspberries, blueberries, elderberries, mulberries, or a mixture

Mix agar flakes with cold water and allow to sit 1 minute. Add 1 cup (235 ml) of boiling water and bring it all to a boil for 2 minutes. Allow to cool and add pineapple juice, honey, and lemon juice. In a glass baking dish pour raspberries, blueberries, elderberries, mulberries, or a mixture. Pour the liquid over the berries and allow to gel in the refrigerator. Makes 6 servings.

genetics, heavy metal toxicity, loud music, fluorescent lighting, and stressful family situations. Though taking prescription medications can be helpful, there are many other solutions you can implement first.

HERBS FOR ADHD

The herb bacopa increases attention span and improves behavior, memory, learning, and motor coordination. It enhances learning new tasks and aids in retention of newly learned material. In one double-blind controlled study published in the *Journal of Research for Ayurveda and Siddha* in 1993, 110 boys ages 10 to 13 took either a bacopa supplement or a dummy wafer (placebo) every day for nine months. The boys who took the bacopa supplement showed significant improvement in math skills and memory. Suggested dose is 50 mg twice daily.

Guarana (250 mg twice daily for kids over 12) helps focus attention and can help calm excessive motor activity, much the same way as Ritalin (which is a stimulant for adults, but a sedative for children) does. Since it contains caffeine, include only in small amounts for younger children like a cup of green tea or yerba maté daily (one half at a time) depending on age. (See page 13 for more information on how to make green tea and yerba mate.)

Lemon balm protects the cerebrum from excess stimuli. It calms anxiety and relieves depression, hysteria, insomnia, nervousness, restlessness, and nightmares. Passionflower quiets the central nervous system and slows the breakdown of neurotransmitters. It is an herb of choice to relieve anger, anxiety, hyperactivity, hysteria, irritability, insomnia, muscle spasms, restlessness, rapid speech, and stress. Look for teas, tinctures, and capsules at natural food stores and take when needed, up to 3 times daily.

Valerian is a strong central nervous system relaxant. It can help poor concentration for those under stress. Tinctures made from fresh plant or capsules are best. Take them twice a day.

Calming herbal baths can relax and center stressed kids (and adults!). Consider adding lavender or chamomile to the bath. (See page 21 for more information on herbal baths.)

CALMING SUPPLEMENTS FOR ADHD

Try these calming vitamins to calm a child with ADHD:

- Calcium and magnesium have muscle-relaxing properties and aid sleep. Recommend dose is 1,000 mg calcium, 500 mg magnesium for adults/half as much for kids depending on size and age.
- 25 to 50 mg of a yeast-free B complex (50 mg daily) can also have a calming effect and improve neurotransmission and appetite.
- GTF chromium helps keep blood sugar levels stable and decreases sugar cravings. 50 to 100 mcg can be taken up to three times daily between meals.
- DHA made from fish oils or algae can be very effective in relieving a wide range of brain-related concerns. Most brands suggest 2 capsules daily.
- Digestive enzymes such as bromelain, papain, and pancreatin can help reduce inflammation and calm moods. Use 2 capsules daily.
- GABA (gamma aminobutyric acid) helps to keep excitatory/anxiety-related messages from bombarding the brain. Recommend dose for kids is 250 mg two to three times daily (see dosage guidelines for kids in "Preparations 101"). It has a very tranquilizing effect and calms anxiety without sedation.

Make sure all supplements are free of artificial color and flavoring.

SOOTHING SMELLS FOR ADHD

Beneficial aromas for ADHD include orange, lavender, peppermint, and rosemary. They can be used as inhalations, with three drops placed on a handkerchief and ten deep inhalations taken. Five drops can be added to the bath or used with an aromatherapy diffuser.

BEST FOODS FOR ADHD

Children and adults who have ADHD may have had digestive, respiratory, and ear disorders early in life, which are all signals of food allergies. Allergies to wheat (as well as gluten also found in rye, barley, spelt, and kamut), dairy, eggs, tomatoes, corn, soy, sugar, peanuts, shellfish, citrus, and yeast can all cause behavioral problems. One of the no-brainer lifestyle changes you can make is to eat differently. It's easier on everyone if the whole family participates!

Besides these problematic foods, you'll want to avoid hydrogenated oils, artificial colorings, chemical sweeteners (even aspartame can cause hyperactivity and behavioral problems), and meats treated with nitrates. It is better to eat a piece of fruit than drink fruit juice, which can elevate blood sugar levels. Refined grains like white flour, bread, many cereals, and potatoes are also high in sugar. Practice a food elimination diet and keep a food journal to determine what the culprit may be.

SOOTHING PRACTICES FOR ADHD

First, try to keep to a schedule of regular mealtimes (and bedtimes). When you eat, encourage a peaceful atmosphere. Turn off the phone, begin with a blessing, speak calmly, listen, and eat more slowly. As much as you can, create a calm loving environment.

Spend one-on-one time daily with the person with ADHD. Physical contact such as hugging and massage can stimulate calming endorphin production. Minimize TV and video games with their frantic messages, constant visual changes, violence, and hyper chatter. (Although there are video games such as The Wild Divine that teaches techniques for exercising your brain in a positive way.) Watch select programs together or not at all and then only after chores and homework are done. Spend more together time reading and playing games.

At school, encourage hands on learning. Seat children away from distractions such as the pencil sharpener and areas of traffic. Consider tutoring or alternative schooling such as home school, smaller classes, or private schools.

Cures from Grandma's Kitchen

Ask your kids to select a produce item for each color of the rainbow to provide a wide array of phytochemicals. Green leafy vegetables, especially celery and cucumbers, are cooling to an overly heated ADHD condition. Sea vegetables can be added to soups in small amounts (without being noticed) to provide many trace minerals. Both green foods and sea vegetables are naturally rich in DHA. Eat wild salmon or sardines once a week for their beneficial essential fatty acids. Raw tahini and chia seeds are a good vegan source of essential fatty acids. Use foods that are as organic as possible to minimize the amount of chemicals the child is exposed to. Drink plenty of pure water to help the body eliminate toxins.

CHAPTER 8

NATURAL REMEDIES
JUST for MEN

Men, like women, have concerns specific to their gender. Here are some ideas to help empower men to care for themselves and promote optimal health.

Overcoming Erectile Dysfunction

Erection occurs when blood rushes in from the penile arteries, engorging the erectile tissue and causing expansion in the penis. In order for a man to have a strong erection, he needs to have healthy blood, muscles, nerves, and bones. It is estimated that about 75 to 85 percent of erectile dysfunction (ED) concerns are physical and between 15 and 25 percent are due to emotional concerns. Performance anxiety is one of the major causes of psychologically induced ED. It may also be nature's way of telling you relationship issues need to be addressed or that you are stressed, fatigued, or working too hard. Find out what might be going on in your relationship and work on healing that. Consider erectile ability a shared responsibility. You may need to heal something in the relationship before you can "connect" again. Love can be deepened by helping each other through difficulties!

NATURAL REMEDIES THAT HELP ED

Herbs that can improve circulatory function and improve ED include ginkgo and ginger . Look for these herbs in capsule or tincture form at natural food stores and use as directed on the bottle, usually twice daily.

In cases of ED, these are some supplements that can help ensure all the bases are covered. Zinc (15 mg) daily indirectly stimulates testosterone production. Nitric oxide (80 mg daily) is the chemical responsible for erection that has the same action as prescription sexual enhancers. It is made from the amino acid precursor arginine. Products containing arginine are delivered transdermally (through the skin) and improve blood flow to the genitals. 125 mg of DMG (di-methyl-glycine) taken sublingually twice a day may be effective for some men. Be sure to get adequate protein, including arginine, to improve erections.

Cures from Grandma's Kitchen

When in season, eat watermelon and chew up the seeds to help clean out the urinary tract. A watermelon won't grow in your belly, despite what your mama told you!

GOOD TO KNOW!

A healthy man will have an average of three to five erections during the night, usually during the REM stages of sleep, some lasting as long as half an hour. If a man doesn't get erect at night, it is wise to get a medical diagnosis. So just how does one know if erection occurs during sleep? Try sticking a strip of postage stamps snugly around the base of the penis before retiring (like Charlotte did to check Trey's ability to have an erection on *Sex and the City*). If the strip is broken in the morning, erection occurred.

SOOTHING PRACTICES THAT HELP ED

Massaging a man's big toes stimulates meridians that boost sexual virility. A Taoist exercise to improve erection capability is for the man to sit in a hot bath and stimulate himself manually to an erection. When erect, he grasps the testicles and squeezes, gently pulling down on them 100 to 200 times. In Japan, men are advised to firmly but gently squeeze the testicles daily, once for every year of age, to maintain potency. Another exercise to improve erection capability is to stroke the perineum and press with the fingertips. These exercises stimulate hormonal production and can be used to regain erectile ability.

Sex therapists suggest that couples experiencing ED "sensate focus," backing off from a focus on pelvic connection and instead touching, exploring, getting naked, and communicating for a two-week period. In fact, 200 years ago, the recommendation for ED was to go home and have six loving connections without coitus. Sexologists even suggest that in cases of ED, it is best to completely avoid intercourse for a month and focus on caressing and other forms of intimacy. It is possible to connect, breathe together, do Kegels (both partners!), and share sensual pleasures without an erection if you use a lot of lubricant.

It's also important to look at what might be going on in one's life or happening in the past when erectile difficulties began. Does ED occur after drinking, with a new or familiar partner or when stressed? Telling your partner beforehand that you have been experiencing ED can remove pressure and help her be more nurturing rather than taking things personally or getting disappointed. Instead she may be pleasantly surprised!

For more information, please check out my book, *The Sexual Herbal.*

Skip This!

Cut out saturated fats, hydrogenated and partially hydrogenated oils, sugar, and icy cold foods and beverages if you have ED. They contribute to blocking the circulation in the body, and if the blood isn't getting to the genitals, erection just won't happen. Correct nutritional deficiencies, environmental chemical exposures, and even constipation that may block the flow of chi to the sex organs.

Improving Prostate Health

The prostate gland is made of both muscular and glandular tissue and shaped much like a chestnut. It is located at the base of the bladder, against the rectum and encircles the urethra, which is the beginning of the urinary tract. This gland is where urine, sperm, and sex hormones meet. Half of the men in America over age 50 will have prostate difficulty at some time. When the prostate enlarges, it can constrict the urethra. Benign prostatic hyperplasia (BPH) is the term for prostate enlargement or adenoma. Signs of BPH include frequent urination, feeling full right after urinating, painful urination, dribbling after urination, and nighttime urination (nocturia). Here's how to treat prostate enlargement naturally.

NATURAL REMEDIES THAT IMPROVE PROSTATE HEALTH

Flower pollen (which is different from bee pollen as it is collected directly from flowers and saves bees a lot of work) can help relieve prostatitis (enlarged prostate). It has anti-inflammatory properties and is antiandrogenic, meaning it helps to counteract some of the effects of excess testosterone. Two 250-mg tablets can be taken twice daily.

The amino acids alanine, glutamine, and glycine (500 mg each twice daily) help shrink an enlarged prostate gland. They can often be purchased in combination with beneficial herbs for reducing enlargement.

An acidophilus supplement will help discourage unfriendly microorganisms from invading the prostate region. Take three capsules daily.

Look for herbal combinations at natural food stores in capsule or tincture form that contain several of the herbs mentioned on page 171.

FOODS THAT IMPROVE PROSTATE HEALTH

Foods that are considered beneficial to the prostate gland include apples, barley, blueberries, brown rice, carrots, fermented soy products, cherries, olives, and yams. Seaweeds such as kelp and kombu have a softening and draining effect on hardened masses in the body, including a swollen prostate. Consume plenty of beta-carotene-rich foods such as carrots, green leafy vegetables, parsley,

℞ WHEN TO SEE YOUR M.D. Diseases that can contribute to ED include atherosclerosis, vascular disease, heart disease, and high cholesterol. High levels of cholesterol can clog the arteries of the penis and impair blood from reaching the penis. Smoking, drug and alcohol abuse, diabetes, kidney or liver disease, endocrine disorders, Parkinson's disease, spinal cord injuries, multiple sclerosis, congenital problems, sickle-cell anemia, cancer and radiation treatments, Lou Gehrig's disease, pain, prostate disease, injury to the penis, and Leriche's syndrome all may contribute to ED. Many medications can adversely affect libido, including antidepressants, antihistamines, antipsychotics, blood pressure medications, and tranquilizers. Consult with a doctor if you have concerns about medications you are taking and to see if ED can be due to an underlying health condition.

tomatoes, sweet potatoes, winter squash, apricots, and peaches that help nourish the tissues of the body, including the prostate. Drink plenty of pure water to make the urine less acidic and irritating. Diluted pure cranberry juice helps to prevent bacteria from adhering to the walls of the genitourinary system, thus preventing the likelihood of inflammation.

In nations where a high-fiber diet and exercise are common, prostate problems are considered rare. A high-fiber diet helps promotes normal elimination. There is only a thin tissue separating the rectum from the prostate gland, so avoiding constipation improves the health of the colon as well as the prostate.

 GOOD TO KNOW!
The prostate gland contains more zinc than any other body part. Zinc is also an important component of sexual fluids. Good food sources of zinc include almonds, beans, sunflower seeds, tahini, oatmeal, nutritional yeast, eggs, and oysters. Pumpkin seeds are also rich in zinc and essential fatty acids. They can help prostatitis and improve difficult urination. You can also take 15 mg daily of chelated zinc.

SOOTHING PRACTICES THAT IMPROVE PROSTATE HEALTH

Alternate hot and cold sitz baths, beginning with hot water for three minutes and ending with one minute of icy cold. Alternate several times to improve circulation and thus move stagnation out of the area.

You can also apply a hot water bottle to the perineal area (between the anus and scrotum). Warm baths relax the pelvic muscles and soften the prostate.

Skip This!

A diet excessively high in fats is believed to be a contributing factor in BPH, or benign prostatic hyperplasia (prostate inflammation). Eating red meat especially can contribute to elevated cholesterol levels, which can impair prostate function and contribute to BPH. Fried foods can contribute to hardening of the arteries and blockage in the genitourinary tract. It's also important to minimize coffee, alcohol, salt, and dairy product consumption, which can irritate the prostate gland. Cadmium exposure from cigarettes, contaminated drinking water and shellfish, and some paints can also increase abnormal prostatic growth.

A slant board or inverted yoga posture such as the shoulder stand can help move blood congested in the area. Avoid sitting for long periods of time. Walking, swimming, and dancing are excellent and nonjarring forms of exercise that do not irritate an already inflamed prostate gland.

Do Kegel exercises to strengthen the muscles in the pelvic floor. Another exercise to help the prostate gland is to lie on your back and put the soles of your feet together. Extend your legs with the soles still together and bring them as close to the chest as possible. Repeat ten times, twice daily.

Finally, keep in mind that when you are struggling with emotional issues about sexuality, imbalances can result in the reproductive system. When working with the prostate gland, do what you can to insure that sexual attitudes are healthy and sexual fulfillment and relationships are in balance.

Take a dropperful of tincture or two capsules three times daily. Herbs to improve prostate health include the following:

HERB	BENEFITS
Cleavers	Helps eliminate wastes from the body — it is rich in silica and vitamin C and soothes prostate inflammation and reduces the urge to urinate frequently.
Corn silk stigmas	Helps relieve prostate inflammation and soothes irritated tissues
Couch grass rhizome	Is cooling to irritated mucus membranes
Marshmallow root	Soothes inflammation due to the presence of mucilage
Nettle leaf and root	Improves metabolism of the prostate gland—it contains sterols, including beta sitosterol, stigmasterol, and campesterol, which decreases DHT (dihydrotestosterone) activity, which when unchecked can increase prostatic enlargement.
Pygeum	Decongesting action that blocks cholesterol buildup in the prostate. Anti-inflammatory—buy only from cultivated sources to avoid endangering this herb.
Saw palmetto berry	Reduces inflammation and frequent urination, lessens pain, and enhances blood flow

CHAPTER 9

NATURAL REMEDIES FOR STOMACH AND DIGESTIVE HEALTH

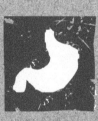

**Using natural remedies is a gentle way to tame tummy troubles.
Herbs and other natural cures also help to ensure optimal digestion,
which is essential to overall good health.**

Taming Colitis

Colitis (irritable bowel) is a chronic inflammation of the colon that manifests as alternating constipation and diarrhea and abdominal pain. It occurs when there is inflammation in the mucosa of the colon. Proliferation of unfriendly microorganisms due to overuse of antibiotics and food allergens can also be contributing factors. Here's how to soothe your digestive system.

Using demulcent (soothing to inflammation) herbs such as marshmallow root, licorice root, plantain leaf, and slippery elm bark in tea form is an excellent way to soothe the digestive system. Drink 2 to 3 cups a day.

A shot glass of aloe vera juice taken 10 minutes before each meal is also soothing to irritated intestines. Juices of carrot, cabbage, and celery can be taken diluted with water for their soothing alkalinizing properties.

Curing Constipation

There are over 700 brands of colon cleansers available in America, which tells you something about our nation's state of inner health! However, most commercial laxatives can destroy beneficial intestinal flora. Constipation can be acute or chronic and can cause not just discomfort in the abdominal region, it can also be a factor in appendicitis, backache, bad breath, headaches, hemorrhoids, kidney problems, pressure on the heart, as well as a number of colon problems such as diverticulitis and colon cancer. Here's how to find relief fast.

Cures from Grandma's Kitchen

Soak 4 teaspoons (16 g) of whole flaxseeds overnight in 1 quart (945 ml) of water. In the morning, strain the liquid off and drink daily to soothe irritated tissues.

HERBS FOR CONSTIPATION

There are many plants that help relieve constipation. Best are fiber laxatives such as psyllium, which is a bulking and lubricating agent. It is best to use the nonirritating husk or seed coatings as they contain mucilage that swells 8 to 14 times their volume when added to water. They gently clean the intestinal walls, speed bowel transit time, and soften the stool. Usually 1 teaspoon (15 g) is taken in a bit of water one to three times daily. Drink it before it gels up or it can be very difficult to get down. Again, it is necessary to drink plenty of fluids to prevent making constipation worse.

Flaxseed is a nonirritating bulking and lubricating agent. It is suitable for long-term use. Simply stir 1 to 3 tablespoons (12 to 36 g) of flax into a cup of applesauce (245 g), yogurt (230 g), or cereal (80 g), The seeds can be crushed (a blender works fine), but they should then be refrigerated and used that same day. It is fine to use them whole, but don't be alarmed if they pass through you unchanged. Soaking flax seeds overnight or making flax crackers are both excellent ways to consume this soothing, slippery food that is high in essential fatty acids.

You can also use a few mustard seeds daily (whole is okay) as a condiment to increase circulation to the bowels.

IRRITANT LAXATIVES

Irritants, also used as laxatives, irritate the wall of the large intestines, causing a reflex evacuation. Examples include cascara sagrada, buckthorn, and senna.

Cascara sagrada (which means sacred bark) is a very bitter inner bark of a tree. It must be aged for one year before it is used. This is one of the gentler irritating laxatives but is best on occasion rather than on a regular basis. Two capsules are usually taken right before bed.

Buckthorn is the next mildest of the anthraquinone (considered a mild stimulant) containing herbs. The dried bark is the part most often used and is only minimally irritating. It can be given for spastic bowel. The fruits are also used and considered gentler

GOOD TO KNOW!
Chicory, dandelion root, and yellow dock root are herbs that stimulate the liver and thus bile production. (Bile helps to make the stool soft by incorporating water into the feces.) These herbs can be used in tea, tincture, or capsule form.

GOOD TO KNOW!
Use an acidophilus supplement (2 capsules 3 times daily) between meals to help establish friendly intestinal flora. Eat small frequent meals rather than large sporadic ones. Blend or puree foods to make them more digestible.

WHEN TO SEE YOUR M.D.
Use a common-sense rule and seek medical advice when physical symptoms recur or persist for any length of time. If you suffer a progression of bloody diarrhea or fever, consult a doctor.

still. Buckthorn is also used as a stool softener. Use this only on occasion. Take two capsules before bed.

Senna is one of the stronger irritant laxatives and is best used for occasional acute conditions. The leaves are a gentler laxative than the pods. Excessive use can cause dependency. Use this only on occasion, two capsules before bed. A study in the *American Journal of Gastroenterology* in 1987 showed that using psyllium and senna together may be more effective.

TIME-TESTED FOLK REMEDIES FOR CONSTIPATION

Folk remedies for treatment of constipation include taking 1 tablespoon (28 ml) olive oil daily, or 2 tablespoons (40 g) blackstrap molasses before bed (brush the teeth after as it is sweet and sticky).

GOOD TO KNOW!
The tissue in the colon is smooth and slippery, much like the tissue in the mouth. During the digestive process, nutrients and fluids are broken down in the small intestines. Absorbed nutrients go into the blood-stream, then into the liver where they are further broken down. The remaining indigestible material then goes to the large intestine to be eliminated. It is in the large intestine that the body absorbs more water and nutrients. Peristaltic action, the "urge to go," is under the domain of the parasympathetic nervous system.

For young children, a gentle laxative tea can be made by simmering 1 teaspoon each of licorice root (5 g) and raisins (3 g) for 20 minutes in 1 pint (475 ml) of water. Babies can also be fed soaked-then-blended prunes, figs, and apricots to treat constipation.

BEST FOODS FOR CONSTIPATION

High-fiber colon-cleansing foods include apples, apricots, bananas, beets, black cherries, cabbage, carrots, celery, chia seeds, dates, figs, grapes (especially with seeds), okra, papayas, parsley, peaches, pears, persimmons, prunes, raisins, rutabaga, sesame and sunflower seeds, spinach, and sweet potatoes. All fruits should only be consumed when ripe or they can cause digestive problems.

If you are constipated, consume foods that promote friendly intestinal flora (especially if you've been on antibiotics, which can kill good bacteria). We need intestinal bacteria to aid

Skip This!

Avoid dairy products, with the exception of yogurt, as a dairy allergy is common in cases of colitis. Many people find when they remove gluten (found in wheat, rye, barley, spelt, and kamut), which is very inflammatory, the bowel irritation goes away. Stay away from coarse fibrous foods, though blending or pureeing them will help these foods be in a more predigested form. Intake of coffee, fried foods, and very spicy foods needs to be curbed as they can be irritating to the digestive tract.

digestion and help in the production of vitamins such as B1, B2, B12, and vitamin K. To do this, eat yogurt with active cultures, kefir, miso soup, blue-green algae, spirulina, and unpasteurized sauerkraut.

BEST BEVERAGES FOR CONSTIPATION

Drink a glass of room temperature water 1 hour before and after meals. Always avoid icy cold beverages as they cause constriction and are not conducive to good digestion. Drinking 2 glasses of warm water (with the juice of $1/2$ a lemon) and then resting in the frog position (laying on the floor on the belly, feet and arms spread out flat on the floor and bent like you were going to hop) for ten minutes is another helpful technique to aid bowel movements.

MASSAGE FOR CONSTIPATION

Massage over the intestinal area is a good way to improve intestinal function. Try using 8 ounces (235 ml) of olive oil that has been scented with 20 drops of any combination of pure essential oils of cumin, fennel, or rosemary. Warm the bottle of massage oil slightly by placing the closed container into a glass of hot water for about 10 minutes.

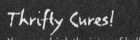

Thrifty Cures!

You can drink the juice of half a lemon in a cup (235 ml) of hot water, which will activate the liver to produce bile, which will then stimulate peristaltic action.

Skip This!

Foods that may contribute to constipation include milk, cheese, ice cream, unripe bananas, white flour products, gluten, alcohol, meat, and blackberries. Coffee also irritates the bowel even though it has a laxative effect.

GOOD TO KNOW!
Soaking a flannel cloth in castor oil, applying it over the abdominal area, and then covering it with a sheet of plastic and a hot water bottle is very effective and comforting.

Cures from Grandma's Kitchen

A laxative candy can be made by mixing together $1/2$ cup (75 g) raisins, $1/2$ cup (88 g) prunes, and $1/2$ cup (84 g) flax seeds. Grind the ingredients in the blender, adding a bit of liquid if necessary. Shape the mix into 2-inch (5.1 cm) balls, which can then be rolled in coconut or sesame seeds. Store in the refrigerator. Eat a couple daily.

The massaging should be done with a kneading action in a circular clockwise motion, going up on the right side, across, and then down on the left. This is the same direction that the intestines function. Another massage technique is to start at the navel and work outwards in a spiral along the pathway of the colon.

ACUPRESSURE FOR CONSTIPATION

Stimulating the indentation between the bottom lip and the chin in a circular motion for a couple of minutes helps to alleviate constipation. Other acupressure points to help normalize bowel function are Stomach 37 (located two hand widths down from the knee and 1 thumb width on the outer side of the tibia, the bone felt on the front of the leg) and Stomach 25 (located two thumb widths on both sides out from the navel). Push these spots deeply and massage in a circular motion for 1 minute daily.

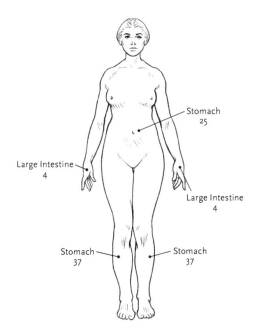

BEST PRACTICES FOR REGULARITY

To promote regularity, take a few minutes at the same time each day to sit on the toilet. Squatting on the toilet or having a low stool available to place under your feet helps ease elimination by lifting the knees and bringing the thighs closer to the abdomen. During the day, spend more time sitting cross-legged on the floor rather than using chairs. As I write this book, I am sitting on a large exercise ball that keeps me gently stretching as I work!

To improve bowel health, take daily walks while practicing deep breathing. Breathing more deeply and fully into the lower belly area also helps to prevent stagnation, while laughter sends healing energy to a congested lower belly.

Another beneficial technique is to lie on your back with your knees flexed to your chest while holding them. Take short rapid breaths and roll to the right then left. Repeat several times.

Another effective practice to ease constipation comes from the yogic tradition called Kapalabhati. Sit cross-legged, take two normal nasal breaths, and then exhale forcefully while sharply contracting the abdomen. Pump the abdomen in and out 10 times. Hold your breath, then exhale. Repeat two times. I find this most beneficial when done 10 minutes after drinking the hot water and lemon mixture mentioned in the beginning of this chapter.

℞ WHEN TO SEE YOUR M.D.
If you've had symptoms for more than three weeks and folk remedies are not helping—even with plenty of fluid, fiber, and exercise—see your doctor. You should also consult your doctor if there is blood in your stool.

Finally, to be more regular, it also helps to have regularity in your life when it comes to patterns of eating and sleeping.

Stopping Diarrhea

Although uncomfortable and inconvenient, diarrhea can be nature's way of eliminating something that probably shouldn't be in the body. Viral or bacterial infections, intestinal parasites, side effects from medication, laxative abuse, eating while stressed, eating too fast, and food intolerance may all be factors. The key is to bring your body back into balance. Here's how.

HERBS THAT EASE DIARRHEA

A teaspoon of carob powder blended into a cup of spring water is an excellent diarrhea remedy that can be used for children as well as adults. Carob contains tannins that are astringent. They may also bind to (and thereby inactivate) toxins inhibiting bacterial growth. The natural sugars make carob gummy, acting as a thickener to absorb water. Carob is also rich in dietary fiber and polyphenols, a type of antioxidant. Research published in the *Journal of Pediatric Gastroenterology and Nutrition* in 1989 showed that carob powder helped to reduce the duration of diarrhea in children. Adding $1/2$ a banana and $1/2$ teaspoon cinnamon (either by itself or in a carob smoothie) and blending in a blender tastes great and also has stool solidifying (banana) and antimicrobial (cinnamon) properties.

Strawberry leaf tea is good even for infant diarrhea as it is, like carob, also mildly astringent. The astringent qualities, due to tannic acid content, have a tightening effect. Other beneficial herbal teas to help stop the runs due to their astringent effects include blackberry leaf (milder) or blackberry root (stronger), cinnamon bark, raspberry leaf, and white oak bark. Drink three to four cups daily.

Psyllium is usually used as a laxative but can also help to solidify the stool. Take two capsules three times daily or stir one rounded teaspoonful (5 g) of psyllium into a bit of water. Slippery elm can also do the trick. Just mix a spoonful of slippery elm powder (to help solidify the stool) with a pinch of ginger powder (antimicrobial) and drink in a cup (235 ml) of hot water.

Two tablespoons of bentonite clay mixed with water can also help relieve diarrhea. Look for it at natural food stores.

BEST FOODS TO EASE DIARRHEA

Think BRAT, an acronym for banana (moderately ripe), rice, apples, and toast (slightly burnt so it provides its own charcoal remedy). These are all traditional foods to stop diarrhea that have a binding and absorbing quality. Other beneficial foods include applesauce (with cinnamon!), blackberries, puréed carrots, rice pudding with cinnamon, yogurt with cinnamon, or miso soup. Most of these foods contain pectin, a natural solidifying agent. You'll also want to increase your fluid intake. Whatever

GOOD TO KNOW

Charcoal can be a powerful antidote to diarrhea. No, not the kind you grill with in the summer time (that can be toxic!). We're talking about charcoal capsules, which are known for their ability to adsorb toxins. Taking 2 charcoal capsules every 2 hours should help stop even the most stubborn cases.

is eaten or drunk, take in small amounts at a time, using only food or beverage that is warm or room temperature.

A time-tested natural remedy is to eat an umeboshi plum, which has antibacterial properties. This popular Japanese alkalinizing paste is made of a pickled fruit (Prunus mume). It can be found in Asian markets or health food stores. Stir about $1/8$ teaspoon of the concentrate or 1 teaspoon (5 g) of the paste into 1 cup (235 ml) of warm water up to three times daily. You can also take this as a supplement.

As an adjunct to help good digestion, it's wise to take a good probiotic supplement. Doing so will recolonize the intestines with friendly bacteria. Look for probiotic pearls as they pass through the stomach and dissolve in the gut, where they are needed. Take one "pearl" three times daily between meals.

Diarrhea also causes loss of minerals, especially sodium, potassium, and magnesium, so take an electrolyte supplement from a natural food store once or twice daily.

Soothing Heartburn and Gastroesophageal Reflux Disease (GERD)

Heartburn is aptly named since it feels like your stomach is on fire! Heartburn is the symptom you feel when acid splashes up and out of the stomach. Heartburn is used interchangeably with acid reflux. Food sensitivities, allergies, insufficient digestive enzymes, yeast overgrowth, bacterial infection, and low stomach acid can all be factors. In pregnant women, heartburn can be due to progesterone having a relaxing effect on the valve at the stomach's end so that the stomach's acids can pass into the esophagus. As the baby grows and pushes the stomach upward, heartburn can be worsened.

GERD is severe or chronic acid reflux. When acid (HCL) builds up in the stomach, it can splash up and irritate the sensitive tissues of the esophagus, causing GERD. Here's how to feel better fast.

WHEN TO SEE YOUR M.D.
Diarrhea can be very serious if it is persistent, and in many parts of the world it is the leading cause of infant mortality. Signs of dehydration from diarrhea include sticky saliva, dark or scanty urine, a temperature of 103°F (39°C) a fast pulse, lethargy, and sunken eyes. Seek medical attention of any of these symptoms occur.

Thrifty Cures!

To soothe heartburn and GERD, add 1 tablespoon (15 ml) of apple cider vinegar to 1 cup (235 ml) of warm water and sip slowly. Though apple cider vinegar is acidic, low stomach acid often causes heartburn.

To soothe and buffer the tummy, stir 1 teaspoon (5 g) of slippery elm bark or marshmallow root powder into a bit of water and drink to buffer any irritation. Or chew on a bit of organic dried orange peel for its bitter digestive properties. One cup (235 ml) of licorice root tea or a shot glass of aloe vera juice will also soothe inflammation when taken 10 minutes before each meal.

Enjoy teas of chamomile to soothe heartburn and GERD but do not drink more than three cups (705 ml) daily to prevent diluting digestive enzymes. Eat more raw fresh fruits and vegetables, which are naturally high in digestive enzymes. Drink fresh cabbage juice for its ulcerative healing balm, vitamin U.

Easing Indigestion

Have you got indigestion? Many people do. Digestive disturbances contribute to bloating, discomfort, gas, halitosis, and heartburn. Incomplete digestion can lead to colitis, diverticulitis, and irritable bowel. Here are a few suggestions for how to ease tummy troubles now:

- Try ume concentrate or umeboshi plum paste. Both can be found in Asian markets or health food stores and are very alkalinizing and have antimicrobial properties. Stir 1 teaspoon (5 g) of the paste or 1/8 teaspoon of the concentrate into 1 cup (235 ml) of warm water and drink it slowly, up to 3 times daily.

- Papaya tablets contain papain, an enzyme that aids in the digestion of protein. Take 1 or 2 after a meal that feels difficult to digest.
- Drink 2 teaspoons each of apple cider vinegar (28 ml) and raw honey (13 g) in a glass of warm water daily for its pH balancing effect.
- Use a probiotic supplement to help colonize the digestive tract with friendly microorganisms.
- You can also massage clockwise over the abdomen with 1 ounce (28 ml) coconut oil scented with 20 drops total anise, fennel, and ginger essential oils (good for several applications).

Skip This!

Gulping cold things may further irritate the digestive tract.

Skip This!

Avoid peppermint and spearmint as they can irritate the gut wall. Sugar, juices, milk, fatty foods, overly spicy foods, and tomato products can all be contributing factors in heartburn, so you may want to minimize or avoid them. Taking baking soda or sodium bicarbonate preparations can also upset the body's acid/alkaline balance. Don't cook in aluminum and copper cookware. Commercial antacids may contain aluminum and bring quick relief, but in the long run, they are not the best choice. Also note that it is best to not lie down when experiencing heartburn to avoid a backflow of stomach acids into the esophagus. If you must lie down, lie on your left side as this position aids digestion and helps remove stomach acid. Sleeping on the right side has been shown to worsen heartburn.

Healing Stomach Ulcers

One in ten people are likely to develop an ulcer at some time in their lives. You're most susceptible if you suffer from stress or exhaustion, work day and night shifts, are exposed to noise from industrial jobs or traffic sounds, have type O blood, or have a history of ulcers in your family. Type A personalities are likely candidates for ulcers. If you drink alcohol, smoke, use lots of aspirin (irritating to the stomach), consume rich foods, and are prone to stomach and intestinal infections, you are also a likely candidate.

GOOD TO KNOW!
Foods that are easy to digest because they tend to be nonallergenic and soothing include apricots, asparagus, avocadoes, bananas, beets, carrots, celery, fennel, fish, green leafy vegetables, kefir, millet, rice, sweet potatoes, wild rice, and yogurt. Eating a small amount of organic orange or grapefruit peel, which are both high in bitter compounds, will stimulate natural digestive secretions.

GOOD TO KNOW!
There are two main types of ulcers: Gastric ulcers make up about 20 percent of cases and occur in the upper stomach and its lining. Peptic ulcers are more common, less dangerous, and may affect the esophagus, duodenum, lower stomach, or small intestine. In general, food makes a gastric ulcer worse, whereas eating brings temporary relief to a peptic ulcer.

The bacteria Helicobacter pylori may also be a contributing factor. Symptoms of ulcers include gnawing pain that reoccurs day after day, nausea, retching, and black stools, which may indicate the ulcer is bleeding. In any case, ulcers are a wake-up call that something in our lifestyle must change! Here's what to do.

HERBS THAT HEAL ULCERS

Many herbs have been used to heal ulcers. Look for combinations that contain several of these herbs and take them as needed, up to 3 times daily. These include the following:

HERB	DIRECTIONS
Aloe vera	Stomach tonic that is anti-inflammatory—Drink 1 shot glass 10 minutes before each meal. You can also blend aloe vera with the herbs mentioned below for extra soothing benefits.
Licorice	Contains carbenoxolone, which protects the stomach lining from gastric acids-Three chewable tablets can be taken daily. Using deglycyrrhizinated licorice (DGL) is safe and effective in healing ulcers, according to a study in the *British Journal of Clinical Practice* in 1972. Consult first with a health practitioner if you have high blood pressure or edema.
Marshmallow root	Rich in mucilage, which reduces inflammation in the digestive tract

Plantain	Rich in mucilage, which soothes inflamed and irritated tissues.
Psyllium	Soothing stool softener, provides mucilaginous intestinal bulk—Drink 1 teaspoon (5 g) in a glass of water or juice three times daily.
Slippery elm	Rich in mucilage and calming minerals that soothe irritated mucus membranes.

SUPPLEMENTS THAT HEAL ULCERS

A number of vitamins can help heal an ulcer:

- Vitamin A (10,000 IU) daily helps to strengthen the mucous membranes, including that of the stomach and intestinal tract.
- Vitamin C (500 mg daily) in a buffered form (often with calcium) that makes the C less acidic helps to promote wound healing and reduce inflammation. When it also contains bioflavonoids, it can strengthen capillaries so they are less likely to ulcerate.
- Vitamin E (400 IU) daily helps promote healing and prevents scar tissue.

 WHEN TO SEE YOUR M.D. In cases of stomachache, get medical attention if pain is severe, is localized in one area, increases, is worse after eating, or if there is blood in the stool (other than slight streaks), there has been a recent abdominal injury, or feces are continuously black.

- Calcium (1,000 mg) and magnesium (500 mg) daily nourish the nervous system, helping one to be less likely to develop ulcers due to stress.
- Zinc (15 mg) daily speeds up healing time and inhibits infection.
- Essential fatty acids such as in fish oils can reduce ulcer inflammation and inhibit H. pylori. Take 1 capsule three times daily.
- Probiotics can inhibit the growth of H. pylori and promote beneficial intestinal flora. Take one capsule three times daily.

AROMATHERAPY FOR ULCERS

Add 5 to 10 drops of essential oil to 4 ounces (120 ml) of olive oil or coconut oil and gently massage over the abdominal region. Oils that are beneficial for ulcers include chamomile, coriander, eucalyptus, frankincense, geranium, jasmine, lemon, marjoram, neroli, rose, and ylang-ylang. The aromas are calming and uplifting, and the massage is nurturing.

Take a relaxing warm bath to which a few drops of these essential oils have been added. Enjoy the beneficial fragrances and when done bathing and imagine all your tensions going down the drain.

Thrifty Cure!

Look to your spice rack to ease indigestion. Use fennel or anise seed, ginger, caraway, dill, spearmint, coriander, cardamom, cinnamon, and cumin liberally in your cuisine to prevent digestive distress. These spices all contain essential oils that increase circulation to the digestive tract. They can even be made into a tea!

BEST FOODS FOR ULCERS

During the acute stage, a bland, low-fiber diet should be eaten. You can later move to more high-fiber fare.

Cabbage has been found to especially helpful in curing ulcers. Research done at San Quentin prison and published in the medical journal, *California Medicine* in 1949 showed that 92 percent of patients with ulcers who ate cabbage were cured in 3 weeks. In fact, there is a vitamin present in cabbage known as vitamin U, named after its ability to help ulcers. Find ways to include it in your diet 3 or 4 times a week.

Other foods that soothe ulcers include avocados, barley, buckwheat, chia seeds, oatmeal, cream of brown rice cereal, sweet potatoes, Irish moss, kudzu, tapioca pudding, bok choy, green leafy vegetables, blended carrots, okra, sea vegetables, turnips, apples, bananas, plantains, persimmons, yogurt, and fresh ground flax seeds.

It is wise to eat small, frequent meals and avoid having the stomach either too full or empty. Be sure to chew food well to allow it to mix with digestive juices. This will help protect intestinal linings from erosion. Drinking water between meals rather than with meals also improves digestion as this avoids diluting digestive secretions.

Thrifty Cure!

Castor oil compresses applied over the abdominal region where the ulcer occurs can bring relief. (See page 18 for directions on how to make a compress.)

Skip This!

To heal an ulcer, it is wise to avoid coffee (even decaf), black tea, and cola drinks, which stimulate stomach acid production. Fried foods, sugar, acidic fruits like citrus, tomatoes, vinegar, alcohol, and carbonated drinks are all best eliminated. Avoid hot spicy foods if they bother you. It was once believed that milk helped neutralize stomach acidity, yet it has been found that milk actually stimulates acid production. If you do consume dairy products, those of a cultured variety are the easiest to tolerate. Studies show that those who don't smoke or who quit smoking, heal faster. Aspirin can have a damaging effect on the stomach lining.

Cures from Grandma's Kitchen

Take 1 tablespoon (15 ml) of aloe vera juice 4 times a day before meals and bedtime to help restrict gastric juices and heal an ulcer. A teaspoon (5 ml) of olive oil taken with each meal helps to soothe the irritated mucosa. Or take 1 teaspoon (5 g) of umeboshi plum extract in 1 cup (235 ml) of hot water and sip slowly.

℞ WHEN TO SEE YOUR M.D.
Bleeding ulcers occur when the ulcer corrodes a blood vessel. Excess bleeding can cause anemia, lower blood pressure, and leave you feeling in a weakened state. If you experience blood in the stool or the vomit or have severe abdominal pain, see a competent health professional.

KEEP IN MIND

Focusing on breathing more deeply and slowly will allow the life force to flow more evenly through your body. Acupuncture, hypnosis, and guided imagery have all provided relief to people who suffer from ulcers. Yoga exercises also help to relax the mind and body. In a study of 40 ulcer patients who took up yoga, 90 percent of them claimed benefit.

It may take 2 to 6 weeks to improve an ulcer, though the symptoms may be relieved in a few days. Initially, bed rest, even for a couple of weeks, may be helpful.

Having an ulcer is an opportunity to find ways to nurture yourself, de-stress your lifestyle, and make the changes necessary for a healthier lifestyle! It Be sure to look at "what's eating you" from the inside.

Thrifty Cure!
Eat a tablespoon of peanut butter! It will change your breathing so your hiccups will stop!

Stopping Hiccups

Hiccups are caused by a spasm in the diaphragm. The hic sound is air being sucked in and then cut short by tightened vocal cords. Folk remedies for hiccups abound, all with the intention of changing your breathing to hopefully get the hiccups to stop. Here are a few of the most common:

- Drink water from the far side of a glass.
- Drink from a glass of water (or lemon and water) while someone pulls down firmly on your earlobes (remove earrings first).
- Breathe into a paper bag without allowing air to escape. Do ten strong inhale and exhalations.
- Drink a tall glass of water.
- Chew on a few mint leaves.
- Put 1 teaspoon (6 g) of salt on half a lemon and suck out the juice.
- Hold your arms above your head and pant like a dog.
- Drink anise or dill seed tea.

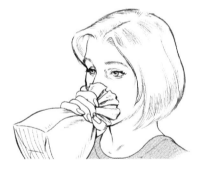

Easing Nausea and Motion Sickness

Nausea is caused by a virus, overindulging, stress, or an imbalance in the inner ear. Traveling can create motion sickness. You can ease both with these natural cures.

GLASS OF NATURAL REMEDIES FOR NAUSEA

Ginger syrup, ginger capsules, ginger soda (I love Reed's Ginger Honey sweetened soda), and candied ginger (wash the sugar coating off) are all helpful in alleviating nausea. In fact, in 2009, researchers at the University of Rochester Medical Center showed that taking ginger supplements with standard antivomiting drugs before chemotherapy can reduce nausea up to 40 percent.

You can also suck on peppermint candies or sip 1 teaspoon of umeboshi plum paste stirred into hot water. The flavors of these plants open different neural pathways rather than the nauseous one. Some find that drinking green tea helps. You can also try sucking on a lemon or olive, both of which have an astringent effect, decreasing salivation.

NATURAL REMEDIES FOR MOTION SICKNESS

Essential oils of peppermint, lemon, and ginger can be inhaled to curb motion sickness. Simply place a few drops on a tissue and take ten deep inhalations. Or just take up to ten deep inhalations at a time from the bottle. You can also get outdoors and breathe some fresh air.

To avoid motion sickness, if you are in a car, sit in the front. Look out of the front window of a car as looking out the side worsens nausea. Keep a window cracked to allow some fresh air in.

When flying, sit toward the front of the plane or over the wings as these sections move less than the back. Turn on the overhead vent.

On a boat, open a window or sit toward the middle of the deck, where there is the least motion.

Sit next to the window on any means of transportation and focus on things that are far rather than close. Keep your head still. Save reading and writing for later. If you must read, slouch down into your seat and hold the reading material close to eye level. Looking down makes some people nauseous.

Getting Relief from Food Poisoning

You had a nice dinner out, but a few hours later you are curled up in a ball suffering from abdominal cramps. You may also feel nauseous and have diarrhea, fever, chills, and a headache, all of which can lead to dehydration and exhaustion. Food poisoning is usually caused by eating organisms or toxins in contaminated food, often including common bacteria such as staphylococcus or E. coli. Here's how to feel better fast!

REMEDIES THAT GIVE RELIEF

Take ume concentrate or umeboshi plum paste. Made of a pickled fruit (Prunus mume) it's both alkalinizing and antimicrobial. Find it in Asian markets or health food stores. Stir about $1/8$ teaspoon of the concentrate or one teaspoon (5 g) of the paste into a cup (235 ml) of warm water up to three times daily.

Thrifty Cures!

To ease nausea, slowly sip peppermint or ginger tea, which is rich in carminative essential oils. This soothes the tummy and eases gas. You can also drink 2 teaspoons (10 ml) each of apple cider vinegar (13 ml) and honey in a warm water.

The acupressure point for nausea is the fleshy area between the thumb and forefinger. Hold firmly for several minutes. You can also rub the tendons on the tops of your feet between the second and third toes.

You can also take 2 charcoal capsules. Charcoal absorbs toxins, thus preventing your body from absorbing them.

Homeopathic Nux vomica helps digestive distress caused by overindulgence. If the food poisoning results in both vomiting and diarrhea, give homeopathic Arsenicum album every 2 hours, up to 3 doses.

REMEDIES THAT SPEED RECOVERY

Taking the herb echinacea (1 capsule two times daily) and vitamin C (500 mg daily) for a few days while you recover can protect you from pathogens by activating the immune system to destroy invaders. Echinacea also increases levels of properdin, which helps your body resist infection. A study in the medical journal, *Alternative Medicine Review* showed that echinacea raised properdin levels by 21 percent.

Garlic, which has anti-bacterial properties, can help kill pathogens acquired from eating tainted food and can prevent their proliferation too. It is used to treat and prevent infections in the digestive tract. It is best raw but can be taken in capsule or tablet form too. You can even blend a few cloves with a tablespoon (20 g) of honey. One dose should do the trick in most cases.

Acidophilus, a probiotic, can help recolonize the digestive tract with healthy bacteria. Take one probiotic capsule three times daily before meals so it doesn't compete with the food in the digestive system (or get killed off by heat, such as from soup).

Keeping hydrated is important. Drink whenever you feel thirsty.

BEST FOODS FOR FOOD POISONING

Chances are you won't feel like eating much when you have food poisoning, as your body might need a rest, but when you do, eat only small amounts at a time. Focus on easy to digest, soothing foods such as miso soup broth, applesauce, baked sweet potatoes, winter squash, or yogurt. Do your best to remember what food caused the food poisoning and remove its availability to others. It is wise to notify any restaurant involved.

GOOD TO KNOW!
Sometimes throwing up gets rid of what was bothering you and you feel better. But to ease a severe case of vomiting, warm half a cup (120 ml) of apple cider vinegar, soak a cloth in it, wring it out, and apply it to the bare stomach. Applying a hot water bottle over it makes this even more effective.

BEST PRACTICES TO AVOID FOOD POISONING

To prevent food poisoning, use clean cutting boards. Wood is the best choice as it is actually the least hospitable to bacteria.

Keep meat products refrigerated and once cooked, do not allow them to come to room temperature again. Avoid eating meat that still has pink in it and cook fish long enough so that it flakes (10 minutes per inch).

Reheating deli food makes it safer to eat in case it sat out longer than it should. Keep in mind that microwaving food can cause food to heat unevenly. Avoid cans that bulge at either or both ends and foods that smell and taste off. When home canning foods, make sure they are boiled at least 10 minutes. And when in doubt, throw it out!

Eliminating Parasites or Protozoa

Parasites. Ick. It's a word that can make your skin crawl. The word "parasite" is derived from Greek para, meaning "besides," and sitos, meaning "food." A parasite can be a plant or animal that lives on or in another organism to obtain sustenance without making contribution to the host's survival.

There are at least 134 varieties of parasites, with two main types. Ectoparasites live on the outside of the body (fleas, ticks, and lice) and endoparasites (giardia and amoebas) live on the inside, primarily in the digestive system. Parasites considered dangerous are known as pathogens. The World Health Organization considers parasitic invasion among the six most harmful diseases.

Thrifty Cure!

Chances are you have apple cider vinegar and honey in your pantry. If you do, just mix a tablespoon (15 ml of vinegar and 20 g of honey) each in warm water and sip it. This effective cure can help deter the replication of unfriendly microorganisms as well as replenish the body with depleted minerals.

R℞ WHEN TO SEE YOUR M.D.

Get medical attention if nausea or vomiting occurs after a head injury, lasts more than three days (unless pregnant or on a boat), if violent retching continues for more than two hours, if you are unable to retain fluids for 10 to 12 hours, if blood is in the vomit or vomit looks like coffee grounds, or if you experience constant severe abdominal pain.

Cures from Grandma's Kitchen

Peppermint tea is very calming to digestive distress and has antimicrobial properties, helping your body get rid of the germs that caused the food poisoning. Drink up to three to four cups (705 to 940 ml) daily.

You can contract parasites from swimming in contaminated water, walking on polluted beaches, taking mud baths, or sitting on sauna benches. Raw meats and fish can carry parasites. Overuse of antibiotics can also leave one susceptible to parasites. Symptoms of parasites include blisters on the inside of the lower lip, bloating, bluish or purplish specks in the whites of the eyes, burning urine, constipation, diarrhea, dizziness, emaciation, extreme hunger, fatigue, gas, immune deficiency, itchy nose, irritable bowel, joint and muscle pain, malnutrition, skin problems, sleep disturbances, night sweats, bleeding from the bowels, colitis, teeth grinding, irritability, weakness, and white coin-sized blotches on the face.

Many microorganisms see the human being as a lovely place to live. Such organisms can block the function of organs. They cause depletion of nutrients as they consume what is valuable to us. They eliminate their own waste products, leaving us overloaded with toxins to break down. Here's how to make your body and home an inhospitable place for such creatures to settle down.

NATURAL REMEDIES THAT ELIMINATE PARASITES

Boiling water for at least 10 minutes at sea level and 15 minutes at higher altitudes is the only sure way to destroy critters. This kills protozoa—microscopic organisms that can take over one's intestinal tract and invade other organs as well. Giardia, a protozoan endoparasite that thrives in the duodenum and small intestines, is the most common. Giardia and amoebas have two main stages of life: the mobile, active form (trophozoite) and the inactive stage (cyst).

Washing food, dishes, or brushing teeth in contaminated water can cause infestation. One half teaspoon of Clorox (not the generic) added to a gallon (3.8 L) of water can be used to soak vegetables and fruits for 15 to 30 minutes. After, soak produce in clean water for 10 minutes. One-fourth cup (60 ml) of apple cider vinegar can also be used per sinkful as a parasite-deterring cleanse for produce.

Grapefruit seed extract can be used to purify water and produce by following label directions. Grapefruit seed extract in its own right combats a wide range of digestive problems including parasites.

Applying petroleum jelly scented with a few drops of eucalyptus, lavender, or tea tree oil to the rectal area of people affected by pinworms every night for six weeks will keep the female worms from being able to lay eggs and help relieve itching.

KEEP IN MIND

Follow meticulous hygiene. Wash hands in hot soapy water before meals and after going to the bathroom. Keep fingernails short and clean to deter scratching.

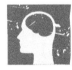

GOOD TO KNOW!
Consider getting a water filtration system as parasitic outbreaks sometimes come through tap water. A water filter with a size no less than 3 microns helps remove the 5-micron size giardia cyst. The Katadyn brand filter is highly recommended for travel.

To avoid infestation, wash laundry, including sheets and towels, in hot soapy water and dry in a hot dryer to kill eggs. Avoid shaking bed sheets out in the morning, which will cause the eggs to spread. Just fold them carefully before washing. Wash toilet seats and vacuum everything including the couch.

For children with worms, have them wear underwear tight enough to keep parasites from spreading to other family members. Wash hands after diaper changes. Toys and water faucets should be sponged down with a mild bleach solution daily.

Skip This!

Coldness in the intestines can cause constriction, so nix ice-cold foods and beverages if you have this ailment. Dairy products, gluten (found in wheat, rye, barley, spelt, and kamut), Brassicaceae family vegetables (such as cabbage, broccoli, cauliflower), improperly cooked beans, eggs, and copious amounts of fruit juice and carbonated beverages can all cause gas.

Fixing Flatulence

Gas is often the result of fermentation in the intestines. Changing your diet, eating too fast, not chewing well, eating while stressed, eating before bed, and overeating all cause gas. These tips can help alleviate gas:

- Use carminative herbs such as anise, caraway, dill, fennel, ginger, and peppermint, which help the body eliminate gas. These can be taken in tea, tincture, or capsule form when needed, up to three times daily.
- Eat foods high in lactic acid such as yogurt, which promote healthy intestinal flora that create an inhospitable environment for parasites.
- Take two charcoal capsules when the need arises. Note that these are best used only on occasion rather than daily. They may interfere with nutrient absorption from food if overused.
- Apply a hot water bottle to the belly if experiencing stomach pain to increase circulation to the area and calm pain.

Cures from Grandma's Kitchen

Aloe vera juice helps repair tissue damage done by parasites. Drink a shot glass four times daily before meals. Parasites will also find you poor company if you drink 1 tablespoon (15 ml) apple cider vinegar with water three times daily.

CHAPTER 10

NATURAL REMEDIES FOR RESPIRATORY HEALTH

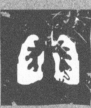

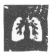

Our lungs connect us to the environment. The ability to breathe deeply and fully can even affect our mental states because our brain depends on oxygen. In this section you will learn how to use food, herbs, and other natural remedies so you can breathe and function to your full capacity.

Easing Allergies

Achoo! Allergies can be caused by animal dander, dust, food, mold, and pollen. Antibodies are produced by the body in response to an allergen. It's these histamines that cause the common symptoms of itchy eyes and sneezing. The best strategies for allergies include avoiding the allergen, strengthening the immune system, and easing the symptoms. Here's how.

SOOTHING HERBS FOR ALLERGIES

Herbs that can soothe allergies include elderflower and elderberry because both are anti-inflammatory, diaphoretic, and expectorants, and they reduce bronchial and upper respiratory phlegm. Ginger improves circulation and respiratory capacity thanks to its anti-inflammatory activity, which can reduce swelling in the respiratory passages. Take in tea, tincture, or capsule form three times a day.

Dandelion root and leaf improve liver and spleen function and are helpful for skin problems related to allergies, including rashes and itchiness. They are also anti-inflammatory, expectorants, and immunosupportive. Take in tea, tincture, or capsule form three times a day.

Marshmallow root contains flavonoids and helps to reduce the inflammation of the skin and digestive tract by moistening dry tissue. For this reason, it is good for coughs and scratchy throats. Take it as a tea up to three times daily.

Nettle is a natural antihistamine and expectorant, so it helps to dissolve mucus in the lungs. It's also naturally high in vitamin C and chlorophyll and relieves allergic reactions. Research published in the German medical journal, *Arzneimittel Forschung* in 1990 showed its effectiveness in treating allergic rhinitis. Take in tea, tincture, or capsule form three times a day.

Cures from Grandma's Kitchen

Eyebright herb (whose tiny flowers resemble a bloodshot eye) contains flavonoids, an antioxidant that strengthens mucus membranes of the nose and eyes. Eyebright clears heat and dries excess mucus. It relieves catarrh, congestion, hay fever, rhinitis, and sinusitis. You can use it as compress over your eyes to relieve swelling.
(See page 18 for instructions on how to make a compress.)

GOOD TO GROW!
Chickweed is an herb that often comes up as a weed in people's garden. Gather this anti-allergenic herb fresh from an unsprayed yard in the early spring and use it as a salad green. It will keep for up to a couple of weeks in the refrigerator.

ANTI-ALLERGY VITAMINS

Nutrients can prevent and minimize allergy symptoms:

- Vitamin A or beta-carotene strengthens mucus membranes and helps prevent allergenic substances from entering cell walls. Take 10,000 IU daily.
- Vitamin C lowers blood histamine levels according to a study in the *Journal of Nutrition* in 1980. It also detoxifies foreign substances and strengthens adrenal glands and immune system. Take 1,000 mg daily.
- Flavonoids, including quercetin and catechin, which are considered antioxidants, stabilize mast cell membranes, thereby decreasing histamine release and are thus an alternative to anti-histamine drugs. Take one 500-mg capsule two to three times daily.

BEST FOODS FOR ALLERGIES

Eat a wholesome diet focusing on fish, seeds (for their essential oil content and adrenal strengthening properties), and antioxidant-rich fresh vegetables. Especially beneficial are green leafy vegetables like kale and collards and dark orange vegetables like carrots and winter squashes for their beta-carotene and flavonoid content, which help promote immunity against infection. Seaweed can help you resist allergens by providing a plethora of minerals. Simply sprinkle a teaspoon (5 g) of kelp or dulse from a shaker on food.

Small amounts of organic lemon or orange peel nibbled throughout the day provide bioflavonoids, which lower histamine response according to the *Journal of Allergy and Clinical Immunology* in 1984. When you eat an orange or squeeze a lemon, just chew on an inch or two. They can even be soaked in some honey for two to three days, and then eaten as a treat.

Consume plenty of fluids. Diluted green, leafy vegetable juices such as carrot, beet, cucumber, horseradish, parsley, and spinach can also bring some temporary relief when allergies are severe. If you have a juicer, you can make these juices at home. Otherwise, visit a juice bar that makes its own juice and dilute the juice with half water so it is less concentrated.

DEALING WITH FOOD ALLERGIES

Food intolerance, allergies, or hypersensitivity is a response triggered by the immune system. The most common food allergens are cow's milk, eggs, wheat, gluten, corn, soy, and peanuts. Allergies can manifest in many ways. Respiratory congestion, excess phlegm, and a runny nose are common symptoms. There are many other ways allergies can affect us, though, including digestive distress, skin reactions, even mental fogginess. Shopping at health food stores can make food allergies easier to deal with as you'll find substitutes for just about every allergen.

Skip This!
Avoid foods that tax the liver, such as fried foods, margarine, chemical additives, caffeine, and refined sugars. The liver helps to break down allergens, and if its function is impaired, it simply can't do its job.

Aspartame sweeteners, monosodium glutamate, and artificial food coloring can be problematic for some people. Many people react adversely to unripe fruit. Don't eat it—it's not good for you and doesn't taste good anyway. Sulfites, which are sometimes added to preserve the color of fruits and vegetables, can cause bronchial spasms in sensitive people.

To diagnose a food allergy, omit suspected foods for at least three weeks to allow allergic symptoms to diminish. Reintroduce a food every three to seven days and see if there is a reaction. Keep a food journal and rate your symptoms as mild, medium, or severe.

Read labels and be careful of the hidden factors. You might know you're allergic to eggs, so you never eat them, but what about that egg-laden salad dressing, mayonnaise in the sandwich, or egg added to a muffin mix? Manufacturers also often use equipment for multiple purposes, which can expose you to soy or peanuts, for example.

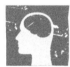

GOOD TO KNOW!

Gluten is used in food products to give elasticity to flour and is present in wheat, semolina, rye, oats, barley, spelt, and kamut. But the gliadin in gluten flattens out the mucosal lining of the intestines and makes it difficult to assimilate nutrients. Instead, use gluten-free grains such as amaranth, buckwheat, corn, millet, quinoa, rice, and teff. Soaking and sprouting grains and beans before cooking can help them be less likely to aggravate allergies and more digestible for anyone.

Breathing Easier with Asthma

Asthma is caused by muscle spasms that make bronchial tubes close and cut off the passage of air and blood supply to the lungs. The result—shortness of breath, coughing, wheezing, chest retraction, flaring nostrils, and rapid heartbeat. In fact, the word "asthma" is derived from the Greek word for panting. An asthma attack can last from a few hours to several days. And one asthma attack can lead to another as the cilia membrane is destroyed, thus lowering resistance. Here's what you can do to feel better.

HERBS THAT LET YOU BREATHE EASIER

A cup (235 ml) of black tea contains the alkaloid theophylline, which works as a mild bronchial dilator and can be helpful at the onset of an attack to open the air passages. Drink a cup of preferably organic black tea up to twice daily (but not in the evening, as it can interfere with sleep).

Lobelia tincture, which is considered an antispasmodic, can help stop the spasms associated with asthma when an attack is occurring. Five drops of lobelia tincture can be taken in a small amount of water up to four times daily during an attack.

℞ WHEN TO SEE YOUR M.D.

In some severe cases, food allergies can cause life-threatening anaphylaxis and even death as airways constrict and breathing is impaired. Immediate medical attention is necessary if this happens. Doctors can also perform skin and blood tests (such as the radioallergosorbent test [RAST] or the ELISA brand) to help you determine whether you have a food allergy.

Applying a ginger compress to the chest and back is also helpful during an asthma attack. Simply take a clean washcloth and dip it into a cup of hot ginger tea. (You can even use herbal tea bags.) Wring it out and apply it to your chest (and later back). Make sure the temperature is not hot enough to burn the skin. Cover with a dry cloth to help hold the heat in. Hot compresses should be left in place until the heat has dissipated. Replace with another compress as soon as removing the first one.

VITAMINS THAT LET YOU BREATHE EASIER

Take supplemental vitamin C (1000 mg) to boost immunity and 10,000 IU beta-carotene daily to help strengthen the mucus membranes of the lungs. This will make them less susceptible to irritation and can help promote rapid healing. A study in the *American Journal of Epidemiology* in 1998 showed that vitamin C improves pulmonary or lung function.

Magnesium helps to open constricted bronchial tubes by relaxing spastic muscles. Take 250 mg twice a day, on a regular basis.

BEST FOODS FOR ASTHMA

The foods you eat can trigger an asthma attack. To help figure out what the cause of your asthma is, try keeping a food journal to track food allergies. See if there is a pattern. Foods likely to contribute to asthma, as they are all common allergens, include dairy products, eggs, wheat, citrus, tomatoes, potatoes, and sulfite preservatives (which are often found in dried fruits, alcohol, and in some salad bars). The yellow food coloring tartrazine can also trigger an asthma attack, as can monosodium glutamate and aspirin (both common irritants). It may take a couple of days for an offending substance to have an affect. Be aware that even trace amounts of a food can be a culprit.

The most beneficial foods for the asthmatic include orange-colored, high beta-carotene lung strengthening and immune boosting foods that are rich in phytochemicals. These include winter squashes, pumpkins, papaya, apricots, and carrots. Include green, leafy vegetables for their oxygen and transporting of chlorophyll.

Make use too of manganese-rich foods such as buckwheat, cherries, beans, and nuts, as studies show that people with low intakes of manganese have an increased risk of bronchial reactivity. Try to eat at least a serving daily.

Pungent condiments known for their bronchodilating properties include garlic, onions, horseradish, ginger, mustard greens, radish, thyme, rosemary, and fennel. Use these condiments liberally in food preparations, such as when flavoring soups and salad dressings.

Lotus root is a traditional Asian medicine that strengthens the lungs and opens the airways. A few root slices can be simmered into a soup or made into a tea.

GOOD TO GROW!

It's easy to grow common herbs such as rosemary and thyme. Just get a big pot at least 2 feet (60 cm) deep and fill it with potting soil. Add plants that you get at your local greenhouse. (You can also grow from seed, it just takes longer.) Put the pot in a place that is exposed to 5 to 6 hours of sun a day. Water regularly.

Cures from Grandma's Kitchen

One of my favorite remedies for treating an asthma episode
(as well as other lung problems) is the following:

½ cup (170 g) raw honey (Note: Never give honey to children under 1 year of age.)
½ cup (120 ml) fresh lemon juice
1 inch (2.5 cm) of fresh ginger root
7 cloves of garlic
¼ teaspoon cayenne pepper

Put all of the ingredients in a blender and blend into a syrup. Pour into a glass jar and give
one teaspoonful as often as needed. Store the unused portion in the refrigerator. This
formula helps to thin mucus secretions, break up congestion, and dilate the bronchioles.

More Cures from Grandma's Kitchen

Steam inhalations can benefit conditions such as asthma, by helping to warm,
increase circulation, and loosen mucus from the respiratory tract.
Try the following when respiration is compromised.

First, boil a quart of water and add 4 heaping teaspoons (25 g) of herbs such as eucalyptus,
pine (break up the needles to better release their properties), and wintergreen,
or add 5 to 10 drops of pure essential oil. One to two tablespoons fresh garden herbs
such as oregano, thyme, or peppermint can also be used for an herbal steam after being
added to a pint of boiling water.

Remove the pot from the stove to a padded kitchen counter. Drape a towel over your head
and the pot, lean over, and breathe in the steam for seven minutes or so. If the steam starts
to cool too much, gently blow into the herb pot to cause more steam to rise.
This can be done up to three times daily.

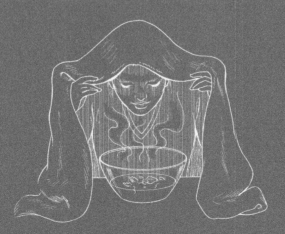

TRICKS TO BREATHE EASIER

Try exhaling forcefully through a drinking straw placed in a large bottle of water to expand the bronchial tubes. It is a good idea to practice deeper breathing all the time, not just when you are sick.

Practice yoga breathing. I have seen this empower people to have control over their breathing rather than have their breathing control them. Learn to do it when not in the throes of an attack so that you'll know how when needed.

One simple method is to practice a deep relaxation breath: Lie on the floor with a pillow supporting your knees. Place your palms over your abdomen, with your fingers gently laced just above your naval. Breathe in to a count of three as your abdomen pushes your fingers toward the ceiling. Exhale to a count of five as your fingers and abdomen move toward the floor. With every third breath, blow out through your mouth as you suck your belly inward.

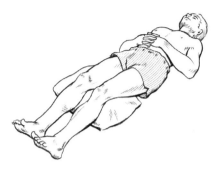

According to color therapists, putting the gemstone citrine under your tongue at the first sign of an asthma attack may bring relief. Visit a gem shop to find this golden stone. You can also visualize breathing in its healing golden ray. Wearing orange clothing or having an orange light in the room may also be beneficial.

Breathing Easier with Bronchitis

Bronchitis occurs when mucous membranes of the bronchial tubes become inflamed and mucous blocks the lungs' airflow. Infection as well as external irritants such as sulfur dioxide, smoke, and airborne pollutants can cause bronchitis. A cold or flu can develop into bronchitis too. Here's how to breathe easier.

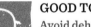

GOOD TO KNOW!
Avoid dehydration and help keep the mucus secretions thin by consuming plenty of fluids. Both lemon in water and cranberry juice will help to thin mucous secretions. Just add the juice of 1/2 lemon once or twice a day to a glass of water. Cranberry juice can be diluted with water as part of your daily beverage intake (about 1/4 cup [60 ml] juice to 1 cup [235 ml] of water).

GOOD TO GROW!
The culinary herb thyme is antiseptic and bronchodilating. Grow it in your flower box and then use it as a condiment to flavor soups and dressings.

HERBS THAT HELP BRONCHITIS

Herbs such as anise, fennel seed, licorice root, marshmallow root, pleurisy root, slippery elm bark, and wild cherry bark relax bronchial spasms by soothing inflammation. Natural food stores carry teas, capsules, syrups, and tinctures that include these botanicals. They can be taken every 2 or 3 hours during respiratory distress.

Fenugreek, ginger, hyssop, juniper berries, osha root, and thyme break up mucus congestion, curb infection, and expectorate mucous so you can breathe better and cough less. They are also available in tea, capsule, syrup, and tincture form. A dose can be taken every 2 or 3 hours during respiratory distress.

BEST FOODS FOR BRONCHITIS

When you have bronchitis, include three to five servings of these foods daily:

- Garlic and onions, which help break up congestion and open the airways
- Salmon, which contains anti-inflammatory oils
- Chlorophyll-rich green leafy vegetables, which help the body better utilize oxygen
- Yellow and orange vegetables high in beta-carotene including potatoes, winter squash, apricots, and persimmons, which help the lungs resist infection

℞ **WHEN TO SEE YOUR M.D.**
If home remedies are not helping, seek medical attention, especially if symptoms worsen and you feel there is nothing else you can do at home. If this is a first attack or you are coughing up yellow, brown, or bloody phlegm, seek proper medical attention immediately.

Soothing Sinusitis

When your sinuses are blocked, fluids collect in the head, causing pain, pressure, and misery. Symptoms of a sinus infection include headache, snoring, cough, earache, greenish/yellow discharge exuding from the nose, pressure, fever, facial pain, and sensitivities in the teeth to sugar and temperature changes. Sinusitis or sinus infections often begin after a bad cold and are often worse in the morning, before mucous has a chance to drain. Other factors that contribute to sinus problems include overexposure to dust, pollen, and airborne chemicals, candida, stress, and poor dental hygiene. Here's how to ease that pressure and congestion.

NATURAL REMEDIES THAT SOOTHE SINUSITIS

Irrigate your nasal passages with $1/4$ teaspoon sea salt with $1/4$ teaspoon baking soda and 1 cup (235 ml) warm water. Stir and pour into a neti pot, spray bottle, or ear syringe. Wash out each nostril one at a time over the sink with the opposite nostril down. When clearing sinuses, it's a good idea to blow one nostril at a time (by covering the other sinus with a finger and tissue) to avoid causing pressure and bacteria buildup in the ears.

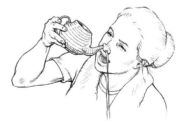

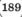

Next, apply a thin film of almond oil or sesame oil into the nose to help protect it from further viruses. If the nasal passages get too raw, apply a small amount of vitamin E oil or a salve made from soothing herbs like comfrey or calendula.

Herbs that help relieve sinusitis include echinacea, (stimulates immunity), eyebright (decreases congestion), and fenugreek (decreases mucus). The Chinese patent formula Bi Yan Pian is also helpful to many people with a sinus infection. Herbal doses are usually taken three times daily.

Essential oils that help relieve sinus congestion include camphor, eucalyptus, lavender, pine, peppermint, and rosemary. Olbas inhalers are available at many health food stores and help clear nasal congestion for up to a couple of hours.

BEST FOODS FOR SINUSITIS

Re-evaluating your diet is a good place to start in improving sinus problems. It may be helpful to decrease consumption of dairy, wheat, eggs, and sugar. Citrus, corn, and peanuts can also be potential allergens causing excessive phlegm. Try eating more foods that are pungent

Skip This!

Cut out gluten and dairy products for a while and you might find that phlegm production decreases.

GOOD TO GROW!
A few nasturtium leaves and flowers from your garden added to salads also help to open the respiratory passages.

GOOD TO KNOW!
You have eight sinuses, four pairs of air-filled hollow spaces lined with mucous membranes located on both sides of the forehead, between the nasal cavities and eye sockets, and in the maxillary cheekbones. All of the sinus openings, which are thinner than a pencil lead, drain into the nasal passages. Our sinuses help to equalize pressure and also warm, purify, and moisten the air we breathe. The sinuses also give the voice resonance.

Cures from Grandma's Kitchen

When sinuses feel especially painful and congested, a ginger compress can be very helpful. First make a tea of fresh chopped ginger root, simmered for 20 minutes. Soak a couple of washcloths in the comfortably hot tea, wring, and apply gently over the afflicted sinus areas. Reapply three or four times daily as needed.

and opening to the respiratory tract such as cayenne, garlic, ginger, horseradish, and onions. (Don't overdo it though, as too much may cause irritation.) Adding some chopped lotus root to soups helps to dissolve mucous. The juice of half a lemon in water helps to thin mucous secretions. Carrots and carrot juice, turnips, winter squash, and dark green leafy vegetables are all rich in beta-carotene and strengthen mucous membranes. Drink plenty of water.

Food allergies, especially to dairy and gluten products, can be a possible cause of sinus problems. Often the food sensitivity comes first, then the germs find a haven in the excess mucous. The mucous can sometimes be acidic in nature, causing more irritation. It can take up to three weeks to see the results of eliminating a particular food.

KEEP IN MIND

Exercise like brisk walking in pure air or gentle aerobics or stretching can help improve circulation in your sinuses. Massaging sore sinuses increases circulation, which helps move stagnation. You can also massage the base of the threesmallest toes, which corresponds to the sinus area.

It is possible to confuse a sinus infection with a toothache. To find out which is which, jump up and down, landing on your heels. A sinus infection will be felt in the sinus region above the teeth or both sides of the upper jaw. A toothache will be felt in the tooth.

CHAPTER 11

NATURAL REMEDIES FOR CIRCULATION AND BLOOD DISORDERS

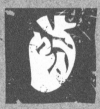

Blood moves through the body, delivering oxygen, nutrients, and immune-supportive chemicals, and it also carries away wastes. Here you'll learn how to ensure that blood is healthy and flows with ease.

Building the Blood for Anemia

Are you feeling tired? You may be anemic. You'll become anemic if you don't get enough iron. Anemia can also be caused by a lack of folic acid or vitamin B12, blood loss (from menses, peptic ulcers, hemorrhoids, or blood donation), red blood cell destruction, or deficient red blood cell production. Addressing anemia will help you to regain your strength and vitality. Here's what to do.

HERBS THAT STRENGTHEN THE BLOOD

Many herbal teas are rich in iron and can help build the blood. These include teas made from alfalfa leaves, burdock root, dandelion leaves, nettles, red raspberry leaf, and watercress. Drink any of these herbs individually or in a combination up to three times daily.

Yellow dock helps improve iron assimilation and has been found to free up iron stores in the liver. It can be used in tea, tincture, or capsule form up to three times daily.

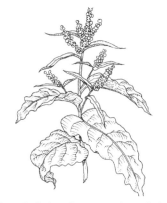

Chlorophyll, found in green plants, helps the body utilize oxygen better. Chlorophyll can also be taken in liquid or tablet form as directed on the bottle.

GOOD TO KNOW!
Though only a blood test known as a hematocrit can determine whether you have anemia for certain, pale fingernails and tongue and lack of color inside the lower eyelid may also be indicators.

VITAMINS THAT BUILD BLOOD

Vitamin B12 deficiency is common in anemics. Dairy products and red meat are important sources of B12. Some fermented foods, such as miso, tamari, and tempeh, also have very trace amounts. Other vegetarian sources of B12 are fortified nutritional yeast, seaweeds, and sunflower seeds. Try to eat a few grams a day of a selection of these foods. You can also supplement with 1,000 mcg of B12 daily.

Note that you can supplement with iron, but it can be constipating and toxic. Ferrous sulfate is often recommended by physicians, but only 10 to 30 percent of it is assimilated. Instead take ferrous fumarate or gluconate, which is less likely to cause digestive problems like constipation.

Taking 500 mg of vitamin C with each meal will help improve the assimilation of iron.

Two products I have long used to improve anemia are Floradix, which is an herbal iron tonic, and Mega Foods Blood Builder, which contains iron, vitamin C, and B12 in appropriate doses as one tablet. Both are available at health food stores.

BEST FOODS FOR ANEMIA

Foods that are high in iron can build the blood and correct anemia. These include almonds, amaranth, apricots, beans, bee pollen, beets, blackberries, blackstrap molasses, burdock root, cherries, eggs, figs, dark green leafy vegetables, liver (organic, please!), mugwort-mochi, prunes, raisins, red meat, and seaweeds.

Lowering Cholesterol

Cholesterol is a white, waxy, crystalline substance that can be good or bad. High LDL (low-density lipoproteins) or "bad" cholesterol can be caused by a diet high in processed fat and sugar or by heredity. HDL (high-density lipoprotein) or "good" cholesterol protects the body by moving LDL cholesterol away from the artery walls and back to the liver where it gets excreted with bile to the intestines. If you have too much "bad" cholesterol, don't despair. Even those with blocked arteries can turn back the progression of the disease. Here's how.

SUPPLEMENTS THAT LOWER LDL

Hawthorn berry can help lower cholesterol by gradually breaking down fat deposits in the body. Clinical trials in Europe have proven that it is safe and effective in helping to treat early congestive heart failure, mild angina, arrhythmia, and hypertension. It also helps you recover from a heart attack. Talk to your doctor about whether hawthorn berry may be right for you. If so, take a dose either in tea, tincture, or capsule form three times daily.

Skip This!
Coffee, black tea, and excess bran can inhibit iron absorption due to their diuretic and laxative effects.

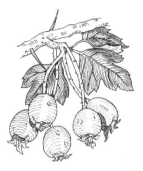

The commonly available Ayurvedic formula Triphala can reduce cholesterol levels and arterial plaque by improving digestion and fat metabolism. Tablets are available at natural food stores and 1 or 2 can be taken as directed on the bottle.

Essential fatty acids can also lower cholesterol, reduce blood pressure, and lower the risk of thrombosis (clot formation). Omege-3 oils taken as a supplement contains eicosapentaenoic acid (EPA), which helps keep the blood from clumping together. Researchers at the Agency for Healthcare Research and Quality recently showed that the omega-3 fatty acids found in fish and fish oil reduce the risk of heart attack. Look for good-quality fish oil free of heavy metal contamination. Good brands include Nordic Naturals and Garden of Life. Take 1 teaspoon (5 ml) daily or aim for three servings a week of salmon, tuna, mackerel, sardines, herring, or blue fish.

Niacin, also known as vitamin B3, increases cardiac output, dilates the blood vessels, and decreases resistance in the circulatory system. Niacin works in the liver to lower "bad" cholesterol. *The Journal of the American Medical Association* in 1986 recommended it as the first supplement to be used after diet to lower cholesterol. However, even though niacin is helpful, it can cause discomfort for about 10 minutes, including itching, flushing, and gastro-intestinal discomfort. A newer sustained release formula prevents this. Excessive use of niacin has the potential to irritate the liver. Talk to your health professional about taking 50 mg three times daily.

Coenzyme Q10 naturally occurs in the heart muscle and has been used to lower high blood pressure and to treat heart failure. It also increases the amount of oxygen received by the heart tissue. Taking statin prescription drugs to lower cholesterol can deplete the body of CoQ10. If you are taking statins, take from 50 to 200 mg daily of CoQ10.

 GOOD TO KNOW!
A normal cholesterol level is around 150 mg/dl or less, and ideally your cholesterol level should be 180 mg/dl or less, with more of the HDL than the LDL. New recommendations by the National Heart, Lung, and Blood Institute say that a desirable level for LDL is 130 mg/dl. HDL is considered at risk if levels are below 35 mg/dl.

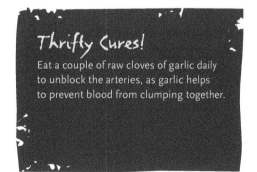

Thrifty Cures!
Eat a couple of raw cloves of garlic daily to unblock the arteries, as garlic helps to prevent blood from clumping together.

FOODS THAT LOWER CHOLESTEROL

Water-soluble fiber such as oat bran and oatmeal lowers cholesterol levels by binding to "bad" cholesterol in the body, according to many studies. Barley, carrots, apple pectin, chia seeds, blueberries, guar gum, and psyllium may also help lower cholesterol by binding with bile acids in the digestive system, which are then eliminated through the bowel.

Other foods than can help lower cholesterol include apples, artichokes, broccoli, cabbage, chili peppers, citrus fruits, dandelion greens, garlic, grapefruit, green leafy vegetables, lemon, lime, melons, onions, rutabaga, seaweed, soybeans, spinach, sweet potato, and turnip. These foods work by improving liver function so the liver can more easily breakdown fatty deposits or because they are high in a fiber called pectin, which binds with cholesterol and carries it out of the body via the bowels.

KEEP IN MIND

To elevate HDL (good) cholesterol, eat lots of onions and garlic and take a daily B vitamin complex. Regular exercise such as walking, dancing, and aerobics elevates the beneficial HDL and lowers LDL.

Improving Poor Circulation

Poor circulation can occur when there is an insufficient supply of blood flowing through the veins and arteries. Stress can cause blood vessels to dilate and contract and can short-circuit circulation. Food allergies can also contribute to frequent cold hands and feet. Here's how to get things moving.

Niacin supplements (50 to 100 mg daily) can be taken for brief periods during extremely cold weather to inhibit spasms of the small arteries.

Culinary herbs that promote circulation include black pepper, cayenne, cinnamon, cloves, garlic, ginger, horseradish, and paprika. This is due to their warming essential oil content, which promotes the movement of chi (energy) in the body. Simply use more of these foods in your cuisine to obtain their benefits.

Ginkgo improves circulation to the body's extremities by preventing the blood from clumping together. Use one capsule 2 or 3 times daily.

Avoid cold by dressing in layers, wearing a hat, and choosing mittens rather than gloves. Wear red or orange long johns, undershirt, and socks as these colors psychologically make us feel warmer. Breathe more deeply to allow energy to move more readily throughout the body. Protect your extremities with quality lotions.

GOOD TO KNOW!
Extreme cold hand syndrome is known as Raynaud's disease. It can cause extremities to turn white, then blue or red. The nose and earlobes may also be affected. Pain and numbness can occur with the white and blue stages and a burning sensation with the red stage. Episodes may last for as long as three minutes and up to an hour. See your doctor if this occurs.

Lowering High Blood Pressure

High blood pressure, or hypertension, is more a symptom than it is a disease. Hypertension can make one a more likely candidate for heart attack, stroke, kidney damage, and vision problems. Symptoms of hypertension include breathing difficulties, dizziness, fatigue, headaches, heart palpitations, intestinal problems, nosebleeds, and numbness and tingling in the extremities. Here's how to lower your blood pressure now.

VITAMINS THAT LOWER BLOOD PRESSURE

Vitamin B6 (50 mg daily) can help lower blood pressure through its diuretic effect. Calcium (1,000 mg) and magnesium (500 mg) both daily have a calming effect on the nerves and arteries and a strengthening effect on the heart muscle.

 GOOD TO KNOW!

High blood pressure is diagnosed with a device called a sphygmomanometer. Two numbers are given in a reading. The first number in a blood pressure reading is systolic—the amount of pressure inside the arteries during the pumping phase. The second number is diastolic—the amount of pressure during the resting phase. A normal reading is $120/70$. Higher than 140 systolic or 90 diastolic are high blood pressure indicators. Readings done at home are often lower than readings taken in a doctor's office. People can elevate their blood pressure simply by worrying about it!

Often people who have hypertension don't have enough Coenzyme Q10 (CoQ10). This antioxidant is especially important to the heart muscle. Research published in the *European Heart Journal* in 2006 showed that CoQ10 improves functioning in people who have advanced chronic heart failure. Take 100 to 300 mg each day.

BEST FOODS TO LOWER BLOOD PRESSURE

Cold-water fish such as bluefish, mackerel, and salmon have blood pressure-lowering properties. Garlic taken as a supplement can expand blood vessel walls and inhibit the blood from clumping together.

Foods that are rich in hypotensive compounds include broccoli, carrots, celery, fava beans, garlic, green leafy vegetables, kiwi, and onions. Hawthorn berries, leaf, and flower can all be used to help normalize high blood pressure, strengthen the heart, and break down cholesterol.

Even chocolate can help lower your blood pressure thanks to the flavonoids it contains, which are antioxidants. A study in the *Journal of Nutrition and Metabolism* in 2006 showed that cocoa and chocolate lower blood pressure. Eat 1 to 2 ounces (28 to 55 g) of dark chocolate, at least 70 percent cacao, each day.

ESSENTIAL OILS FOR BETTER BLOOD PRESSURE

Essential oils that promote a strong and healthy vascular system and can calm blood pressure include basil, bergamot, citronella (increases heartbeat), geranium, jasmine, lavender, neroli, orange, rose, and rosemary. Use them as inhalations, in the bath, or with massage. (For ideas on using essential oils, see the section on "Aromatherapy" on page 23.)

HEALTHY BLOOD PRESSURE PRACTICES

For a healthy heart system, keep blood pressure levels normal, reduce cholesterol, lose weight if necessary, don't smoke, and exercise more. Get aerobic exercise at least three times a week for 15 to 30 minutes. Dancing, cycling, jogging, swimming, jump roping, and rowing are all considered aerobic heart-healthy exercises.

Yoga, stretching, brisk walking, deep breathing, meditation, and verbalizing one's feelings are all beneficial for a healthy heart. Some find watching fish in a fish tank lowers blood pressure.

Music that has 60 beats per minute, such as Baroque music, can lower high blood pressure and reduce anxiety. Also consider playing the soothing sounds of the ocean. Slow down your speech to help lower blood pressure and take in more oxygen. Interestingly, your blood pressure elevates when you are talking and decreases when you are listening.

Meditation can lower blood pressure as effectively as drug therapy. Biofeedback training can help people achieve a state of calmness.

At the end of your day, take a short tepid bath, between 92 and 98°F (33 to 37°C) for 10 to 30 minutes to gently dilate blood vessels and lower blood pressure. When sleeping, use only a small pillow so your head is not too high above your heart, making it easy to get blood to the brain. Body alignment is important day and night.

Use visualization. Picture your heart beating regularly, pumping a healthy amount of blood with each beat. See your arteries gently dilating, allowing the blood to flow, and imagine your blood vessels growing and supplying oxygen and needed nutrients to your heart.

Happiness also helps lower blood pressure, so open your heart to love.

Skip This!

Caffeine elevates blood pressure and strains the heart. High sodium intake retains fluids in the body so that blood volume will be higher, thus raising blood pressure. Most people with hypertension have too much sodium retention and not enough potassium. Losing weight can help reduce high blood pressure. Cut back on refined carbohydrates, including sugar, which can cause elevated levels of insulin.

 WHEN TO SEE YOUR M.D.
If you have cardiovascular health concerns, consult with a health practitioner to help you lower your medication as you improve your health with diet, herbs, supplements, and other natural methods. But never stop taking heart medicine suddenly.

GOOD TO KNOW!
Good supplements for gout include a vitamin B complex 50 mg), vitamin C (1,000 mg), and vitamin E (400 IU) once daily. Tablets made from alfalfa leaf (12 daily) are also helpful. A multienzyme tablet can also be helpful in reducing inflammation. Take it three times daily between meals so it can help reduce inflammation rather than focus on food digestion.

Reducing Gout Inflammation

Gout, a type of arthritis, used to be considered the disease of royalty and the upper classes because of their consumption of meat and wine, which makes people more susceptible. Gout is most common in men. It happens when high levels of uric acid that are not properly broken down by the kidneys result in sodium urate crystals that cause joint inflammation in the toes, ankles, insteps, heels, knees, and wrists. Elevate the joints during periods of inflammation to reduce swelling. Here are some natural remedies that will make you feel better.

Eating cherries is especially helpful in treating gout. That's because they contain nutrients called anthocyanins, which reduce inflammation and relieve gout pain. Research at the University of California-Davis showed that eating just one serving of fresh cherries a day reduced uric acid by up to 15 percent in women. You can also benefit from dried cherries and cherry juice.

Apples, burdock root, celery juice, blueberries, green leafy vegetables, and strawberries are also beneficial. All of these foods help break down excess uric acid.

Turmeric root in capsule form is also excellent for reducing inflammation. Two capsules can be taken 2 or 3 times daily. Bromelain, the enzyme found in pineapple, also reduces swelling in gout. Take 500 mg three times daily.

Skip This!

A diet low in animal foods can greatly help gout. That's because meat is high in uric acid and its consumption increases uric acid in the body. Alcohol can also inhibit the body's ability to secrete uric acid through the kidneys, so avoid it if you are prone to gout as well. Avoid excess beans, which also become purines, natural substances found in all of the body's cells and foods. However, purines are excessively high in anchovies, brains, kidneys, game meats, herring, liver, mackerel, meat, mussels, sardines, scallops and sweetbreads, and purines can increase uric acid levels. Cut down on fats, dairy products, restrict alcohol, and drink plenty of fluids. A yeast free diet may help as well. Visit www.yeastconnection.com for more information.

Cures from Grandma's Kitchen

During a gout attack, soak the afflicted area in warm water to which 5 drops of essential oil of celery has been added. Essential oil of celery helps decrease uric acid buildup and reduces inflammation. You can also soak your feet in warm celery seed tea.

CHAPTER 12

NATURAL REMEDIES to BOOST URINARY TRACT HEALTH

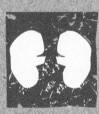

The urinary system controls what remains in the body and what is eliminated as urine. This delicate system requires the right amount of nutrients for optimal functioning. Here you'll learn which herbs, vitamins, minerals, and other natural cures can help.

Curing Incontinence

Incontinence (also called enuresis) refers to a lack of bladder control. Weak kidneys are often the source. Food allergies (often dairy), overconsumption of diuretic foods such as citrus products and coffee, and certain prescriptions can also be factors. Use these tips to bring this problem under control.

Teas that help incontinence include soothing buchu, chamomile, corn silk, and plantain leaf. Drinking cranberry juice can be helpful as it tonifies the bladder with its high flavonoid content. Two teaspoons each of apple cider vinegar (10 ml) and raw honey (13 g) stirred into a cup (235 ml) of hot water three times daily will work as a urinary tract antiseptic and curb the urge to go.

Kegel exercises will also help improve muscle tone in the area.

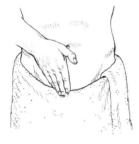

Remember, kidneys need warmth, nourishment, and preservation to continue their constant job of cleansing and balancing. Time alone, quiet, good sleep, the sound of nature and running water, and peaceful music all benefit the kidneys.

Curtailing Urinary Tract Infections

If you feel like you have to urinate all the time, and when you do, it burns, you may have a bladder infection. Actually, urinary tract infections can affect the urethra (urethritis), bladder (cystitis), or kidneys (nephritis). Usually Escherichia coli is present. Here are some ways to soothe the irritation.

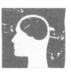

GOOD TO KNOW!
Some find that urinating, then standing up, then urinating again helps them more fully empty their bladder. Empty the bladder more completely by pressing on it (just above the pubic bone) while bending forward at the waist or leaning slightly forward when urinating. During the day, try to establish a routine for urinating, such as every three hours. If you feel the urge to go after having just urinated, relax your bladder. However, if you really do need to go, heed nature's call.

NATURAL REMEDIES THAT EASE BLADDER INFECTIONS

Vitamin C helps prevent bacterial infection by directly fighting infection and boosting immunity. Take 1,000 to 3,000 mg daily.

Vitamin E can help prevent scarring of bladder tissues due to its hydrating effect. Take 400 IU daily.

Another time-tested cure if you feel a bladder infection is coming on is to drink a glass of water to which you add 1 teaspoon (15 g) of baking soda. This helps alkalinize the urine. Repeat only once every 8 hours and only when needed for short periods as it can cause bowel problems and overexcite the nervous system. You can also drink 1 teaspoon (5 ml) apple cider vinegar in a glass of warm water to help acidify the urine and inhibit bacterial growth.

Essential oils that are good to use in a diluted base for massage over the bladder include eucalyptus, lavender, lemon, and juniper. Add 25 drops total of essential oil in $^1/_2$ cup (120 ml) extra virgin olive oil and apply a few teaspoonfuls over the area. The antiseptic properties of the essential oils will be absorbed through the skin. You can also add a few drops of these oils to a bath.

WHEN TO SEE YOUR M.D.

If you are plagued with repeated infections, see a health professional to make sure you do not have a sexually transmitted disease or another disorder. It's also important to see your doctor if you have back pain, fever, and chills because the infection may have spread to the kidneys.

BEST FOODS AND BEVERAGES FOR BLADDER INFECTIONS

When dealing with bladder infections, eat cooling anti-inflammatory foods such as asparagus, barley, carrots, celery, cucumbers, grapes, lotus root, millet, mung beans, parsley, pomegranates, red beans, squash, string beans, strawberries, vegetable juices, water chestnuts, and watermelon. Blueberries, cranberries, and prunes all help to prevent bacteria from adhering to the walls of the urinary tract.

Drinking cranberry juice helps to ease common bladder infections because it inhibits the adhesion of bacteria to the urinary tract so that the infection can't proliferate. Drinking 8 ounces (235 ml) of this juice as needed works better than 4 ounces (118 ml), according to research presented at the 42nd Annual Meeting of the Infectious Diseases Society of America in 2004.

Skip This!

Avoid excessively spicy food, alcohol, and carbonated beverages, which can irritate the bladder if you are struggling with incontinence. Also, citrus juice is very diuretic, and coffee can be irritating to the bladder and contribute to leakage. Constipation can put pressure on the bladder, so see the section on constipation if that seems to be part of the problem.

A shot glass of aloe vera juice three times daily between meals also cools bladder inflammation and deters infection.

Drink eight tall glasses of pure water a day to flush out bacteria in the urinary tract.

KEEP IN MIND

If you can, wear only natural fiber underwear. It is important that the body can breathe, and synthetic fibers cause a sweaty, moist environment where bacteria love to thrive.

Tampons can obstruct the neck of the bladder, so women may want to use smaller tampons, change them more frequently, or better yet, use external protection during their menses.

Skip This!

Avoid fried foods, heavily spiced foods, alcohol, artificial sweeteners, fruit juices (except cranberry), coffee, sodas, and tomatoes, all of which can irritate the ladder.

Eliminating Kidney Stones

Having a kidney stone has been compared to giving birth. Yes, it's that painful. Kidney stones are a common problem affecting people in their 30s to 50s. Men are more likely to get them than women. Stones form when mineral salts from the urine clump together and grow. Stones not only can form in the kidneys but other parts of the urinary tract as well. The stones are usually composed of phosphates, calcium, oxalates, struvites, and uric acid. They often go unnoticed until a stone becomes trapped in the urinary tract, causing excruciating sharp pain that may cause a person to double over. Chills, fever, blood in the urine, decreased urination, and vomiting may also accompany the blockage. Here's how to get rid of this common, yet very painful, complaint.

 GOOD TO KNOW!
It is important to urinate completely to prevent residual bacteria from being trapped. Try to urinate at three-hour intervals. Be sure to wipe yourself front to back using undyed and unscented toilet paper. Also urinate before having intercourse and right afterwards, even if it means having to drink a large glass of water. Then you can go back and snuggle!

NATURAL REMEDIES FOR BEING STONE FREE

People with kidney stones are often deficient in magnesium. A supplement of magnesium (500 mg daily) with 50 mg of B6 (which helps make the magnesium more effective) will help to bind with oxalates and prevent the precipitation of calcium oxalate and calcium phosphate. If you take calcium as a supplement with meals, it will minimize the likeliness of stone formation. Planetary Herbals makes an excellent formula called Stone Free.

GOOD TO KNOW!
Apply a castor oil compress to the kidneys to help ease the passage of kidney stones.

Using some of the following herbs can also help to be beneficial:

HERB	BENEFITS
Buchu	Soothes and strengthens the urinary system
Cleavers	Clears heat and reduces inflammation
Corn silk	Regenerates and soothes irritated tissue; eases passage of stones
Couch grass	Soothes renal tissue due to high mucilage content; eases passage of stones
Goldenrod	Cleanses kidneys; helps dissolve stones
Gravel root	Aids removal of uric acid and breakup of small stones in bladder and kidneys
Marshmallow root	Eases passage of stones
Parsley root	Eases kidney inflammation and stones
Uva-ursi	Diuretic and antiseptic; helps eliminate kidney stones

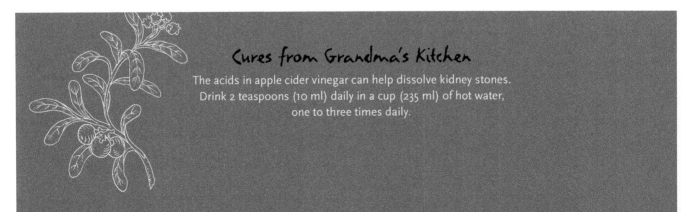

Cures from Grandma's Kitchen
The acids in apple cider vinegar can help dissolve kidney stones. Drink 2 teaspoons (10 ml) daily in a cup (235 ml) of hot water, one to three times daily.

BEST FOODS AND BEVERAGES
FOR KIDNEY STONES

Consuming beta-carotene–rich foods such as apricots, broccoli, carrots, winter squash, and sweet potatoes all benefit the urinary lining. Drinking diluted carrot juice also help.

Asparagus contains a substance called asparagin, which helps the body eliminate excess uric acid.

Kale, lettuce, and parsley provide vitamin K, which helps urinary glycoprotein to prevent the growth of calcium oxalate crystals.

Foods with a favorable magnesium/calcium ratio such as avocado, banana, barley, buckwheat, lima beans, oats, and rye can also be consumed.

Drink plenty of fluids, especially non-carbonated pure (you don't need the phosphates) water. This will help to prevent buildup of components that cause stone formation. Cranberry juice, without sweeteners, can be diluted and added to pure water to reduce the amounts of ionized calcium in the urine. Cranberry inhibits the adhesion of bacteria to the urinary tract, perhaps due to a polymer in the plant, thus allowing bacteria to be eliminated.

Thrifty Cures!

Add 1 cup (235 ml) of apple cider vinegar to the bath one to two times daily to inhibit infection. A sitz bath of baking soda (1 whole box) can also be helpful in reducing microbes. Simply add the baking soda to the bath and soak for about 20 minutes. Make sure the bathtub is very clean.

Skip This!

If you eat a lot of refined carbohydrates, low-fiber, high-fat, high-salt foods, and consume a lot of alcohol, this can cause mineral imbalances in the body and lead to a kidney stone. It's also a good idea to avoid foods with a high oxalic acid content such as beans, beets greens, black tea, chocolate, nuts, rhubarb, spinach, strawberries, and Swiss chard, as oxalic acid can contribute to stone formation. Also eat lower amounts of meat and dairy products, which can elevate levels of uric acid. Cut down on salt and alcohol. Foods that are fortified with vitamin D can cause excessive retention of calcium in the urine. Limit intake to about 400 IU daily. Also limit intake of antacids and aspirin, which can be a factor in stone formation due to their content of calcium carbonates and silicates.

CHAPTER 13

NATURAL REMEDIES THAT ENCOURAGE EMOTIONAL HEALTH AND WELLNESS

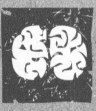

According to Asian medicine, emotional health can contribute to physical problems, and physical problems can contribute to emotional imbalances. When you take a whole body approach, it's important to deal with both aspects. Here's how.

Diffusing Anger

Anger often occurs when we resist change, when someone disappoints us, or when our expectations are unmet. In Asian medicine, anger is characterized as Liver Fire Rising. Anger stimulates a contraction of chi (energy) that causes stress to the liver. Anger can cause shallow inhalation and strong panting exhalation, dizziness, contribute to high blood pressure, elevated cholesterol levels, tight shoulders, stiff upper back, jaw tightness, eye problems, increased hydrochloric acid production, and ulcers. But what is more dangerous than the experience of anger is the repression of it. Pent up angry feelings can be a factor in hemorrhoids, migraine headaches, cancer, rheumatoid arthritis, and heart disease. Here's how to calm down now by safely defusing anger.

CALMING SUPPLEMENTS
According to traditional folklore, herbs that help cool the liver and thus soothe anger include blessed thistle, dandelion root, licorice root, oat straw, and skullcap. Take them as a tea two to three times a day.

Along with behavior counseling, the amino acid 5-HTP (5-hydroxtryptophan) can help curb anger and violence by elevating serotonin levels. Take 50 mg twice daily.

A good daily supplement of calcium (1,000 mg) and magnesium (500 mg) helps to quell an angry countenance by nourishing the nerves and relaxing the muscles.

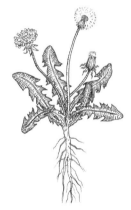

Cures from Grandma's Kitchen

What you eat can change how you feel. So try eating yogurt, which is high in calming calcium, green, leafy vegetables provide nerve-nourishing magnesium. Lettuce also helps to calm anxiety, being high in the calming alkaloid lactucin. Include whole grains such as buckwheat, millet, quinoa, and wild rice and veggies such as sweet potatoes and winter squash. These will help keep your blood sugar on an even keel. Avoid stimulants like caffeine, sugar, and fruit juice that rev you up and put your body into panic-alert.

CALMING FOODS

Foods that benefit the liver and thus mellow the emotion of anger include artichokes, barley, berries, daikon radish, dandelion greens, green leafy vegetables, lentils, mung beans, rye, and sour green apples. Dandelion root tea helps to cleanse emotions of anger stored in the liver, according to traditional folklore.

CALMING ESSENTIAL OILS AND FLOWER ESSENCES

Essential oils that can be used to diffuse anger include basil, cardamom, chamomile, coriander, frankincense, geranium, hyssop, jasmine, lavender, lemon balm, lotus, marjoram, neroli, pine, rose, and ylang-ylang. Essential oils can be used as inhalations, in the bath, or diluted and used in massage. (For guidelines, see the section "Aromatherapy Preparations" on page 23.)

Flower essences are made by soaking flowers in spring water. Though subtle, they can be effective in helping to balance the emotional body. To learn more about flower essences, read any of the books about Bach Flower Remedies. Placing four drops of the following flower essences on or under your tongue or in a glass of water is also recommended:

- Cherry plum: For those prone to temper tantrums
- Heather: For those easily irritated
- Holly: For jealousy and sibling rivalry
- Impatience: To help you be more patient
- Walnut: For those going through big life changes

SOOTHING PRACTICES THAT DIFFUSE ANGER

In a journal, make a list of what aspects of the anger you are accountable for. Focus on what you can do about it. Avoid blaming.

It has been said that "art is toxic discharge." So get out there and paint, write, create music, or find some way to express yourself and contribute to your own therapy.

Some people say that anger makes them "see red." Try counting to 10 while you visualize the color blue. There may be some occasions where counting to 100 is what is takes.

Learn what triggers your anger and try to avoid those situations. Consider writing up a disaster scale and rating the things that make you angry from one to ten. You may find that some of them are not as important. Consider humor a more valuable ally than profanity.

In dealing with anger, it helps to affirm that you are angry. Be clear about what it is that is really bothering you. Take a breather and then discuss the conflict. Without attacking, let your feelings be known. Avoid statements like "you always" or "you never." Listen to what the other person has to say and do your best to understand. If you need to, give yourself a "cooling off" period first. Finally, be willing to forgive!

Skip This!

Excess garlic and onions can aggravate the emotion of anger. Coffee and sugar can also make one more likely to fly off the handle. Be aware that allergens such as gluten, corn, and soy may cause inflammation, a sense of unease, and anger in some people.

Taking the Edge Off Anxiety

Anxiety is fear, plain and simple. It can happen when we are stressed or afraid and the "flight or fight" mechanism is triggered. It can occur when we are out of harmony within ourselves and with the people and things around us. Anxiety can cause shortness of breath, heart palpitations, chest tightness, trembling, sweating, dizziness, numbness, shaking, and muscular tension. If you have panic attacks, you may feel as if you're dying or going crazy. Though panic attacks rarely last longer than 10 minutes, they can be very disabling. Here's how to calm down now.

HERBS THAT EASE ANXIETY

Choose nervine mineral-rich herbal teas such as California poppy, catnip, chamomile, hops, lemon balm, oat straw, and passionflower. Drink 3 cups (705 ml) daily.

Hops and valerian tincture are not so lovely to taste but have strong sedative properties to calm anxiety and relax tight muscles. Put 4 drops in water and sip.

Kava kava extract was recently approved in Germany for its anti-anxiety effects. A study in the German medical journal, *Arzneimittel Forschung* in 1991 showed that this herb significantly reduced anxiety levels. Take 100 mg 3 times daily.

VITAMINS THAT EASE ANXIETY

Taking calcium (1,000 mg daily) and magnesium (500 mg daily) can help ease anxiety. So can taking a good B-complex vitamin (50 mg daily). These nutrients help calm and restore the nervous system.

GABA (gamma-aminobutyric acid) helps protect the brain from excitatory messages so one is less likely to feel overwhelmed. Take 250 mg up to three times daily.

The amino acid 5-HTP (5-hydroxytrytophan) is a precursor to serotonin, which has a calming effect. Take no more than 50 mg twice daily.

FLOWER ESSENCES THAT EASE ANXIETY

Have Rescue Remedy, a combination of five Bach Flower Remedies, with you in several convenient places such as your briefcase, desk, purse, and glove compartment and use it when anxiety starts to come on. Take four drops under the tongue or in a glass of water as often as needed, up to every 15 minutes.

You can also take Aspen flower essence if you feel fearful and anxious but don't know why. Take four drops under the tongue or in a glass of water. Mimulus flower essence and Agrimony flower essence also ease restlessness and anxiety. Take four drops under the tongue or in a glass of water three times daily.

AROMATHERAPY THAT CALMS ANXIETY

The brain is in very close proximity to the nasal passages, so taking ten deep inhalations from an opened bottle of pure essential oils changes neural pathways in a moment. Inhale the anxiety-relieving essential oils of basil, bergamot, cedarwood, chamomile, cypress, geranium, jasmine, juniper, lavender, marjoram, melissa, neroli, petitgrain, rose, rosemary, or ylang-ylang. You can find these in your health food store.

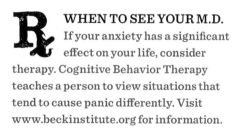

WHEN TO SEE YOUR M.D.
If your anxiety has a significant effect on your life, consider therapy. Cognitive Behavior Therapy teaches a person to view situations that tend to cause panic differently. Visit www.beckinstitute.org for information.

SOOTHING PRACTICES TO CALM ANXIETY

Remember to breathe and feed your brain the oxygen it craves for serenity. Deep diaphragmatic breathing can actually help relieve anxiety. For this reason, exercise is a good way to reduce anxiety.

Use a peaceful mantra to calm the spirit. Say "OM" (the sound of everything in the universe all at once), "the Universe supports me," or any other centering phrase over and over. I've always liked "Om Mane Padme Hum," which means "God is a lotus in my heart." Repetition gets you to breathe more slowly and calms a racing heart.

Write about what has triggered your anxiety. Are there any common denominators such as a food, place, theme, a certain person, or a situation? Ask what the anxiety is trying to protect you from. Make a list of the people and places you typically encounter. Ask which of those feel safe and which don't. Put a mark by all those that feel threatening. Try to avoid those situations to reduce anxiety until you feel strong enough to face them.

GOOD TO KNOW!

Massage can help release tension and, in turn, anxiety. Hold the thumb of one hand with the other as a calming technique. Rub the third eye (center of the forehead) to calm the spirit. Holding your toes, especially the middle toe, helps to bring the energy down from the head and ground it so you feel calmer.

Alleviating Depression

Depression is more than feeling down. It's like living under a cloud all the time. In Asian medicine, liver stagnation is at the core of depression. That's because a healthy liver is needed to maintain even blood sugar levels, filter blood, and remove waste products as well as negative emotions. If the liver is impaired, the filtration process becomes weakened; toxins circulate throughout the body and affect the brain. Of course, life can present us with difficult circumstances that leave us depressed. Many people also find that during the grayer months (from October to April), they experience Seasonal Affective Disorder (SAD), which includes depression, lack of energy, weight gain, and decreased libido. Here's what you can do to clear those clouds away and feel better.

HERBS THAT BOOST YOUR MOOD

The following herbs have been traditionally used to lift people's spirits. Use one to three times daily in tea, tincture, or capsule form:

- Saint-John's-wort slightly inhibits both A and B monoamine oxidase, thus slowing down the breakdown of neurotransmitters norepinephrine and serotonin. It also appears to inhibit serotonin reuptake and is good for mild to moderate depression. Many studies, including one published in the German medical journal, *Fortschritte der Medizin* in 1993, show its benefits on mild to moderate depression.
- Lemon balm is useful for depression, homesickness, insomnia, nervousness, nightmares, and coping with difficult life situations. The famous Arabian physician Avicenna said of this herb, "It causeth the mind and heart to be merry." It makes a lovely tasting tea.

- Motherwort is effective for depression, anxiety, exhaustion, gloom, and hysteria.
- Oat straw is high in the nerve nutrients calcium and silica, which means it helps soothe the nervous system.

A popular remedy that contains several of these herbs is Phyto-Proz by Gaia Herbs. It can be found at many health food stores.

BEST FOODS FOR DEPRESSION

Eating the right foods can help ease the blues. Consume raw, soaked chia seeds daily for their omega-3 brain-nourishing properties. Fish is especially beneficial for depression because it contains essential fatty acids that are excellent brain food. Eat several servings a week of cold-water fish such as salmon, tuna, or mackerel, or supplement with 1 teaspoon (5 ml) of a good-quality fish oil each day.

When blood sugar elevations shift from extreme highs to low, emotions might also seem like a rollercoaster ride. Avoid refined foods like white sugar, white bread, white flour, and white rice, which contribute to high blood sugar levels. The pancreas tries to compensate by secreting extra insulin, giving you a temporary lift with an undesirable let down feeling later. Instead, consume small frequent complex carbohydrate meals that keep blood sugar levels even. Eat whole grains such as brown rice, buckwheat, quinoa, millet, and oatmeal. Foods like beans, tempeh, root vegetables such as carrots and dandelion root, green leafy vegetables, miso soup, onions, and scallions are also stabilizing to the blood sugar. Use basil, ginger, and oregano as condiments, which are herbs with high essential oil content that can invigorate the brain.

Chew your food well, breathe deeply, and try to be in a relaxed state when dining. A blessing before a meal can help put you in the right frame of mind.

ESSENTIAL OILS FOR DEPRESSION

Using essential oils has been shown to enhance moods. This is due at least in part to the close proximity of the nerve endings in the nasal cavities and the brain. Essential oils used to lift one's spirits include basil, bergamot, cedar wood, cinnamon, clay sage, clove, coriander, geranium, jasmine, lavender, neroli, palmers, patchouli, peppermint, rose, rosemary, rosewood, sandalwood, thyme, vetiver, wintergreen, and ylang-ylang.

Thrifty Cures

Two ripe bananas a day help production of serotonin and norepinephrine, brain chemicals that can make you feel happier.

GOOD TO KNOW!
It has been estimated that between 15 and 20 percent of all depressed people have low thyroid function or hypothyroidism. If you do have hypothyroidism, eat mineral-rich sea vegetables such as dulse, kelp, or wakame to nourish the thyroid and boost a sluggish metabolism. For more information on thyroid disorders, visit www.thyroid-info.com.

You can use these oils in diffusers to scent an entire room, or add a few drops to bath water or massage oils. Massage is an excellent way to improve circulation and wake your mind and body. You can also simply open the bottle and take 10 deep inhalations. Repeat as necessary. Note that you should never ingest essential oils.

SOOTHING PRACTICES TO ALLEVIATE DEPRESSION

Exercise stimulates endorphin production. It also increases the brain's intake of the essential nutrient oxygen. Spending time near a river, ocean, or even a fountain can also boost serotonin levels. The negative ions in running water will also improve your mood. A brisk walk in the radiance of nature or gardening and helping things grow will also lift your spirits. You'll also be exposed to the sun, which will elevate your mood if you have SAD.

Delight your senses with color, beauty, and aromas. Wear uplifting colors to make your mood brighter. Pleasing pinks, scarlets, and oranges may well have a beneficial effect on your outlook. Brighten your living environment too. A clean, comfortable space with pleasant colors, art, and flowers will do a lot more for your head space than dirt, dreariness, and clutter. Yoga and t'ai chi stimulate one's life force too. Listen to beautiful and rhythmic music and dance!

Here are a few other ways to improve your mood:

- Choose ten activities to accomplish every day (even if it is as simple as getting dressed and making the bed).
- Write down goals that you can accomplish.
- Learn a new skill to build your self-esteem.
- Listen to uplifting and motivating tapes.
- Enjoy books and movies that are inspiring.
- Get counseling and share your feelings.
- Let go of old scripts from the past and other peoples' opinions.
- Start loving and forgiving yourself.
- Spend time with happy uplifting people.
- Pray or meditate to reconnect with our Source.
- Find some creative outlet such as writing poetry, working with clay, or music. Creativity helps to counteract depression.
- Count your blessings!

Skip This!

Alcohol is in itself a depressant and is the last thing a depressed person needs. Food allergies, sensitivities, and food additives such as chemical sweeteners and colors may be perceived by the body as foreign particles, thus causing a brain allergy and mood changes. Yeast in food, sugars, fruits, and juices can aggravate yeast overgrowth, which can lead to the blues. Keep a food journal to help correlate dietary patterns to moods.

℞ WHEN TO SEE YOUR M.D. If you are seriously depressed, see a mental health professional. Don't try to go it alone. If you are suicidal, temporary hospitalization may be necessary.

Quelling Grief or a Broken Heart

Good Grief! This is a favorite lament of Charlie Brown, but if you are grieving, you know it's not funny. When we grieve, our heart rate increases and adrenaline and hydrochloric acid production are increased. It is not unusual to experience a sensation of numbness, pain along the breastbone, and sinus congestion when grieving. In Asian medicine, the lungs and large intestines are associated with grief. Being grief stricken for extended periods can lead to a weakened immunity. But crying can be a great release, so don't fight the tears. Crying helps provide emotional release that lowers blood pressure and muscular tension. Chemicals released in tears include endorphin, which helps relieve pain. Suppressing tears can make us more vulnerable to disease. You can also support the body with these strategies.

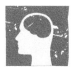

GOOD TO KNOW!
Vitamin B complex (50 mg daily) is a great ally during times of emotional distress, as our supply of B vitamins is quickly diminished.

GOOD TO GROW!
A formula for heartbreak-type sorrow is made with 2 parts hawthorn leaf, flower, or berry, 1 part motherwort, 2 parts lemon balm herb, and 1 part violet leaves. Make them into a tea and drink 3 cups (705 ml) daily.

HERBS THAT PROVIDE COMFORT

Herbs can provide comfort during times of grief. Consider the benefits of calming hops, lemon balm, and passionflower. Saint-John's-wort is beneficial when you are worn out from sobbing. Gardenia can cheer you. It is known in Chinese medicine as "the happiness herb." Use these herbs in tea, tincture, or capsule form three times daily.

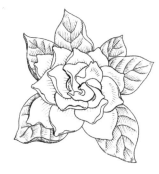

SOOTHING HOMEOPATHIC REMEDIES

A good homeopathic remedy for sorrow is Ignatia. Use it for grief, loss, and hysteria and for disappointment in love or the death of a loved one. It's also indicated if you can't sleep or are nervous and shake. Also, it helps for those bereaved individuals who strongly identified with the person lost and feel they cannot exist without them. Take 3 pellets under the tongue 3 times daily as needed.

ESSENTIAL OILS AND FLOWER ESSENCES THAT PROVIDE COMFORT

Essential oils can stimulate chemical changes in brain chemistry by opening different neural pathways. Adding some essential oils to a bath can be a good way to let the tears flow. Helpful essential oils include cedarwood, clary sage, cypress, frankincense, geranium, ginger, grapefruit, hyssop, lavender, lemon balm, jasmine, marjoram, neroli, orange, rose, rosemary, or ylang-ylang. Let the water out and visualize your sadness going down the drain as you stay in the tub for a few moments.

Essential oils are absorbed through the skin and when used topically can be a way of nurturing and relaxing specific parts of our being. You can also make an essential oil blend by putting two drops of essential oil in one ounce (28 ml) of vegetable oil and massaging over the heart and lungs. Apply some rose oil gently over the solar plexus to dispel grief and bring comfort. Melissa oil is good for heartbreak over a love relationship. You can also use these oils in a diffuser.

Flower essences have been used since the research of Dr. Edward Bach in the early 1900s. They have been found to have subtle though transforming properties for the emotional body. Take 2 drops in a glass of water 3 times daily if needed. Flower essences that are helpful include the following:

- Bleeding heart: For grief related to the loss of a love or separation; helps to foster peace and detachment.
- Mustard: For deep gloom that comes on strong then suddenly leaves.
- Star of Bethlehem: For great physical shock and trauma such as rape, injury, robbery, and accidents—it can also be used when one is having a difficult time coping with death of a pet or loved one. Dr. Edward Bach calls this "the comforter and soother of pains and sorrows."

SOOTHING PRACTICES THAT ALLEVIATE GRIEF

Besides crying, groaning is a sound you can use to help dissipate sadness and pain. While groaning, think of the reason for your suffering. When you exhale, visualize the sorrow being exhaled from your body. Stand facing the rising sun and let its rays beam on your heart. Visualize the sun healing the grief. Breathe!

Rest is always an important healer of grief. As we heal from the trials of grief, travel can also help the heart and give us new perspectives. The color violet is a good color to wear, visualize, and surround yourself with when needing to heal feelings of grief. Practice deep slow breathing to cleanse the emotions of grief. Exercise can also raise dopamine levels. Time is a great healer.

SOOTHING PRACTICES THAT ALLEVIATE HEARTBREAK

We often assume that the jubilance of love can carry us through life and conquer all problems and differences. But when one partner has completed the lessons needed and the other hasn't, the partner wanting to end the relationship can feel sad and guilty and the one being left can feel heartsick. If you are the one being left, loss and separation can cause feelings similar to death of a loved one. Here's how to move on.

You may want to have a closing ritual. Place a photo of your ex, a sprig of rosemary (for remembrance), and a candle in a bowl filled with sand or dirt. Anoint the candle with a fragrance that reminds you of your ex and etch his or her name into the candle. Light the candle with a prayer of thanks for the lessons learned in the relationship and as it burns down reflect or write in your journal about the relationship. Make a list of what you have learned.

Make a list of all the reasons the relationship could not have survived. Write about how each of you benefited one another. Be willing to look at any part of you that may have contributed to the ending; then let go of it. Write about what you will look for in a new partner. This is very soul cleansing. Give your story a title. Allow the candle to burn itself out.

It can also help to write your ex a letter, for your eyes only. Use this as an opportunity to collect your thoughts, getting everything off your chest. Vent venomously! Include a list of all their flaws. Eventually you may want to send a modified version (without the bad language) to them. Or burn it. The important thing is to clear it out of you.

Here are some other suggestions for mending a broken heart:

1. Avoid calling or running to your ex-partner when you are sad, scared, or depressed. Calling just to "check in" should be minimized. Listening to the same music and hanging out where you hope you will run into him or her keeps you thinking too much of the past and causes you to avoid new experiences.

2. Remove mementos. Put your ex's belongings into a box and return things with a minimum of drama. Be fair about giving back heirlooms and expensive things that were not gifts. It is not worth fighting over CDs or books that can easily be replaced.

3. Clean everything. Feng shui your home. Burn some sage or artemesia to clear the air.

4. Get busy. Enjoy new experiences. Improve the way you look. Get into health. Exercise helps lift depression. Practice yoga.

5. Quit bad habits. Overdoing alcohol, drugs, and junk food will only make this time more difficult.

6. Put energy into your career. Develop talents and work on personal growth. Take a class. Read self-help books. Learn a new language. Start enjoying all the things you were unable to while in the relationship.

7. Call a few of your best friends over and allow them to cheer you up. Seek out those who want to see you happy and avoid negative people. Call friends you neglected during the relationship.

8. Tell your friends not to give you constant gossip reports about who your ex has been seen with and where (unless you really need to know). Ask friends who invite you to gatherings to inform you if your ex will be there to avoid surprises and so you can choose whether you still want to attend. Go dancing with friends. Get out there and flirt!

9. Make an appointment with a spiritual counselor or therapist to process unexpressed feelings and help resolve them.

10. Next time you run into your ex, let him or her see the new improved version! If he or she is with a new love, walk over and introduce yourself, making it sweet but brief. Show you have class! If you are at a party and you are both alone, say hello but refrain from leaving and having sex. Continuing to sleep with someone when the relationship is really over prolongs pain.

KEEP IN MIND

Time is a great healer. Be glad for the happiness and lessons you shared. Hopefully you have learned things that can be of value in other aspects of life and future relations. Sometimes the one who was left fares better than the one who left, as the hurt person has to look at him or herself and do emotional healing. Let go of the old to make room for the new!

For ideas on finding and keeping new love, please check out my book *The Sexual Herbal.*

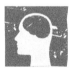 **GOOD TO KNOW!**
According to color therapists and gemologists, the color violet is good to wear and visualize when you are experiencing grief. Sleep with a rose quartz in your hand and your dreams may have a healing effect on your heart.

Improving Memory

Are to-do lists scattered all over your house? Are you constantly forgetting or losing things like your keys or your phone or missing appointments you need to keep? Natural remedies can help you focus. Here's how.

HERBS AND SUPPLEMENTS THAT BOOST BRAIN POWER

Ginkgo is an ancient herb that improves the brain's ability by enhancing peripheral blood flow. Bacopa herb enhances neurotransmitter function and serotonin production. Gotu kola herb improves the movement of impulses from the left and right brain hemispheres. Ginseng root increases cerebral circulation. Take them in tea, tincture, or capsule form three times daily.

Also good is DHA (docosahexaenoic acid), which is a primary component of brain structure. A new study in the *Journal of Neuroscience Research* (2010) showed that DHA (found in fish oil) helps preserve brain function in rats as they age. Take 300 to 500 mg daily.

Phosphatidylserine enables brain cells to metabolize glucose and to release and bind with neurotransmitters. Take 500 mg daily. Choline is part of the B vitamin complex and is a precursor of acetylcholine, a stimulatory neurotransmitter. Take 250 to 500 mg daily.

Inositol, another component of the B vitamin complex, helps maintain proper electrical energy and nutrient transfer across the cell membrane. Take 100 to 300 mg daily.

SCENTS TO HELP YOU REMEMBER

The nasal cavities are in close proximity to the brain. Perhaps this is why ancient Greek scholars wore laurels of rosemary when taking examinations. When receiving important information, inhale up to ten breaths of pure essential oils like basil, lemon, lemon grass, lime, peppermint, or rosemary to help imprint the information into the psyche. When you need to recall something, smell the same scent.

FOODS THAT BOOST MEMORY

Green foods are high in chlorophyll, which transports oxygen to the brain. Make at least one daily meal a salad of leafy greens, even wild ones like dandelion. Eat a handful of raw sunflower seeds daily. Drink 1 teaspoon (5 ml) of raw apple cider vinegar in water three times daily before each meal to improve memory.

High cholesterol clogs arteries, decreasing blood supply to the brain. So use good fats such as extra virgin olive and cold pressed coconut oil. When you prepare food, use liberal amounts

WHEN TO SEE YOUR M.D. Many medications affect your brain. If you are experiencing memory problems, learn about prescriptions you are taking (visit www.rxlist.com, type in the drug name, and click on Side Effects) and talk to your doctor. Also when memory loss starts getting you into dangerous situations, seeing a neurologist can be a good idea.

Skip This!

Avoid excessive exposure to substances such as tobacco, alcohol, pollutants, MSG, and toxic body- and house-cleaning products. Food sensitivities and allergies, addiction, and nutritional deficiencies can also contribute to memory impairment.

of brain-enhancing antioxidant herbs like basil, cilantro, mint, oregano, rosemary, sage, and thyme.

High-carbohydrate foods such as pasta and bread are more for feeling serene and stuffed rather than sharp. Go for protein with greens rather than carbs with protein. Saturated fats and heated oils can lead to feeling soggy, foggy, and groggy.

PRACTICES THAT IMPROVE BRAIN FUNCTION

Exercise increases the body's intake of oxygen and speeds up nerve impulses. Working up a sweat at least three times a week can open the receptor sites. Make exercise fun—go for a walk with a friend. Even walking a different direction inspires new thoughts as we take in various sights. In classrooms, sit closer to the front but move to different spots to increase perception by seeing from a different angle.

Exercise the brain too. Learn two new vocabulary words a week, using them soon after, do puzzles, play challenging games, or journal. To remember names, associate the name with a picture. Eileen has big blue eyes and is leaning. Visualize Bob becoming a bobcat. Soon after being introduced, use their name. If you don't catch their name, say, "Spell it, please?" Or picture all the people you know named Eileen or Bob standing together.

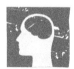

GOOD TO KNOW!
Using the opposite hand a few minutes daily on simple tasks help to open neural pathways.

When you want to remember something, repeat it aloud. Visualize it being imprinted upon your brain and file it. Then practice retrieving and refilling it.

The following are some other ideas on how you can improve your memory:

1. Hang with intelligent folk. Have deep discussions. Ask questions. Get answers.

2. The color yellow is cerebrally stimulating. Use yellow to highlight important passages when reading. Try a yellow legal pad. Wear accents of yellow or use it in décor where mental work is being done.

3. Read things that are challenging and give new insights. If fiction is usually your thing, try a biography, self-help, spiritual, or even science fiction book.

4. Think positively. Success is most likely when affirming, "I can do this" rather than "I'll never make it."

5. Record flashes of brilliance and words of wisdom! You never know when you may get a great idea. Meditate to expand calmness and consciousness.

6. Try different foods and things wherever you are on the planet.

7. Learn and practice handicrafts. Take classes. (I just learned to crochet!)

8. Practice the art of brainstorming to lead to fruitful concepts.

9. Break blockage and negativity with diversion. Go for a walk. Call a friend. Go to a film. Take a bath.

10. Wearing an amethyst crystal, according to gem therapists, improves memory.

Alleviating Stress

We all know that life is full of stress. Stress can be caused by anything disturbing the serenity of our lives, including change, pressure, emotions, and physical trauma. Even activities such as skiing down a mountain, aiming for higher goals, or falling in love can take a toll on one's nerves. Unfortunately, during difficult times, people often take worse care of themselves. Though stress may be unavoidable, we can come through most ordeals if our lifestyles are balanced by faith, rest, good nutrition, and exercise. Here are some natural ways to take care of yourself.

HERBS THAT RELIEVE STRESS

Nature's floral pharmacy provides many herbs that nourish and support a frayed nervous system. Taking the time out to savor a cup of soothing herbal tea made out of one of these herbs is a wonderful way to nourish your nerves:

- Valerian calms nerves without dulling the mind and relaxes the muscles, leaving you less uptight.
- Catnip contains nepetalactones, which are chemically similar to valepotriates in valerian, both calming chemicals. It calms anxiety, hysteria, insomnia, and restlessness.
- Chamomile is a great nerve restorative for exhausted systems. Use it for anxiety, hysteria, insomnia, nervousness, and nightmares.

GOOD TO KNOW!
Good posture promotes the best brain function because the oxygen and nutrients the body needs all get delivered where they need to be.

- Hops is helpful for anxiety, hysteria, insomnia, irritability, nervous heart, nightmares, and stress.
- Kava kava is good for anxiety, stiff muscles, and tension that prevents sleep.
- Oat straw calms anxiety and nervous exhaustion.

Natural food stores carry herbal combinations of calming plants in tea, tincture, or capsule form. Use when needed, up to three times daily, though some prefer these remedies at night as they can make you too restful during the day.

ESSENTIAL OILS THAT RELIEVE STRESS

Essential oils that relieve stress include anise, basil, cardamom, chamomile, clary sage, cypress, fennel, frankincense, geranium, juniper, lavender, lemon, marjoram, melissa, neroli, nutmeg, orange, peppermint, pine, rose, rosewood, sandalwood, spearmint, and ylang-ylang. You can take up to ten deep inhalations from the bottle or add five to seven drops to bath water.

BEST FOODS TO RELIEVE STRESS

During tense times, you owe it to yourself to choose nutritious foods. Small, frequent whole-grain meals rich in complex carbohydrates help to keep the blood sugar on an even keel as well as provide important B vitamins. Oatmeal and yogurt are two foods that are easy to digest and rich in calming calcium. Other good stress foods include almonds, beans, raisins, and sunflower seeds, as they are rich in nerve-nourishing minerals like calcium and magnesium as well as B vitamins. Onions contain tension-relieving prostaglandins.

SOOTHING PRACTICES TO RELIEVE STRESS

Here are a few other ideas to enhance the serenity of your life.

1. Exercise improves respiration and circulation, sends nutrients to the cells and stimulates endorphin production. Yoga and t'ai chi can help relax the mind and body.

2. Every day, do something you really enjoy. Read books that are uplifting. Act like a kid. Throw a Frisbee. Read fairytales. Play with clay.

3. Get a massage or massage your own hands, face, and feet.

4. Reach out to someone. Hug your child, love your mate, pet your dog or cat, get in touch with an old friend, lend a hand to someone in need.

5. Breathe more deeply and slowly. Oxygen nourishes the brain. Alternate nostril breathing is an excellent technique to relieve stress.

6. Slow down your eating, talking, walking, and driving. Do whatever you need to do, but do it slower. Even speaking more calmly can have a calming effect.

7. Psychotherapy can be essential for releasing pent-up feelings that cause stress.

8. Wear comfortable clothing that allows your skin to breathe and allows freedom of movement. Some people find that wearing the blue and green is calming. Avoid yellow as it contributes to anxiety.

9. When choosing music, select that which is calming and contemplative.

10. Get out of bed 15 minutes earlier to allow time to take care of what's needed. Prepare your clothes, paperwork, and perhaps lunch the night before rather than starting your morning in a frenzy.

11. Rather than letting your mind carry around so much, get an engagement book and write down numbers, errands, and appointments.

12. Write down all your problems and brainstorm possible solutions for solving them. Remember that you don't need to be perfect.

13. Learn to say no to the things you really don't want or have time to do.

14. Get rid of clutter in your life. Clutter causes confusion.

Skip This!

Foods that increase the negative effects of stress include alcohol, caffeinated beverages, fruit juices, and sugar.

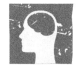

GOOD TO KNOW!

Stress depletes the body's reserves of vitamins and minerals, so it's wise to take daily supplements during stressful periods. Consider a vitamin B complex (50 mg) with C (500 mg) to replenish the water-soluble nutrients. They not only can nourish the nervous system but also give you the energy you need to deal with life's problems. Calcium (1000 mg) and magnesium (500 mg) help to ease tension and irritability.

 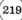

15. Practice visualization. There a many tapes available where you close your eyes and visualize yourself floating on a cloud or lying by a trickling brook. Visit these tranquil places in your mind.

16. Learn to do a craft. To create things of beauty is great for self-esteem.

17. Get a set of Chinese hand balls, available at many natural foods stores. Learn to use them.

18. Be prepared for lines that keep you waiting. Have something to read so you don't have to feel like you are wasting time.

19. Smile. Relaxing your face helps the rest of your body as well as putting those around you at ease.

20. Spend time in the beauty and quietude of nature. Go outside and look at the sky. Sit by a stream.

21. Pray for guidance and/or meditate. Have some alone time every day.

22. Take a short nap when you can.

23. Make two lists: one of the stresses in your life you can change and the other of the stresses you can't.

24. Plan something to look forward to.

25. Remember to count your blessings!

Treating Trauma

Unfortunately, many people experience trauma on planet Earth. Trauma may be verbal, physical, psychological, sexual, and/or violent. Rape, miscarriage, robbery, and accidents are all traumatic. Though females are the most often affected by sexual abuse, abuse occurs to many males. In some cases, both partners have been victims of sexual trauma. If abuse issues are never brought up, they can continue to affect current relationships in subtle ways. If abuse occurred via the opposite sex, feelings of hurt, anger, and grief can be transferred to others of that sex. Counseling can help even

if the trauma occurred years ago. It's important to ask for what you want and need to heal completely. Here are some natural remedies that also help.

AT EASE TRAUMA

Herbs that ease trauma include oat straw, motherwort, and Saint-John's Wort, all of which nourish the nervous system. Oat straw makes a lovely tea, but the last two can be found in tinctures and capsules and 1 or 2 can be taken up to 3 times daily.

Schizandra berries are beneficial following trauma and eleuthero can also support the body during times of stress. Both are adaptogens, helping the body adapt to difficult situations, and are available in tea, tincture, or capsule form, taken as directed on the package up to 3 times daily.

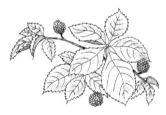

Raspberry leaf, which is mineral rich and targets the reproductive centers, can be taken in tea, tincture, or capsule form 3 times daily to help heal sexual trauma.

ESSENTIAL OILS AND FLOWER ESSENCES THAT EASE TRAUMA

Flower essences for trauma include Star of Bethlehem, which is beneficial for great physical shock and trauma such as rape, injury, robbery, and accidents. Rescue Remedy is a combination Bach Flower remedy good for panic, shock, grief, despair, and other crisis. Take two drops in a glass of water 3 times daily.

It can also help to smell lavender oil or even take a bath in it. Rose essential oil can be inhaled to soothe emotional traumas.

SOOTHING PRACTICES TO EASE TRAUMA

Soak your feet in warm water to which a bit of cayenne pepper has been added and stirred. The warmth infuses the body with a feeling of safety and security.

Apply acupressure to point two thirds up from upper lip to nose.

Eat soothing nutrient-dense foods, seaweeds, wild rice, black sesame seeds, and especially chia seeds, which can be soaked and consumed as a raw breakfast cereal. (Flavor with blueberries, apples, raisins, and/or honey.) According to Asian medicine, foods that are black in color are high in minerals that affect the kidneys, the organ system associated with fear.

GOOD TO KNOW!
A Chinese patent formula to use for stress resulting from bad fright or severe shock to the emotional body is Ding Xin Wan, also called Calm Heart Pill. It can also help relieve posttraumatic stress. Follow the directions on the bottle.

Surround yourself with the healing color green. Green clothes, green bedding, green foods, and green plants all have a calming presence.

When you allow the pain of old emotions to resurface, after you feel them, you can release them. It can help to discuss your wounds with a trusted friend. Don't be afraid to express feelings of hurt, anger, and grief. It's okay to feel! You can also benefit by writing about your feelings.

Another way to heal is to take two deep inhalations, allowing hurt feelings to leave the body with each exhalation.

GOOD TO KNOW!
Homeopathic Ignatia helps when sexuality has been altered by grief or trauma. Take 3 or 4 pellets slowly dissolved under the tongue as needed, up to four times daily. For more information, see my book *Sexual Herbal*.

GOOD TO KNOW!
If you are providing comfort to someone experiencing trauma, offer words of encouragement, such as "It's okay. I'm here for you. I care." Offer a tissue. Avoid correcting or analyzing. Don't tell the person to get over it or put it behind them.

 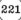

CHAPTER 14

NATURAL REMEDIES FOR BEAUTIFUL SKIN, HAIR, AND NAILS

The condition of our skin, hair, and nails not only adds to our beauty but can also be a reflection of our true inner health. Rather than using only cosmetic fixes, learning about nourishing foods and herbs can help us reflect our most beautiful self.

Alleviating Acne

The dreaded zit—also known as *Acne vulgaris*, or simply pimple outbreaks, is an inflammation of the skin that results from clogged pores. Acne is likely to occur when sebum, a waxy substance that lubricates the skin, and keratin, a skin protein, block the sebaceous glands. Acne can have many causes, including allergies, poor circulation, constipation, food sensitivities, medications, nutritional deficiencies, smoking, stress, yeast overgrowth, inadequate sloughing off of the skin's cells, overactive oil glands, and lack of fatty acids (which reduce inflammation). Excess sebum production can be partly genetic or hormonal, thus acne is most likely to occur on oily skin. Stress can cause the skin to produce more oil. These tips can help.

ANTI-ACNE HERBS

Herbs that can be used in tea, tincture, or capsule form that can help improve skin quality include burdock root, raw dandelion root, Oregon grape root, and yellow dock root. These herbs are available in combinations at health food stores and help improve liver function, bowel action, and help the body metabolize fats. Burdock and Oregon grape root also have mild antibacterial activity.

Herbs to apply to an impending breakout include tea tree oil or lavender essential oil. Either can be applied undiluted to a problem area. A study published in the *Medical Journal of Australia* in 1990 showed that tea tree oil was just as effective in treating acne as benzoyl peroxide lotion, with less dryness, stinging, burning, and redness.

Spirits of camphor, available at drugstores, is also effective for spot treatments. Just dab this on an impending pimple and it will help dry it up quickly.

The company Desert Essence makes a blemish stick (available at health food stores) that contains tea tree oil and is a favorite product for those who suffer occasional breakouts.

Cures from Grandma's Kitchen

To encourage healthy skin, drink the juice of half a lemon in a glass of water one to three times daily to help the liver break down toxins. You can warm the water up slightly but not so hot that it destroys the vitamin C in the lemon.

BEST FOODS FOR CLEAR SKIN

Foods that are most beneficial for improving acne include apples, apricots, artichokes, barley, beets, carrots (with the skins), celery, cucumbers (organic with the peel), flaxseeds, green leafy vegetables, lemon in water, parsley, radishes, sweet potatoes, raw sunflower seeds, and winter squashes. All of these foods are cleansing yet high in minerals or beta-carotene that can help the skin be more resistant to outbreaks.

A raw high-fiber diet, without heated oils, refined carbohydrates, dairy, sugar, and wheat, is the ultimate.

Foods to minimize include peanuts, peanut butter, wheat, high-fat dairy products, sugar, heated oils (this includes commercially bottled salad dressing and oils like canola, soy, and safflower oil), fried foods, and hydrogenated oils. Not only is eating fried foods a possible problem, but heated oils in the air (such as those around a fryer) can also clog the pores. Acne can be inflammation related to a food allergy. By removing the offending food, the problem can go away.

BEST PRACTICES FOR CLEAR SKIN

Here are some additional clear skin tips:
- Consider changing your pillowcase every other night to minimize exposure to bacteria.
- Wash hands frequently during the day and avoid touching the face unnecessarily, and only touch with clean hands.
- Keep hair off the face and be aware that hair products such as sprays, gels, and mousses can contain pore-clogging ingredients. Be aware that products that are used on the skin (make up, cleansers, moisturizers, even sun screen) can also contain pore-clogging mineral oil, allergens, or chemicals that cause reactions.
- Keep in mind that holding a telephone receiver against your face can contact you with bacteria that causes acne. Wipe the phone down with alcohol daily.

Erasing Age Spots

Age spots, also known as liver spots, sunspots, solar lentigines, and senile keratosis, are changes in the skin's pigmentation, usually of light to dark brown or light to dark gray coloring, and may appear on the face, neck, V of the neck, and backs of the hands. Though they often come on as we age, that does not have to be the cause. Age spots can also be brought on through nutritional deficiencies, free-radical damage, elevated blood sugar levels, sun exposure, and topical alcohol contacts (such as cologne and some cosmetics). To prevent age spots, protect the skin from the sun, even if it means wearing a hat and cotton gloves. Natural food stores carry sunscreens made with quality ingredients that can offer sun protection.

Age spots take years to form and eliminating them will take time too, so don't give up! Try a remedy for a few months, and if the condition hasn't improved, try another one.

Thrifty Cures!

At the first sign of an acne outbreak, apply an ice cube wrapped in a washcloth for several minutes at least twice daily to reduce inflammation. After cleansing the face, apply a cotton ball soaked in equal parts apple cider vinegar and water to restore the skin's proper pH.

NATURAL REMEDIES THAT REJUVENATE THE SKIN

Things to apply topically twice a day for at least a month include aloe vera juice, apple cider vinegar, plain yogurt, castor oil, lemon juice, fresh papaya, or pineapple slices. Just rub any of these items on the area you have spots, leave on for 15 minutes, rinse off, and dry. All of these remedies, many of which are high in alpha-citric acid, help heal damaged tissue, lighten the skin, or cause the dead layers of skin to easily exfoliate, so new skin will be healthier and visible.

BEST FOODS TO PREVENT AGE SPOTS

Eat more blueberries and vitamin C rich foods, which help increase collagen production, making the skin more resistant to free radical damage. Eat at least five servings daily of tart apples, berries, red pepper, and fresh fruit in season.

Eat fresh raw leafy greens daily and dark orange vegetables, such as carrots, winter squash and sweet potatoes, which are all high in beta-carotene, which makes the skin more resilient to damage.

GOOD TO GROW!

You can even use dandelion sap for age spots. Just pick a dandelion, break open the hollow stem, and apply the white juice inside on the spot. It contains enzymes that help break down spots.

Skip This!

To avoid age spots, avoid refined sugar, caffeine, alcohol, tobacco, junk foods, and heated or rancid oils. All of these foods are stressful for the body and rather than being health giving can expose the body to free radicals that show up eventually as skin damage.

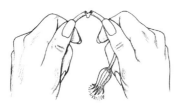

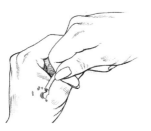

℞ WHEN TO SEE YOUR M.D.

If you have irregular dark spots that increase in size or change color or texture, have them checked immediately by a doctor.

Moistening Dry Skin

Is your skin as dry as the Sahara desert? Weather, sun exposure, and the heating and cooling of homes, cars, and workplaces can all exacerbate dry skin conditions. It's important to protect your skin from the elements, especially when outdoors in the summer (or year round in temperate climates) between the hours of 10 am and 4 pm. Avoid sunburn, tanning booths, and excessive heat such as sitting close to a fire. Keep the heat lower in your house, especially at night. Use more blankets! You'll not only save energy and reduce your power bill, you'll also save your skin. For more skin soothing tips, read on.

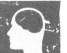

Skip This!

Caffeine, alcohol and tobacco are all dehydrating to the skin.

GOOD TO KNOW!
The best time to apply a moisturizer is right after cleansing as water helps keep the skin's outer layers from drying out and oil seals it in. Avoid poor-quality cosmetics that contain mineral oil, chemicals and artificial colors and fragrances. Some of my favorites include Astara, Weleda and Aubrey Organics. A massage done with a good-quality massage oil can be both relaxing and moisturizing.

HERBS THAT MOISTURIZE

Moisture-providing herbal teas that can be drunk up to a cup three times daily include fennel seed, marshmallow root, plantain leaf, red clover blossoms, and violet leaves.

BEST PRACTICES TO AVOID DRY SKIN

Avoid using soaps and cleansers that contain deodorants and detergents. Cleansers made of oatmeal, white clay, vitamin E, coconut oil, shea butter, or olive oil are least drying. Cleanse the face with warm water (not hot) and rinse with at least ten splashes of cold water to remove any residue of cleanser.

During the day, rehydrate the skin, especially the face, which is most exposed to the elements. One half cup (120 ml) each of rose water and mineral water can be used as a moistening mister. Another easy spray can be made with 8 ounces of spring water and 10 drops of chamomile, geranium, lavender, neroli, or rose essential oil. Shake before spraying. If you fly in airplanes, keep in mind that cabin air is very drying and a small spray mister is great to use for external hydration.

The best way to hydrate the skin is from the inside. Drinking at least a quart of pure water a day is essential to being moist on the outside. If you are dry inside, your skin will reflect that fact.

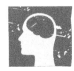

GOOD TO KNOW!
Showers that are short and not too hot are less drying than baths. If you do like to soak in a tub, mix up a rich bath oil with 2 cups (475 ml) cold-pressed coconut oil and 1/2 ounce (15 ml) of pure lavender oil. Shake the oils together and add 2 tablespoons (28 ml) to the bath.

BEST FOODS FOR MOIST SKIN

Foods that improve skin quality include the dark orange and green beta-carotene-rich foods like apricots, carrots, green leafy vegetables, parsley, pumpkin, sweet potatoes, winter squash, as well as moistening almonds, apples, avocados, barley, buckwheat, millet, oatmeal, pumpkin seeds, sesame seeds, sunflower seeds, and yogurt. Beta-carotene protects the cell membranes and stimulates the growth of new skin cells.

It is essential to consume the right kinds of fats. Commercial oils such as soy, corn, and canola contain omega-6 fatty acids, which can contribute to inflammation. Use instead skin-beautifying extra virgin olive oil, even to make your own salad dressing.

KEEP IN MIND

Exercise delivers oxygen and nutrients to the skin and increases collagen production. These are important reasons to be active!

Easing Eczema and Psoriasis

Eczema, also known as contact dermatitis and allergic dermatitis, can be chronic or temporary and is characterized by abraded, cracked, blistered, weepy, crusted, patchy dry skin along with intense incessant itching, inflammation, and a tendency for anything you touch to make it worse. It most often occurs in the autumn. It is worse at night. Psoriasis is a chronic inflammatory skin condition characterized by small scaly silvery pink and red patches, commonly occurring on the knees, elbows, chest, scalp, lower back, and buttocks. Psoriasis can be mild to disabling and is considered more stubborn than eczema. Here's how to soothe the skin you're in.

HERBS THAT SOOTHE ECZEMA AND PSORIASIS

A dose of tea or tincture taken 3 times daily of burdock root, calendula, chickweed, cleavers, raw dandelion root, nettle leaf, Oregon grape root, plantain leaf, prickly ash bark, red clover blossoms, and/or yellow dock root improves skin health. Look for a combination in natural food stores that contains some combination of these herbs designed to improve liver, lung, and colon function, all helping to reflect clearer skin.

Turmeric root in capsules is a potent anti-inflammatory agent to help clear up skin condition. Take three times daily.

Cures from Grandma's Kitchen

Cold pressed coconut oil is also a nourishing emollient for the skin. Here's one way to include it in the diet:

VEGAN BUTTER

1 cup cold pressed coconut oil
½ teaspoon turmeric
¼ teaspoon Celtic salt

Mix together and serve on dehydrated crackers.

SALVES AND ESSENTIAL OILS THAT SOOTHE ECZEMA AND PSORIASIS

Salves to apply topically include those made from aloe vera, burdock, calendula, chickweed, comfrey, echinacea, goldenseal, plantain, and Saint-John's-wort, green tea, and/or tea tree oil. Apply three times daily, especially after bathing. Use only the best and more natural quality moisturizers for elsewhere on the skin.

Essential oils that best clear up eczema and psoriasis include bergamot, Roman chamomile, geranium, jasmine, lavender, lemon, lemon balm, (aka melissa), neroli, rose, sandalwood, or tea tree. Apply these oils topically in a jojoba-, olive-, or coconut-oil base 2 or 3 times daily.

BEST FOODS AND BEVERAGES FOR ECZEMA AND PSORIASIS

Eat plenty of green leafy vegetables to get more alkaline to your skin. Soak chia seeds to make a moistening raw porridge that lubricates the skin from the inside. Use extra virgin olive oil as your main fat. Eat 3 tablespoons (21 g) of freshly ground flaxseeds daily or learn to make flaxseed crackers.

Drinking an ounce of aloe vera juice after each meal can help calm inflammation.

Drinking a diluted vegetable juice daily made of celery, cucumber, beet, and parsley provides skin supporting trace minerals. Taking 1 tablespoon (28 ml) daily of organic hemp seed oil might be helpful in providing healing moisture for the skin.

SOOTHING PRACTICES FOR ECZEMA AND PSORIASIS

Many chemicals are irritating and harsh on the skin and can contribute to eczema and psoriasis. Soaps, bubble baths, shampoos, hair dyes, lotions, cosmetics, nail polish, laundry soaps, pet dander, and chlorinated and overly hot water are common examples of skin irritants. Avoid scrubs, harsh cleaners of any sort, overly hot water, bubble baths, loofahs, or anything else that might aggravate these conditions. Use fragrance-free products and avoid contact with chemicals on the skin. Remember what gets on your body can be absorbed by as much as 60 percent. Don't pollute your body or the planet!

Be aware of what you wear. Avoid wearing elastic, nylon, spandex, suede, wool, and synthetic fibers. Dry cleaning fluid residue and synthetic laundry soaps can irritate the skin. It may be helpful to add 1 cup (235 ml) of apple cider vinegar to the final rinse of a laundry load to neutralize possible irritants.

GOOD TO GROW!
Houseplants are moisturizing to the air and body. They take in atmospheric toxins and use them as food, while releasing fresh, clean oxygen into the air we breathe.

Thrifty Cures!
A folk remedy worthy trying on either eczema or psoriasis is to apply raw potato juice (made from a juicer) to the affected area 2 or 3 times daily. It can be left on until your next bath.

Climatherapy indicates that brief exposure to natural sunlight can improve or even clear psoriasis. Swimming in the ocean may be helpful to both eczema and psoriasis.

Get plenty of fresh air and exercise to ensure good circulation. Saunas can also be a way to clear internal toxins.

Anger, anxiety, fatigue, frustration, grief, and worry can also be contributing factors to eczema and psoriasis. Slow down. Practice stress reduction. Massage is also a good way to soothe the tension from the body.

Skip This!

Avoid chocolate, dairy products, citrus, tomatoes, meat, eggs, peanut butter, potatoes, wheat products, gluten, soy foods, fried foods, food additives, and hydrogenated and even heated oils (which can include bottled salad dressings). Any food allergen can be a contributing factor to a skin condition.

Nixing Warts

Warts are caused by viruses, not toads! The proper medical name for warts is *Verruca vulgaris*. These hard pale protrusions often occur in groups and are considered benign skin tumors caused by strains of the papilloma virus. They are contagious and can be transmitted through contact with a person who has warts or by using their towels or clothing. It's important to treat the warts so they don't continue to spread. Here's how to get rid of them naturally.

NATURAL REMEDIES THAT GET RID OF WARTS

Herbs to use internally to get rid of warts include burdock root, cleavers herb, dandelion root, echinacea root, nettles leaf, and peppermint herb, all of which help detoxify the body. Look for a tea, tincture, or capsule combination that is considered a natural detox agent and consume a dose three times daily.

GOOD TO KNOW!
Daily doses of beta-carotene or vitamin A (10,000 IU), vitamin C (1,000 mg), vitamin E (400 IU), and zinc (15 mg) may be helpful for skin resiliency and repair.

Cures from Grandma's Kitchen

Add 1 pound (455 g) of baking soda and 1 cup (235 ml) of apple cider vinegar or 2 handfuls of oatmeal tied into a cloth into the bathtub to ease eczema and psoriasis. (See the section on therapeutic baths on page 21 for more ideas.) You can also apply black tea with a clean cloth to affected skin as the tannic acid helps dry the eczema blisters.

Essential oils that can be applied topically to get rid of warts include bergamot, cedarleaf (also known as thuja), cinnamon, clove, eucalyptus, garlic, lavender, lemon, niaouli, oregano, patchouli, and/or tea tree.

Salicylic acid is a substance that occurs in nature and is available in over the counter anti-wart preparations. But avoid using over the counter wart remedies on the face or genitals as they can irritate the delicate surrounding tissues.

SUPPLEMENTS THAT GET RID OF WARTS

Supplements that help get rid of warts include daily doses of vitamins A (10,000 IU), B complex (50 mg), C (1,000 mg), E (400 IU), and zinc (15 mg). You can find them all in an antioxidant formula. Also include 500 mg of lysine daily as an antiviral agent.

BEST FOODS TO GET RID OF WARTS

To get rid of warts, eat more apples, asparagus, avocados, barley, carrots, celery, cucumbers, endive, garlic, millet, onions, pineapple, radish, seaweed, and winter squash. All of these foods invigorate the blood and disperse stagnation. Avoid fried foods and hormonally treated animal products, which congest the body, overload the liver, and make it more difficult to break down other toxins.

GOOD TO KNOW!
Taking homeopathic Thuja (30c, four pellets under the tongue four times daily) will help the body's immunity against warts.

OTHER REMEDIES TO TRY

Here are some other remedies you may want to try to get rid of a wart:

- Cover the wart (including plantar warts on the soles of your feet) with any kind of medical or first aid tape or a bandage and leave on around the clock for three weeks, removing only to change the tape.
- Gently file the wart down with an emery board.
- Moxibustion, usually done by an acupuncturist (until you learn to do it yourself), can help a wart to atrophy and fall off within several days.
- Apply duct tape to a wart for up to six days. Remove the tape and gently rub with a pumice stone or emery board. Leave the tape off for a night and reapply in the morning, continuing for six more days.

Skip This!

Plantar warts, those on the soles of your feet, are contagious and are frequently picked up in moist areas such as bathrooms, locker rooms, and around swimming pools. Avoid going barefoot in these areas and keep your feet dry. To get rid of them, first use a pumice stone to remove any dead skin. Next, make a paste of baking soda and castor oil, apply it, and cover it with a waterproof band-aid. Plantar warts are difficult to get rid of and may take three to six weeks before any progress is noted.

- Consider drawing a picture of the body with the warts and then throwing the drawing in the fire. Warts have been demonstrated to be susceptible to the power of suggestion. When working on getting rid of a wart, tell it, "You will be gone by August 21 (or other date several weeks in advance)."
- Warts can be emotionally related to harboring anger and resentment. Forgive the past and protect yourself with thoughts of joy and peace.

GOOD TO KNOW!

As with any virus, warts are contagious, but not in the normal sense of being contagious as in catching someone else's cold. The other person needs to be susceptible to the virus. Only genital warts and those around the anus are especially contagious through contact, and care must be taken not to spread them to others. If they are in an area you shave, stop shaving. If you scrape them or use a hair removal cream, the scraping will spread the wart virus.

Thrifty Cure!

Make a compress from the inside of a banana peel to get rid of that wart! You can also take some green (not fully ripe) black walnuts and make a few incisions in the outer shell and rub the juice on the warts. There may be a slight stinging sensation or the area may turn brown, but this is only temporary. It's a very effective cure!

Cures from Grandma's Kitchen

Some of the most effective topical folk remedies for warts include applying the fresh juice of dandelion stem or flower, castor oil, fresh elderberry juice, raw potato, garlic oil, milkweed juice, or a paste of baking soda and enough apple cider vinegar to moisten. You can also apply a fresh slice of garlic daily to the affected area, but cover up the nearby skin with some Vaseline to prevent it from becoming irritated from the garlic. You can also prick a vitamin A (2,500 mg) capsule and apply it topically.

WHEN TO SEE YOUR M.D.

See your doctor for the following:

- You are not sure whether a skin growth is a wart.
- You are older than 60 and have never had warts.
- Home treatment is not successful after 2 to 3 months.
- Warts are growing or spreading despite treatment.
- Infection develops, including increased pain, swelling, redness, tenderness, or heat.
- Red streaks extending from the area or the presence of pus.
- You have a fever.

Repairing Wrinkles

As we age, our bodies produce less collagen and elastin, circulation decreases, and sebaceous glands function less actively, resulting in wrinkles. Both smoking and drinking can cause you to wrinkle more easily, as can exposure to the sun. But you can repair the damage. Here's how.

HERBS AND SUPPLEMENTS THAT FIGHT WRINKLES

To keep your skin moist and deter wrinkles, drink mineral-rich herbal teas of marshmallow root, Irish moss, plantain leaves, and violet leaves. All of these herbs are rich in soothing emollient compounds that help provide lubrication to the body. Aim for 3 to 4 cups each day. Drink plenty of water too, at least 8 to 10 glasses daily.

 GOOD TO KNOW!

Slant boards are a wonderful way to de-stress on a daily basis, and lying on one for 10 to 20 minutes daily helps prevent wrinkles and improves skin quality by improving circulation to the face. I bought one as a present to myself a few years back and love it. However, don't use slant boards if you have had a recent stroke, have high blood pressure, or have a detached retina without consulting with your physician.

 GOOD TO KNOW!

Repetitive facial movements and extreme facial expressions, such as frowning, squinting, wrinkling the nose, and propping one's face in one's hands, pull on the skin and weaken its supportive structure. Avoid squinting and frowning, as this will edge unnecessary lines in your face. Use a small hand mirror to watch yourself speak on the phone sometime to observe just how many face-wrinkling movements you might be making.

 GOOD TO KNOW

If you smile, you're more likely to have smoother skin than those who frown constantly. When you smile, you only use thirteen muscles. Frowning uses many more. So get grinning!

Vitamin C (1,000 mg daily) is necessary for collagen production. Vitamin E (400 IU daily) helps our bodies utilize oxygen better, balances hormonal production, and preserves the skin's elasticity. Zinc (15 mg daily) helps synthesize collagen and is essential in restoring dry flaky skin into balance.

ESSENTIAL OILS THAT FIGHT WRINKLES

Essential oils against wrinkles include chamomile, frankincense, lavender, and neroli and can be found in many natural cleansers and moisturizers. You can also make your own, here's how:

Magic Moisturizer

$3/4$ ounce (21 g) beeswax

1 cup (235 ml) vegetable oil such as almond or coconut

15 drops essential oil of frankincense

15 drops neroli essential oil

15 drops lavender essential oil

1 cup (235 ml) water

Grate the beeswax, add the vegetable oil, and gently melt them together in a double boiler. When the wax has melted, allow it to cool for a few minutes, but not long enough for it to harden. Pour the water into a blender. Turn the blender on to high speed and slowly add the beeswax and oil mixture. After about $3/4$ of the oil has been added, the mixture will begin to harden. Turn the blender off and stir. With the stirring implement removed, restart the blender, adding the rest of the beeswax/oil mixture. Then add the essential oils. Don't over blend. Put moisturizer into clean, wide-mouth containers. Store any extra in the refrigerator. Use it on your face and body.

For directions on making other cosmetic preparations, please check out my book *Beauty by Nature* (Book Publishing Company, 2006).

BEST FOODS TO FIGHT WRINKLES

Fruit, yogurt, and buttermilk contain the much-touted alpha-hydroxy acids that stimulate new cell growth, are humectants, and result in younger-looking skin. Eat these on a regular basis. Moisture-rich foods include avocados, chia seeds, freshly ground flax seeds, oatmeal, barley, sweet potatoes, and winter squash. Also consume antioxidant-rich colorful fresh fruits (like blueberries and cherries) and vegetables. Do your best to eat at least three servings of some of these foods daily.

BEST PRACTICES TO FIGHT WRINKLES

Don't scrub or rub your face as this causes wrinkles. So does over cleansing the face with harsh soaps that contain deodorants and detergents. This can strip the face of moisturizing oils. Choose soaps with white clay, oatmeal, or olive oil. These are the least drying. Better yet are gentle nonsoap cleansers available with dry skin-soothing ingredients such as calendula. After you wash your face, apply moisturizer. Water helps to keep the skin's outer layers from drying out and oil seals it in. You know better than to suntan or use tanning booths!

During the day, rehydrate your skin with a mineral water spray, even over makeup. Reapply moisturizer faithfully. The keratinized protein of the top layers of skin requires water to look and feel supple.

Before bed, massage a small amount of serum, which is concentrate of potent substances that nourish the skin (containing less water than a cream or lotion) and then moisturizer in any lines you want to reduce.

Sleep on your back, as sleeping all crunched causes creases leading to permanent lines. Sleep with an open window. Not only does fresh air encourage sleep, it provides oxygen to your body.

Getting Rid of Dandruff

Snow on your shoulder can be embarrassing when it comes from dandruff. Dandruff can be caused by an excessively dry or oily scalp, by sensitivity to hair and scalp products (color, perms, sprays, conditioners, etc.), by fungal overgrowth, and by stress, trauma, and illness. Simple dandruff (pityriasis) manifests as dry, flaky scalp, especially when the hair and scalp are brushed. Seborrheic dermatitis results from overactive sebaceous glands causing an oily scalp and can range from small scaly dandruff to large patches. The best remedies for dandruff are good nutrition and hygiene.

BEST SHAMPOOS FOR DANDRUFF

Look for shampoos and conditioners that contain tea tree, lavender, or rosemary essential oils, all of which are antifungal. Selenium in dandruff products helps remove scalp buildup and control itching and flaking. Sulfur when used in dandruff products can help restore damaged hair. Zinc is often included in shampoos to relieve dandruff, as it is immune enhancing.

A folk remedy to treat dandruff is to mix the juice of ginger with an equal amount of cold-pressed coconut oil. Apply before bed and shampoo it out in the morning. Jamaicans rub aloe vera juice into the scalp until the dandruff disappears. In Burma, coconut oil is used in the same way.

GOOD TO KNOW!
Dandruff that is fungal-related can be contagious, so avoid sharing towels, combs, hats, or other materials that come in contact with the head.

GOOD TO KNOW!
The following anti-dandruff aromatherapy rinse works great!

2 tablespoons (10 ml) apple cider vinegar

5 drops essential oil of rosemary

1 cup (235 ml) pure water

Mix together the ingredients and apply to the scalp after every shampoo. Leave on for at least five minutes, but ideally just leave it on.

Cures from Grandma's Kitchen

Make a facial mask with mashed ripe avocado, banana, or carrot pulp. Just mash up the fruit, apply to the face, and leave on for 5 to 10 minutes. Rinse well and apply moisturizer.

Jojoba oil helps to dissolve imbedded sebum in the scalp, so look for jojoba-based hair care products.

BEST FOOD FOR DANDRUFF

It is normal to experience some flaking of the scalp, but if it's excessive, your diet may be too rich in sugar, fat, dairy products, and fried foods. A tablespoon (15 ml) of cold-pressed hemp seed oil or two omega-3 oil capsules daily will help the body better metabolize fats and help balance both dry and oily scalp conditions. Broccoli and onions are both high in selenium and sulfur, which help curb dandruff from within. Drink a quart (950 ml) of nettle herb tea daily for its high antifungal sulfur content.

Remedying Hair Loss

Alopecia totalis is the loss of all scalp hair. Sometimes hair loss is genetic (androgenic alopecia), but it can also occur from stress, psoriasis, a variety of drugs (those for blood pressure and cholesterol, for example), hormonal imbalances, kidney disease, thyroid deficiency, and more. Nutritional deficiencies (including anorexia and bulimia) can also impede the cell proliferation and division of hair. One frequent cause of male balding is excessive production of the hormones androgen and testosterone. Both of these hormones can cause the hair follicle to shrink. In men, hair loss patterns typically follow the maternal rather than paternal side. Though it is most common in men, hair loss can also be experienced by women. Here's how natural remedies can help minimize hair loss.

HERBS THAT PROMOTE HAIR GROWTH

Many herbs have been used to improve hair growth and diminish hair loss. For all of these herbs, mix a blend of your choice and drink three cups of tea from them daily:

- Nettles and oat straw, with their high mineral content, are good for women and men with hair loss.
- Burdock root is a nutritive herb that helps break up fatty deposits that can obstruct bodily functions, including hair growth.
- Horsetail is rich in the minerals silica and selenium, which helps promote good scalp circulation.
- Rosemary improves circulation to the scalp and all other parts of the body.
- Licorice root prevents testosterone from becoming dihydrotestosterone, which is a substance believed to damage hair follicles, thus curbing hair loss in men.
- Saw palmetto also prevents the conversion of testosterone into dihydrotestosterone.

 GOOD TO KNOW!
Schizandra berries were widely used among the royalty of ancient China as a youth preserver, beautifier, and sexual tonic. They nourish the kidney essence, calm the liver, purify the blood, and promote radiant skin and hair. They are both astringent and demulcent, having the ability to both dry and moisten the system as needed.

FOLK REMEDIES FOR HAIR LOSS

If the hair roots are still alive, rubbing a clove of garlic or a piece of onion (preferably when sleeping alone!) over the scalp before bed increases circulation and encourages hair growth. The scalp can be first warmed with a steaming towel to be even more effective. Shampoo and condition in the morning..

You can also take fresh-peeled ginger dipped in brandy and rub it over the balding area, or mix castor oil with equal amounts of fresh onion juice, cover with a scarf and leave on overnight. Do this for two consecutive weeks.

Applying tincture of cayenne to the balding area of the scalp also increases circulation and stimulates hair growth. Keep it away from the eyes and mouth.

Aloe vera gel can be applied to the scalp until it tingles fully. This stimulates the hair follicles and promotes thick, full hair.

℞ WHEN TO SEE YOUR M.D. Sudden hair loss can be a sign of serious health changes and should be discussed with a competent health professional.

Other folk remedies to use to stimulate hair growth and stop hair loss include applying fresh stinging nettles to the balding area by lightly beating them on the head. Be aware that this can cause a rash and irritation that lasts up to 24 hours, yet can be very helpful. I would never suggest such a harebrained idea, except it is valid part of European herbal practice, and my own husband since 1978 has done this many times and still has beautiful hair.

I personally know of three men who have told me the following remedy worked for them: Buff your fingernails against each other in a circular motion. Do this five minutes at a time, three times daily. This sure beats biting your nails and is also said to help slow down hair loss and graying.

BEST FOODS FOR HEALTHY HAIR

Soybeans help to block the formation of dihydrotestosterone, a hormone associated with hair loss. They are best when fermented in the form of unpasteurized miso or nama shoyu tamari.

Eat a diet that tonifies the kidneys such as black and kidney beans, chia seeds, black sesame seeds, wild rice, and sun cured olives, all rich sources of trace minerals.

Eat silicon-rich foods such as kelp and onions. Also eat the outer (organic) skin of cucumbers and red peppers for their high silica content, a nutrient needed for healthy hair.

Cures from Grandma's Kitchen

Use an apple cider vinegar rinse ($^1/_3$ cup [80 ml] vinegar, $^2/_3$ cup [160 ml] water). Pour on after rinsing your shampoo off and leave on. The vinegar smell will leave when your hair dries. This works as a great antifungal agent.

Other good foods include cabbage, kale, watercress, cauliflower, raspberries, parsnips, cranberries, Brussels sprouts, oats, onions, nuts, buckwheat, barley, nutritional yeast, almonds, seaweeds, and seeds such as pumpkin and sunflower. These foods are high in hair-healthy nutrients such as sulfur, protein, B vitamins, and zinc.

Finally, drink juices of beet, carrot, nettle, and spinach with a bit of onion to help improve circulation to the body (including the scalp) and provide a variety of trace minerals.

KEEP IN MIND

To preserve hair, don't shampoo every day as it causes more hair to fall out. Wear the hair loose to avoid pulling at the scalp.

Spend about 20 minutes daily lying on a slant board to allow increased blood flow to the scalp. You can also consider yoga postures such as the shoulder stand or headstands as they improve blood flow to the scalp. However, note that these are advanced poses and should not be attempted unless you are familiar with yoga.

Let go of negative thought patterns. Rather than saying, "I'm losing all my hair," try "I'm taking better care of myself. My hair will grow thick." Bald can also be beautiful!

Thrifty Cure!

Coloring the scalp in thin areas of hair with a soft eyebrow pencil can minimize the visibility of hair loss until natural remedies have a chance to take effect.

Skip This!

Avoid a diet high in heated fats and refined sugar. Hydrogenated oils are likely to clog the pores. Minimize alcohol, caffeine, sugar, and refined carbohydrate consumption, which all cause the body to become overly acidic and unhealthy.

Cures from Grandma's Kitchen

Here is a super smoothie you can drink daily to help promote hair growth:

1 cup (235 ml) raw almond milk
1 ripe banana
1 tablespoon (6 g) nutritional yeast
½ cup (32 g) raw pumpkin seeds
½ teaspoon bee pollen
½ teaspoon sea kelp
1 tablespoon (20 g) blackstrap molasses

Whiz in the blender until smooth and then enjoy.

Getting Rid of Body Odor

Body odor comes from sweat, which is made up of water, sodium salts, lactic acid, sulfuric acid, potassium, phosphorus, iron, and urea. Sweat is secreted by the exocrine glands, which are located in the armpits, face, chest, pubic area, and anal regions. Sweat actually has a purpose, moisturizing the skin, maintaining a healthy acid balance, and preventing unhealthy proliferations of microbes. But too much can be off putting. Here's how to smell sweeter!

HERBS THAT ABSORB BODY ODOR

Add a 1/2 teaspoon of an essential oil such as lavender, sage, or rosemary to an ounce of baking soda and apply a bit to the underarm area after bathing or when getting dressed to absorb mild to moderate perspiration. Aloe vera juice can be applied directly as an antibacterial, antifungal, and deodorizing ally.

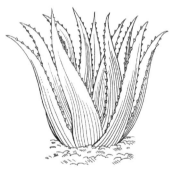

BEST FOODS TO FIGHT BODY ODOR

To smell sweeter, eat plenty of greens and radishes and drink lemon in water, all of which are naturally detoxifying. Use super green foods like wheat grass, spirulina, barley grass, or chlorophyll, which are available in capsules, three times daily. Chlorophyll is regarded as a natural deodorizer.

KEEP IN MIND

Many deodorants contain aluminum chlorohydrate, a manufactured form of aluminum that many believe contributes to Alzheimer's disease. It is known to accumulate in the tissues, especially when applied to broken skin. This is a real problem as many people apply it just after shaving. Yikes! Many deodorants also contain synthetic fragrances and methyl- and propylparabens, both of which have been implicated in breast cancer. Instead, look for deodorants that contain ingredients such as coriander and tea tree oil. You can find some good deodorants in natural food stores. Weleda's spray deodorants work great.

Another practice that can help is to wear natural-fiber clothes so the skin can breathe. Certain synthetics produce an unpleasant smell soon after wearing and do not allow sweat to evaporate naturally.

GOOD TO KNOW!

In order to make themselves more alluring, harem women ate fenugreek seeds to produce a seductive smell. You can eat fenugreek sprouts or make a tea of this herb, available at health food stores.

Strengthening Weak Nails

We use our hands to express ourselves, so healthy nails are important. Nails are made of keratin, a strong fibrous protein that is produced by cells beneath the cuticle at the nail's base. Nails grow about $1/250$ of an inch daily (about $1/3$ to $1/2$ as fast as hair). Nail growth is generally faster during the summer and between the ages of 18 and 28 for some yet-undiscovered reason. Here are some natural ways to strengthen weak nails.

NUTRIENTS THAT STRENGTHEN NAILS

The best nail hardeners are nourishing foods, rich in trace minerals and phytochemicals: fresh fruit and vegetables, especially green leafy vegetables, sea vegetables, nuts, and seeds. Drink mineral-rich teas of nettles, horsetail, and oat straw, one quart (950 ml) daily individually or mixed together.

Gently massage the cuticles whenever applying hand lotion to keep them pliable and less likely to crack. Polishing nails with a buff gives them a natural shine.

STRATEGIES FOR STOPPING NAIL BITING AND OTHER BAD HABITS

Biting your nails and cuticles can cause swelling and redness and make one prone to infections of the hands. Nail biting can also cause dental problems. Biting the nails can be an indication of stress and/or a calcium deficiency. So as a start, take a daily supplement of calcium (1,000 mg) and magnesium (500 mg). You can also use tea tree oil topically on the fingers as the pungent taste is a bitter deterrent to nail biting.

To stop biting your nails, start by making a list of the reasons why you should stop. Put it where you will read it—above a sink, on a mirror, on a bookmark, or in your wallet. Being clear about why you want to give up a habit is important.

If you do catch yourself indulging in the habit, say "Stop" aloud to yourself and later under your breath. Every time you catch yourself engaging in a bad habit, write it down in your calendar or journal. Wear a loose elastic band around your wrist and snap it hard every time you indulge.

Cures From Grandma's Kitchen

To reduce body odor, look in your fridge. Rub lemon peel (not the juice) or fresh sage leaves on skin to inhibit bacteria and odor. When using sage leaves, simply grab a handful of the leaves from the garden, crush them between your fingers, and rub the pieces on potentially odiferous areas of the body such as under the arms. You can even rub a piece of cucumber into potentially smelly body portions.

Have someone photograph you indulging in your addiction or habit while you look into the camera. When you get the photo back, look at it carefully and ask yourself what it is trying to tell you. Put all that extra energy into doing something good that helps society and yourself.

Whatever part of the body is involved in the habit (nails, hair, skin, etc.), do something different and more positive. Instead of biting your nails, buff them. Instead of picking at your face, massage it. Play with toys for a few minutes such as modeling clay or Chinese handballs. Keep these tools where you are likely to need them.

Be consistent and keep track of your progress. Consider showing your progress chart to someone you really trust. Tell them you are not asking them to nag at you, but ask them in what ways they can best help you. Reward yourself. For example, if you go all day or week without engaging in a habit, put some money in a piggybank so that you can buy something special.

Decide to change. Refuse to be enslaved by anything. Learn to deal with any lapses in a positive healing way. Be a free conscious being. Habits are automatic and the way out of them is to remember the way out.

Skip This!

Nail polish removers are hard on the health of nails. Of all the cosmetics available, nail polish is one of the most allergenic. Acetone is more harmful than acetate. Avoid using cuticle removers or pushing them back as the cuticle helps protect the fingers.

CHAPTER 15

NATURAL REMEDIES FOR ORAL HEALTH

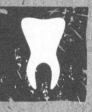

Oral health is key to healthy teeth, gums, and fresh breath. Here's how to care for this gateway into our internal health.

Freshening Bad Breath

Bad breath is at least embarrassing and at worst offensive to others. It can be caused by eating a food you are allergic to (like dairy products), constipation, detoxifying the body, some medications, tooth or gum problems, poor health in the lungs, as well as eating garlic. When the mouth is dry, such as in the morning from not having had any water in several hours, salvia production decreases and can contribute to bad breath. Here's how to freshen up now!

BREATH-FRESHENING HERBS

Drink a tea using anise seed, cardamom, cinnamon, cloves, fennel, orange peel (if organic), parsley, or peppermint or let the tea cool and use it as a breath-freshening mouthwash. They are all high in antimicrobial essential oils.

FRESH BREATH PRACTICES

Bacteria can collect on the tongue. Brushing your tongue or using a tongue scraper gets rid of twice as much bacteria as simply brushing your teeth. You can even use a soup spoon instead of a tongue scraper. Just insert the spoon upside down and press the edges into the tongue. Rub it across the surface several times and then follow with a rinse of cool water.

If you still suffer from bad breath, take three chlorophyll capsules daily, which act as a natural deodorizer.

Soothing Canker Sores, Cold Sores, or Fever Blisters

Canker sores are an irritation inside the mouth that can make eating difficult and painful. Cold sores or fever blisters are painful ulcerations caused by viruses that appear on your lip, mouth, or nose. Too much sugar and stress can all make you more prone to both. Here's how to soothe those sores right now.

Cures from Grandma's Kitchen

It's easy to make an instant breath freshener. Just take ¹/₂ cup (120 ml) of water and add 4 drops anise, fennel, cinnamon, peppermint, or tea tree essential oil.

For cold sores, do a warm salt-water swish (1 tablespoon [18 g] of salt in 8 ounces [235 ml] of water) every hour. Though it will sting, it will help heal the cold sore more quickly. It can also help to apply ice held in a white handkerchief. Leave it on as long as you can and do it as often as possible.

Salves that contain combinations of soothing and antiviral substances including the amino acid lysine (which inhibits the virus's replication), anti-inflammatory licorice, and antiviral melissa (aka lemon balm) essential oil can help heal cold sores. Look for these salves at a natural foods store and apply them 3 or 4 times daily.

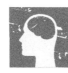

Thrifty Cures!

Chewing on whole cinnamon bark pieces, cloves, fennel seed, or peeled cardamom pods will give your mouth an alluring flavor your lover will want to kiss. My favorite breath-freshening remedy is to suck on a whole clove for a long-lasting, inexpensive breath freshener. Even if you take a few bites of food, you can tuck the clove between your cheek and gum with your tongue and then bring it back in your mouth after eating. You can also eat a sprig of parsley or a small piece of lemon peel to freshen the breath. Apples and celery are natural breath fresheners too. Eat them liberally!

You can also apply aloe vera gel, a pinch of baking soda, apple cider vinegar, calendula salve, goldenseal powder, or tea tree oil to help combat bacteria.

Finally, take probiotics (1 capsule three times daily) and lysine (550 mg 3 times daily) to boost immunity when feeling vulnerable. You can also find lysine in flounder, nutritional yeast, and potatoes.

Improving Gum Health

Healthy gums can mean the difference between keeping your teeth or not. Unfortunately, one in three people over the age of 30 has some form of periodontal disease but are unaware of it because it is a problem that develops silently and painlessly. Periodontal disease occurs when bacteria in plaque infect the gums and bones that anchor the teeth. Bleeding gums, inflamed gums, loose teeth, change in bite, and recession are all indicators of periodontal disease, which accounts for 70 percent of tooth loss. Bacterial toxins are also released into the bloodstream, beginning a cascade of health problems. Recent research has revealed a relationship between periodontal infection and more serious health problems, such as cardiovascular disease, diabetes, respiratory diseases, and preterm low birth weight babies. So it's important to do all you can to make your gums healthy. Here are some natural remedies for your gums.

 GOOD TO KNOW!
It's important to replace your toothbrush after a canker sore or cold sore episode because the virus thrives in a damp environment.

Both sage and sea salt have antiseptic properties that reduce inflammation and promote healing. They are also astringent, which helps tighten the gums. Just pour 1 cup (235 ml) of boiling water over 1 tablespoon (2.5 g) of sage leaves, cover and steep for 15 minutes, strain, and add 2 teaspoons (10 g) of sea salt. Use twice daily after brushing your teeth. Refrigerate between uses.

You can also add a drop of tea tree oil to your toothbrush on top of your toothpaste and brush as usual. Tea tree oil, derived from the leaves of the native Australian Melaleuca alternifolia tree, contains antiseptic compounds which help prevent gum disease. Make sure the product label says it is 100 percent pure tea tree oil.

Chewing burdock root massages the gums and improves stomach activity. You can also massage bleeding gums with a piece of inner lemon rind. Or try my plaque fighting, gum strengthening solution:

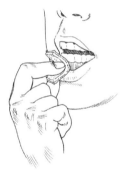

Take $^1/_8$ ounce of coconut oil; add 8 drops oil of myrrh, 8 drops tea tree oil, and 2 drops peppermint oil. Shake before using and massage a few drops into your gums to promote healthy teeth and gums.

Another formula to massage into receding gums to increase circulation, tighten tissues, and decrease microbes as follows:

2 parts yerba mansa
$^1/_2$ part myrrh
2 parts echinacea
2 parts prickly ash bark

For bleeding gums, you can make a mouth rinse or use herbal tea of some of the herbs mentioned above to run through a Water Pik oral irrigation type device that shoots out a gentle stream of water to clean and massage teeth and gums. This is a great way to clean out any missed places, stimulate circulation, and get an herbal treatment at the same time! Use once a day.

Soothing Toothache

A toothache usually indicates it is time to visit the dentist. Do not delay! But if it's the middle of the night or the weekend and you can't get an appointment, natural remedies can ease the pain temporarily. Here's how.

Apply a few drops of clove oil to the area with your finger. It's a natural anesthetic and germicide containing the active ingredient eugenol. For children, dilute the clove oil with equal amounts of olive oil. After applying, keep your mouth open a few seconds to allow it to dry and minimize the strong clove blast on your mouth and tongue. A plantain poultice or resin from a pine tree can also be applied to draw out infection.

Another good idea? Place a piece of garlic on the area of the painful tooth for twenty minutes. It will increase circulation to the area and combat infection. A hot ginger compress applied to the cheek area over the afflicted tooth will also help relieve pain.

GOOD TO KNOW!

Several studies have shown that chronic dental infection is associated with a significant increase in the risk of stroke. Here's why: bacteria from dental plaque, including *Streptococcus sanguis*, can enter your bloodstream and cause blood platelets to clump together and clot abnormally. Normally, the bacteria are cleared from your body by the immune system, but if your immune system is compromised, as is the case with any infection, the bacteria create a major risk factor. Gum infections lead to chronic inflammation and the buildup of arterial plaque, which reduces circulation. The result is atherosclerosis, or hardening and narrowing of the arteries, which can lead to a heart attack or stroke.

In addition, a hot ginger or mustard footbath will help to draw pain away from the head. Just soak your feet for three minutes in hot tea and then plunge them into icy cold water for a minute. You'll want to alternate back and forth for about 15 minutes. Start with the hot and end with the cold.

Every couple of hours, add 1 teaspoon (6 g) of salt to 1 cup (235 ml) of water (hot or cold) and swish it around to help remove bacteria. Apply cold compresses or ice in the mouth for numbing qualities as needed. A hot water bottle can also give comfort. You'll need to decide whether warm or cold applications make the pain worse or better.

Take 50 to 100 mg of niacin to help move congested blood at the site of a toothache. Goldenseal and myrrh in capsule or tincture form and applied topically can help clear up an infection.

Achieving Total Tooth Health the Natural Way

As children, most of us had 20 teeth. As adults, the norm is 32, including 8 incisors, eight premolars, 4 canines, and 12 molars. Some people who lose their second set of teeth get a third one—from their dentist! Even though Americans have checkups, fluoridated water, and new improved toothpastes, about 35 percent will have full or partial dentures by age 60. Some tooth problems are hereditary, others aggravated by lack of care. Many tooth problems can be helped with good nutrition and proper care. Here's how.

NATURAL WAYS TO KEEP TEETH HEALTHY

Cultures that use chewing sticks for oral hygiene have lower instances of dental disease. Pick a twig from a bay, beech, birch, dogwood, fir, eucalyptus, juniper, maple, neem, oak pine, poplar, or sumac tree. Peel off the bark. Use your teeth to chew the twig end until it is bristly.

GOOD TO KNOW!

If you lose a filling (which can make your tooth ache) keep any broken tooth part, especially if it is gold or porcelain, and bring it with you to the dentist. Fill the hole temporarily with a piece of beeswax so you don't scratch your tongue.

Then use this to gently massage your teeth and gums. You can also dip the twig in water and baking soda.

Herbs that provide nutrients for strengthening the teeth include alfalfa, horsetail, nettles, and oat straw. Try drinking a tea of various combinations of these plants three times daily. Bilberry and hawthorn are high in flavonoids, which may be helpful in protecting the periodontal ligaments.

BEST VITAMINS AND MINERALS FOR TEETH

Calcium, the main element of which teeth are composed, is a necessary nutrient for teeth and gums. Calcium can help prevent bone loss and teeth grinding. Be sure to use a calcium supplement that is either a chelate, citrate, or hydroxyapatite. Calcium is best assimilated with some magnesium, so take 1,000 mg

℞ WHEN TO SEE YOUR M.D.

If your tooth is knocked out, get to a dentist within half an hour! If the tooth is loose but doesn't fall out of your mouth, keep it in your mouth (place it into the socket), cover with sterile gauze, apply slight compression, and get to a dentist or an emergency room where dentists are on call.

If the tooth falls out of your mouth, rinse off any dirt and blood and replace it in the socket. The roots of the tooth must be kept moist. Don't hold the tooth by the root! If it does fall out and can't be kept in the mouth due to other injuries, store it in milk wrapped in a cloth or piece of gauze as you hasten to the dentist. Or simply hold the tooth under the tongue until dental health has been obtained.

Take two drops of Rescue Remedy and homeopathic arnica (3 or 4 pellets under the tongue four times daily) to help deal with the trauma of the event.

calcium and 500 mg magnesium daily. Note that excess soft drinks and meat can contribute to calcium loss.

Vitamin C (100 mg daily) with bioflavonoids (500 mg daily) can help prevent and treat sore and bleeding gums since they help collagen production. Vitamin C deficiency can contribute to breakdown of connective tissue that produces blood vessel walls, bone matrix, cartilage, collagen, and dentin. However, it is best to avoid chewable vitamin C, especially for adults, as the ascorbic acid can be corrosive to dental enamel.

Deficiency of B vitamins, especially folic acid, can cause weakened gums. Birth control pills can create a need for more B complex. Take 50 mg B complex and 400 mg folic acid daily (which is likely to be contained in the B complex tablet). Coenzyme Q 10 (take 50 to 100 mg twice daily) has been found helpful for gingivitis. It improves circulation and increases oxygen levels in the tissues.

Vitamin E (400 IU) and selenium (50 mg) are both natural antioxidants. Rub them on gums to tonify the tissues, after pricking the capsule with a pin. Vitamin D (1,000 IU) helps bone formation. Zinc (15 mg) inhibits plaque formation and inflammation. These last two supplements are taken orally daily.

Essential fatty acids can also help reduce inflammation. Take 2 or 3 capsules of a good quality fish oil each day.

Thrifty Cure!

Rub a fresh cut raspberry or strawberry over the teeth for its natural whitening action due to their high concentration of acids. Or use this tooth whitener you can make at home. Just add 1 teaspoon (5 g) baking soda to enough hydrogen peroxide to make a paste. Use it to brush teeth for two minutes.

Cures from Grandma's Kitchen

Make a simple tooth-cleaning powder with 1 cup (221 g) baking soda, 2 tablespoons (30 g) sea salt, and 5 drops essential oil such as anise, cinnamon, peppermint, rosemary, spearmint, or tea tree. The essential oils will freshen the breath and they taste good!

Baking soda cleans teeth, removes stains, and does not damage tooth enamel. It also is antibacterial and neutralizes plaque acids.

Salt helps to draw out agents that contribute to decay. Salt also helps to lessen the reactions of sensitive teeth from hot or cold and curbs bleeding from the gums. Use this mixture a few times a week. It can be abrasive if used excessively.

BEST FOODS FOR HEALTHY TEETH

Teeth are nourished through their roots, building and renewing from the materials we eat. Foods considered beneficial for the teeth include yogurt (calcium and probiotics inhibit bacterial growth), tomatoes (lycopene, an antioxidant), shiitake (lentinan combats plaque), green tea (catechin inhibits plaque), onion (combats mouth bacteria), celery (cleans teeth), and kiwi (vitamin C strengthens gums). Fluorine in moderate doses can help prevent tooth decay and occurs naturally in avocados, cabbage, black-eyed peas, brown rice, cheese, rye, sea vegetables, green tea, green leafy vegetables, and goat's milk.

Snacks of crunchy foods like raw carrots, celery, sunflower seeds, and apples massage the gums. Eating fresh corn helps to strengthen the teeth and gums. The French tradition of eating some cheese at the end of a meal helps counteract mouth acids and is beneficial. Snacks considered okay for the teeth include eggs, fish, raw vegetables, popcorn, and plain yogurt. Chewing all food well helps seat the teeth more firmly.

BEST PRACTICES FOR HEALTHY TEETH

Flossing first allows you to brush away dislodged particles later. Flossing is even more important than brushing. Take 18 inches (46 cm) of the floss of your choice and wrap it around the middle fingers of both hands. While holding the middle of the floss between the extended thumb or forefinger, insert it gently between two teeth in a "C" fashion. Press the floss toward the back of one tooth while you gently bring it into the gum and move the floss up and down several times. Pull the floss forward against the other tooth and floss up and down several times. Avoid forceful flossing that can cut into the gums. If you use waxed floss, look for brands using beeswax or jojoba rather than petroleum products and dye.

After a thorough flossing, use a soft brush and brush at a 45-degree angle at the gum line, pressing gently. Jiggle the brush back and forth, and then rotate it downward to wipe off the tooth. Do this a few times in each location before moving on. This is known as the "modified bass technique." Ask your dentist for a demonstration. Brush not only the teeth for about two minutes but also the gums and tongue with

GOOD TO KNOW!

Use this tooth powder to keep teeth healthy:

Brigitte's Tooth Powder
- ¹/₄ cup (55 g) baking soda
- 20 drops peppermint essential oil
- 20 drops tea tree essential oil

Combine ingredients and sprinkle on a damp toothbrush. Store the remainder in a clean glass jar with a lid. Remember the oil folk saying: "Be true to your teeth or they'll be false to you!"

toothpaste or baking soda. Brushing too hard can cause gum recession and tooth destruction. Give yourself five minutes to do a good cleaning job. Natural bristles can be too rough and sharp. Rounded bristles are gentler. Change your brush about every six weeks to three months.

Brush after eating sticky foods such as dates and raisins as their sugars can stick to the teeth. Sugary foods produce acids that cause tooth decay and decrease the ability of white blood cells to destroy bacteria. Use a disclosing tablet on occasion to note the areas that are being missed. There are a plethora of gadgets to clean your teeth. Talk to your dentist about what she suggests.

KEEP IN MIND

Some dentists may also offer acupuncture or relaxation tapes. A headset of beautiful music can help mellow the dental drilling sounds. You may find valerian tincture relaxing before a dental appointment. Taking a 500 mg supplement of bromelain, an enzyme derived from pineapple, can help lessen swelling from dental surgery. Take some before and for a few days after major dental work, up to three times daily.

Health food stores have selections of beneficial products for mouth care. Some natural toothpastes contain xylitol, a sweet-tasting substance derived from birch trees. It has anticavity properties. You can also find chewing gums made with xylitol that are used to increase saliva production and reduce cavities. Green tea helps inhibit plaque buildup.

Skip This!

Refined carbohydrates, which break down quickly, also feed the bacteria that cause tooth decay. Many respected health authorities deplore the use of fluoride in our water supply. Though it does help prevent decay, a lifetime of use can mottle the teeth and bones.

Foods likely to stain teeth include coffee, tea, red wine, blueberries, and tobacco. Smoking also contributes to the buildup of tartar and decreases the body's supply of vitamin C. Even milk and rice can cause a buildup of yellowish plaque on the teeth.

Abrasive substances to be careful of using to extreme on the teeth include calcium carbonate (made from stone), dicalcium phosphate (which is bone), and silica, which is a sand substance. They can be damaging to tooth enamel over the years.

Saccharin and artificial colors are not great things to put into your mouth. Harsh chemicals in dental products can aggravate teeth sensitivity. That's why it's important to read the labels on your tooth care products.

CHAPTER 16

NATURAL REMEDIES FOR HEALTHY SLEEP

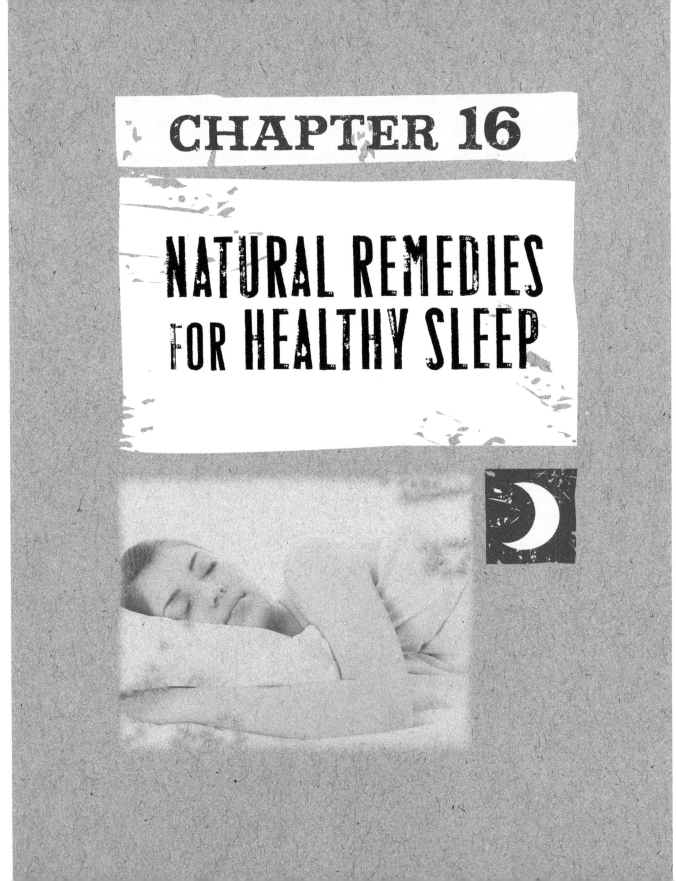

Blissful sleep is that rejuvenating, recharging repose in which about one third of our lives is spent. Only during rest do bone marrow and lymph nodes produce substances to empower our immune systems. It is during the beginning of our sleep cycle that much of the body repair work is done. But for many of us, the peace of sleep may be elusive. Here are natural ways to get those zzzzzs.

Solving Insomnia

When sleep escapes you, there are remedies from the realm of lifestyle, diet, herbs, and supplements that can help you to rest more deeply. Get to the cause of the condition and try a natural cure.

HERBS FOR SWEET DREAMS

Many herbs can be consumed in the evening to aid sleep. Take a dose of herbal tincture or two capsules an hour before bed. Avoid tea because drinking tea before bed is likely to cause you to awaken to urinate!

Chamomile

Chamomile has long been used as a remedy for sleep. It is considered a nerve restorative and helps calm people with anxiety and stress. Chamomile is high in nerve- and muscle-relaxing calcium, magnesium, potassium, and some of the B vitamins known to aid relaxation. Chamomile is also known for its anti-inflammatory and antispasmodic properties that can help a tense person unwind.

Add some chamomile tea to a child's bath before bed to help them sleep peacefully. Taken before bedtime, chamomile is also a traditional remedy to help those prone to nightmares.

Hops

Hops help to induce sleep and provides a pleasant numbing sensation. Hops contain lupulin, which is considered a strong but safe sedative. Hops can help mellow a person with a quarrelsome nature and is an anodyne, meaning it can help pain. Though its taste is bitter, it is safe for children.

Kava kava

Kava kava is an ancient Polynesian remedy for insomnia and nervousness and is reputed to induce vivid dreams. It is often used in the islands ceremoniously as a religious ritual to welcome guests and honor births, marriages, and business deals. It helps foster open communication and a feeling of "letting go." It is an analgesic, antispasmodic, and sedative.

Cures from Grandma's Kitchen

A folk remedy is to cut a piece of yellow onion and place it in a jar. Cover and set on the nightstand. If you wake up or can't fall asleep, open the jar and take several deep inhalations. Recover the jar, lie back down, and you should fall back to sleep within 15 minutes.

Passionflower

Passionflower helps to relax the mind. It is useful for worried insomniacs. It slows down the breakdown of serotonin and norepinephrine, allowing one to maintain a more peaceful state of consciousness. Passionflower has traditionally been used to treat hysteria, nervousness, and to aid recovery in nervous breakdown. It is an antispasmodic and sedative.

Skullcap

Skullcap is considered one of the best tonics for the nervous system. It has long been used to calm teething babies and reduce convulsions, delirium, insomnia, neuralgia, restlessness, and even help emotional upsets. It is rich in calcium, magnesium, and potassium. Scutellarin, one of its active ingredients, gets transformed into scutellarein, which stimulates the brain to produce more endorphins. Use skullcap to help rebuild a nervous system that is exhausted. Skullcap is best when used over an extended period of time.

Valerian

Valerian helps sleep disorders that are the result of anxiety. There are some individuals who find valerian works for them as a stimulant rather than a sedative. When this occurs, it is often because their bodies are unable to transform the essential oils in valerian into valerianic acid, one of the main calming components.

For many people, though, valerian calms fear, anxiety, and panic. During World War I, valerian was used to treat shellshock. In Germany, valerian is used for childhood behavioral problems yet still gives the children good reaction time and muscle coordination. Research published in the medical journal, *Pharmacology, Biochemistry and Behavior* with 128 volunteers showed that valerian helped people fall asleep faster.

Skip This!

Sleeping pills are often habit forming and paralyze the part of our brains that control dreaming. They can leave us feeling less than rested and impair clarity of thought. Many prescribed drugs can leave us unable to sleep. Antibiotics, steroids, decongestants, cold remedies, appetite suppressants, contraceptives, and thyroid medications all can make sleep difficult. However, always see your doctor before stopping any medications you are on now.

You'll probably find the smell or taste of valerian objectionable, so use it in a capsule or tincture form rather than as a tea. Valerian is best used for two- to three-week periods or when needed rather than on a daily basis. If you are prone to depression though, check with your health care practitioner first.

HOMEOPATHIC REMEDIES FOR INSOMNIA

A homeopathic remedy that can help induce sleep is Hyland's Calms Forte. You can also use these remedies as needed and indicated:

- Arsenicum album: For insomnia caused by fears, worry, and anxiety—Take this if you wake up in middle of the night and feel the need to walk around or if you are too tired to sleep.
- Chamomilla: For young and old, especially when the cause of insomnia is physical, such as pain

- Coffea cruda: For sleeplessness due to excited mental energy and dreams—Feeling groggy in morning is another indication that this might be the right remedy for you.
- Nux vomica: For sleeplessness due to overindulgence of food, coffee, alcohol, or drugs, and for mental strain and work worries

MELATONIN FOR BETTER SLEEP

Melatonin is produced by the pineal gland and made from the neurotransmitter serotonin. It helps the body regulate circadian rhythms. Getting out in the sun for a bit during the day and turning off the lights earlier at night can help trigger our natural production of melatonin.

Food sources that stimulate natural melatonin production include bananas, barley, and rice. Also eating foods that contain tryptophan, such as bananas, cottage cheese, dates, figs, milk, tofu, and turkey, can boost melatonin levels. The pineal gland converts tryptophan into melatonin. You can also use melatonin sublingually to promote a restful night's sleep. Take 0.03 to 3 mg in the evening for bed.

Melatonin, because it is a hormone and has not been evaluated for its safety during these conditions, should not be used by children, pregnant women, or nursing mothers as well as people with hormonal imbalances, depression, autoimmune disorders, or those on steroids.

GOOD TO KNOW!

Another way to use herbs to help you sleep is to make a 5 by 5 inch (13 x 13 cm) sachet and fill it with hops, lavender, chamomile, woodruff, or lemon balm and put it in your pillowcase. The calming aroma will help you slumber. Both King George II and Abraham Lincoln are said to have used hops pillows to help them sleep. Other pleasant smells like lavender and myrrh will soothe your spirits. Use them in aroma lamps, diffusers, on your pillow, or simply inhale these essential oils.

A warm bath before bed is also comforting. Add 7 drops of essential oil of chamomile or lavender to the bath water. Adding a pound of baking soda makes the water alkalinizing and sedative. When done bathing, remain in the tub for a few minutes while you let the water out and visualize all your tensions going down the drain. A sauna before bed can also help produce a state of calmness.

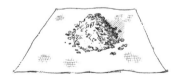

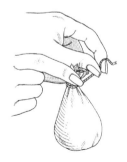

FOODS FOR BETTER SLEEP

It has been said that "Sleep doesn't interfere with digestion, but digestion interferes with sleep." Avoid eating late at night as many foods stimulate the adrenal glands and elevate blood pressure. However, if you insist on eating late at night, the few foods that can actually help sleep include bananas, lettuce, oatmeal, and yogurt. A cup of plain yogurt is naturally rich in calcium and the calming amino acid tryptophan. For some insomniacs, caffeinated food and drinks such as chocolate, coffee, black tea, and sodas may be too stimulating even when consumed early in the day.

BEST PRACTICES FOR BETTER SLEEP

Studies show that people who are more active in the day are less likely to have problems with sleep. But don't exercise too close to bedtime. The hours between 4 pm and 8 pm are ideal. Take a walk after dinner instead of watching TV.

GOOD TO KNOW!

As we get older, our requirements for sleep actually decrease. If you lie awake for more than 30 minutes, get up and write a letter or read something that is not too action packed. If you wake up, don't snack (or your body can get used to demanding 3:00 am munchies). Return to bed after urinating and breathe deeply, thinking of nothing but the in and out of your breathing.

Yoga postures that help to relax the mind and body and that aid sleep include the corpse, cobra pose, shoulder stand, and mountain. T'ai chi, meditation breathing exercises, biofeedback, and guided visualizations can all be effective noninvasive methods to aid sleep.

If your thoughts are keeping you awake, why not download your mental baggage onto a piece of paper before bed and then rest easily knowing that the cares of tomorrow will not be forgotten.

When trying to sleep, allow no thoughts except the in and out of your breath. You should soon be able to bore yourself to sleep. Try some sort of visualization, such as with one breath relax your toes, with the next breath your feet, and moving slowly up your body to help you slumber.

Another sleep technique is to get comfortable in bed and take 8 breaths while lying flat on your back. Then take 16 deep breaths while lying on your right side; then take 32 breaths while lying on your left side. Most people are asleep before completing the exercise.

KEEP IN MIND

The following are some additional tips for getting a good night's sleep:

1. Establish a regular sleep and awakening time and do your best to stick with it.

2. Sleeping with one's head to the magnetic north is said to improve sleep and dream quality.

3. Sleeping on the back is said the give one's internal organs the most room for optimum function. Sleeping on one's left side can put excess pressure on the heart.

4. Paint your bedroom a calm color, like blue. Keep your bedroom space sacred and don't use it as a place to do homework, business,

or carry out arguments. Also, try to put your bed in the quietest and darkest corner of the room.

5. Keep the bedroom between 60 and 66°F (16 and 19°C). Allow a bit of fresh air into the bedroom at night, though not directly by the head.

6. Make sure your bed is comfortable and fabrics that are as natural as possible are used as bedding to allow the skin to breathe. If you don't suffer from allergies, you may find a feather bed a comfortable addition to place on top of your mattress.

7. Be aware that electromagnetic pollution too close to your body can stimulate your nervous system as well as weaken your immune system. Avoid having clocks, stereos, or electric blankets as your nighttime companions.

8. Remember that light is a stimulant. If there is light shining brightly through your windows at night, consider getting heavier curtains. Many mechanical gadgets such as clocks also emit light that can encourage wakefulness.

9. Avoid excess mental activity right before bed, such as action packed TV or page-turning novels. Sex, however, can be a pleasurable prelude to sleep.

10. You may need to use earplugs or eye masks to help shut the world out for a while.

Chasing Away Nightmares

Nightmares can make you afraid to go to bed at night. Often, the sensation you get when you have a nightmare follows you into wakefulness, leaving you feeling strange. Here's how to erase nightmares.

For those prone to nightmares, herbal teas and sachets made of basil, chamomile, dill seed, and rosemary provide a pleasant aroma and are said to dispel disturbing dreams. These herbs can also be hung as sprigs over the bed. Rubbing garlic briefly on the soles of the feet can end night fears and repel evil influence. (Hey, it works to ward away vampires!)

The flower essences Aspen, Rock rose, and Rescue Remedy also help alleviate nightmares. Take 2 drops under the tongue or in a cup of water when needed.

Using the color violet helps calm the spirit. Finally, keep in mind that nightmares are a way of getting your attention, and you may want to explore what their significance is.

Stopping Snoring

If your mate snores, it can keep you from sleeping. Most snorers breathe through their mouth. An obstruction of the airways, usually the tongue, is the cause of this nocturnal noise. Often, when a snorer relaxes into deep sleep, the tongue falls back against the soft palate and tissues at the back of the throat. As one breathes, air enters the throat and causes the tongue and tissues to vibrate against one another. Heavy snorers may even have their tongue sucked into their airway and thus block their breathing!

Skip This!

Avoid eating sweets after dinner or right before bedtime. Excess rich and spicy or oily foods as well as food allergens can provoke nightmares.

When breathing temporarily ceases, survival instincts kick in and the snorer awakens to pull the tongue in before falling back to sleep and repeating the process. This is known as sleep apnea. A person with sleep apnea can be more susceptible to strokes, high blood pressure, and heart attack, not to mention feeling fatigued from lack of sleep. Doctors will may suggest surgery to fix it. However, here are some gentler alternatives you may want to try first:

1. Sew a marble or golf ball into your pajamas at the back of the neck area. This will encourage you to sleep on your side, which usually minimizes snoring.

2. Elevate the head slightly, ideally by placing a brick or two under the bed head. Extra pillows will just give you a sore neck. Special pillows are available that help deter snoring. Look for them in catalogs or bedding supply stores.

3. Try the devices now available in grocery stores and drugstores that you tape to your nose to keep nasal passages open.

4. Natural food stores carry homeopathic drops and sprays that help snorers breathe more easily.

Ask your dentist or doctor about a tongue-retaining antisnoring device.

Have a friend, lover, or spouse record your snoring to see if you need to seek medical attention.

Skip This!

Avoid alcohol for at least three hours before bed as it is a central nervous system depressant and can increase episodes of apnea. Avoid heavy eating and smoking before bed as they both contribute to congestion. Ditto sleeping pills, tranquilizers, and antihistamines as they can also cause the throat muscles to be overly relaxed. Nix foods such as dairy and wheat products that cause mucous congestion. It is worth going a few weeks without any dairy or wheat (as well as gluten) products to see if this makes a difference. Food allergies and sensitivities can cause throat swelling and nasal blockages that lead to snoring. Lose weight if you can. If weight is excessive, the excess bulk in the throat can block airways.

Thrifty Cure!

Put a drop of sesame oil into each nostril, which moistens the tissues and decreases their tendency to vibrate loudly.

R WHEN TO SEE YOUR M.D.

If home remedies are not effective, get evaluated by a medical doctor for the possibility of apnea or obstruction in the respiratory passages.

CHAPTER 17

NATURAL REMEDIES FOR ADDICTION

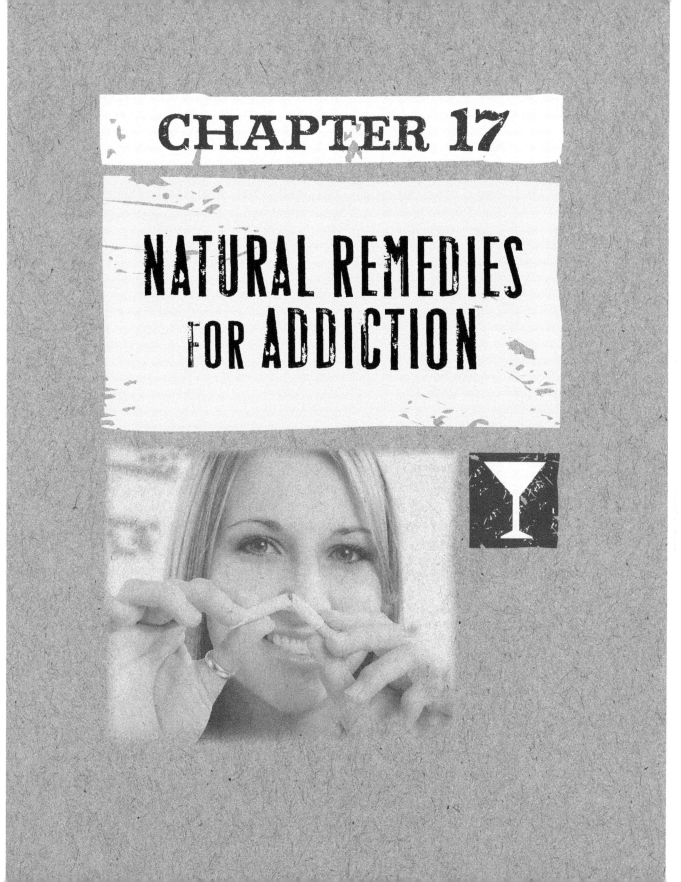

Despite all our attempts at healthy living, such as eating right and exercising, an addiction can get in the way of ultimate well-being. Here are a few ideas to liberate yourself from addiction.

Quitting Smoking

It may take several attempts to quit smoking may before you succeed. That's because nicotine in cigarettes is extremely addictive. When you smoke one cigarette, it sets you up to want another and so on and so on. Nicotine is a mild central nervous system stimulant and a strong cardiovascular stimulant. It even stimulates digestive secretions and shortens bowel transit time, thus decreasing nutrients available to the body. For some people, though, it acts as a sedative, settling nerves—but at a high cost. Quitting smoking enhances the senses of smell and taste, benefits breath, and provides whiter teeth and healthier respiratory and circulatory systems. Help save lives, money, and the environment with one hand! Here's how to quit for good.

HERBS TO HELP YOU QUIT

The following herbs can help you quit:

1. Lobelia contains the alkaloid lobeline, which helps to satisfy the body's craving for nicotine. Oat straw helps to nourish and calm the nervous system when you are giving up tobacco. There are several preparations for both these herbs available in natural food stores in tea, extract, or capsule form. Use them when you crave a cigarette, up to six times daily.

2. Using garlic as a supplement (one capsule three times daily) during the period of quitting helps open the lungs.
3. Chewing on about five juniper berries a day helps to open and detox the lungs.

You might also want to try smoking the nontoxic herb mullein (Verbascum thapsus) instead. It can be put in a pipe or rolled with cigarette papers for a non-nicotine smoke that helps you let go of the habit. Some people mix tobacco in with the mullein and gradually decrease the amount of tobacco they use.

AROMATHERAPY TO HELP YOU QUIT

Helichrysum aids tobacco detoxification and black pepper essential oil will help alleviate nicotine withdrawal. Lemon, lime, grapefruit, and orange are other essential oils that can be used in aromatherapy to alleviate the desire for a smoke. Whenever you feel a strong craving, open a bottle of essential oil and take a few deep breaths from the bottle.

BEST FOODS TO HELP YOU QUIT

Many addictions like smoking have their roots in low blood sugar. Most addictions temporarily elevate blood sugar, but when the effects wear off, blood sugar drops, leading you to feel like indulging again. Eat smaller, frequent meals with adequate protein like wild fish, beans, green leafy vegetables, nuts, seeds, and olives to keep blood sugar levels stable.

When you are overly acidic, you also experience more cravings. Get alkaline with apples, berries, carrots, celery, dandelion greens, figs, raisins, and spinach.

Include high-chlorophyll vegetables like kale to better utilize oxygen. High beta-carotene foods like carrots and winter squashes and high sulfur vegetables such as broccoli and cabbage nourish the lungs and boost immunity.

Chew on licorice roots or cinnamon sticks—they are hollow and you can even inhale a sweet flavor from them.

Enjoy raw sunflower seeds in the shell to keep that hand to mouth connection busy and out of trouble.

Suck the juice from an organic juicy orange, poking a hole in it about the size of a cigarette. Enjoy the sweetness and vitamin C rich succulence!

Drink lots of fluids, especially water, and sip liquids through a straw.

BEST PRACTICES TO HELP YOU QUIT

The following are some tips for best practices to help you quit:

1. Make a list of all the reasons you want to quit and have it somewhere you can look at frequently.
2. Set a target date a month in advance in case you need to gradually wean yourself off. Switch to a brand you don't like. Once you have reached your target date, cease saying, "I'm trying to quit," but instead say "I quit." Get rid of smoking accessories like ashtrays and lighters and make an appointment to get your teeth cleaned.
3. Wrap cigarettes packs in several layers of paper or perhaps in a beautiful cloth to give you pause when you want to light up.
4. Stop smoking between certain hours and extend the time by one half hour progressively. If you smoke when you are bored, stressed, in certain social situations, or drink certain beverages, change those patterns.
5. Only smoke half the cigarette, where tars are least concentrated, using the hand you usually don't smoke with. Avoid inhaling.
6. Make a list of other small pleasures in life, such as taking an aromatherapy bath, reading a great novel, or trading foot massages with your partner, and try to engage in these activities instead.
7. Go for a brisk walk after a meal rather than lighting up. It will get more oxygen into your lungs. Aerobics also help reduce stress and increase energy.
8. Take up a craft or activity that keeps your hands occupied. Use Chinese handballs, sketch, knit, crochet, do origami, or journal.
10. Put money saved from smoking less into a special fund to buy something nice. This small bank can be kept in the Wealth Corner of the feng shui bagua (furthest left corner from the entrance). Fill it with every bit you save, even if it's just a tuppence at first!

Thrifty Cures!

Chewing on pieces of ginger slices or candied ginger (wash off the sugar) can helpful curb cravings. Or you can suck on a whole clove.

11. When desiring a smoke, take deep diaphragmatic breaths, inhaling deep and slow, letting the abdomen fill with air, and expand. When exhaling, pull the abdomen in, sending out old stagnant energy. Feed your head and body oxygen. You don't have to smoke to breathe more deeply.

Overcoming Alcoholism

Drinking a glass or two of wine each day can improve health, stimulate the appetite, and ease stress. But if you abuse alcohol, it can have disastrous effects on your life. Next to sugar, alcohol is the oldest and most prevalent addiction in America. Here's what you can do to overcome your addiction.

HERBS THAT HELP

Important note! When it comes to using herbs, you'll want to stick to tea or capsules rather than use herbs in alcohol tincture form. (You can use herbs in a vinegar or glycerin tincture.)

Start with kudzu flowers, a long-standing remedy in Chinese medicine for drunkenness and alcoholism. Research published in the *Proceedings of the National Academy of Sciences* in 1993 showed that when mice were given kudzu, they decreased their alcohol consumption by 50 percent. That's because kudzu root contains daidzin, a substance that helps reduce the craving for alcohol. It's available in capsules at natural food stores. Take two capsules three times daily.

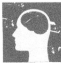

GOOD TO KNOW!

When smoke is inhaled, the body responds to the stress by producing adrenaline to help eliminate the toxins by speeding up the metabolic process. Tobacco stimulates mucous production and promotes glucose release into the blood stream. The "high" that people initially experience from smoking is caused by increased adrenaline levels, elevated blood pressure, blood vessel constriction, and elevated heart rate, as well as increased production of fatty acids. It increases salivation and heart palpitations and constricts the blood vessels of the skin. Tobacco leaves are usually cured with sugar and thus when smoked they increase the rate of glucose released into the blood stream.

After 20 minutes without a cigarette, heart rate and blood pressure fall to normal levels. After eight hours, carbon monoxide levels drops to normal. After only 24 hours, the risk of heart attack decreases. 48 hours after the last smoke, the sense of smell and taste improve. After two weeks, lung function improves and circulation is bettered. Going without cigarettes for one year allows the natural cilia of the lungs to regrow and reduces the risk of lung infections.

Milk thistle seed capsules help prevent and repair alcoholic-induced liver disease. A study in the *Journal of Hepatology* in 1989 showed that it helps to treat cirrhosis of the liver. One to two capsules can be taken daily.

Angelica when used as capsules or tea is said to help create a distaste for alcohol due its own presence of natural sugars. One capsule three times daily can be used or brewed into a tea if you enjoy the flavor of celery and spice.

The antioxidant herb chaparral helps to eliminate drug and alcohol residues from the body. Use for no longer than 21 days consecutively as it is high in resins that can stress the liver if used too long.

Cinnamon helps keep blood sugar levels stable as it is naturally rich in mannitol.

GOOD TO KNOW!

Milk thistle seed helps detoxify the liver and repairs damage to this organ. Sesame seeds are high in nerve-calming calcium. You can also make this to sprinkle on food:

Milk Thistle Seed Gomashio

$1/2$ **cup (32 g) milk thistle seeds**
1 **cup (144 g) sesame seeds (black, if you can find them)**
$1/4$ **cup (60 g) Celtic salt**

Grind the ingredients in a blender, or use a mortar and pestle. Keep in a glass jar in the refrigerator to season soups and vegetables.

SUPPLEMENTS THAT REDUCE CRAVINGS

Supplements of essential fatty acids like hemp, fish, evening primrose, or borage seed oil can reduce alcohol cravings and help restore brain and liver function and minimize withdrawal. One capsule can be taken three times daily.

The amino acid L-glutamine can deter alcohol cravings, possibly by protecting cells in the appetite regulation portion of the hypothalamus in the brain. Take 500 mg four times daily between meals and at bedtime.

The sedative valerian root, in capsule form, can also help during the first few days of withdrawal. Take 1 or 2 capsules up to 3 times daily, when feeling very stressed.

Vitamins B (50 mg daily), C (1,000 mg daily), and the amino acid cysteine (500 mg daily) can help protect against cellular damage from alcohol consumption.

AROMATHERAPY TO CHANGE THE BRAIN

When you are giving up alcohol, the following essential oils are helpful: bergamot, clary sage, eucalyptus, fennel, juniper, lemon, marjoram, rose, and rosemary. Simply smelling them affects the brain directly, opening neural pathways away from "I want a drink" to "I am breathing deep and accessing plant memories." (See page 11 for suggestions on using essential oils.)

BEST FOODS AND BEVERAGES
TO STAY SOBER

A high-protein, low-carbohydrate diet with nutritional supplements can help you stay sober. Tomato juice with lemon squeezed into it can ease the urge to drink since it contains fructose and helps satisfy the body's desire for alcohol. Drinking plain water with the juice of half a lemon will help detoxify the liver. Drinking plenty of water when getting off alcohol will help diminish cravings.

Alcoholics need to beware of moving into sugar addiction. Avoid sugar, fruit juices, and caffeine, which will keep the blood sugar on a rollercoaster ride. Get your sweets from fresh fruits that contain fiber, like an apple, instead. Miso is a great way to keep blood sugar levels stable. Small frequent meals will also help stabilize blood sugar levels. For more information about sugar addiction, read *Beat Sugar Addiction Now!* (Fairwinds Press 2010), and *Addiction Free Naturally* (Inner Traditions 2001).

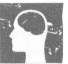

GOOD TO KNOW!

If you feel you are drinking too much or those around you say you are, get help from Alcoholics Anonymous. You'll find it in the yellow pages or at www.aa.org. It is inexpensive and available worldwide. It has changed many people's lives for the better!

Cures from Grandma's Kitchen

A folk remedy that can create a distaste for alcohol is to eat apples three times daily. This helps by cleansing the liver and keeping blood sugar levels stable. Bananas, unsweetened fresh coconut, and romaine lettuce are other folk remedy foods to deter alcohol desire, perhaps due to their calming properties. The minerals in celery help to neutralize the body's pH balance so it's considered an antidote for alcohol. Eat three to four stalks daily.

APPENDIX A:
A Closer Look at Herbs

Here you will find in-depth information about the herbs mentioned in this book (including when they are safe to use and some that aren't) that you may want to explore using. This will help you better understand the vast array of benefits plants offer! For more in-depth information on the herbs mentioned here and how to use them, check out my book, *The Desktop Guide to Herbal Medicine* (Basic Health Publications).

ALLSPICE *(Pimenta dioica, P. officinalis)* is a member of the Myrtaceae (eucalyptus) family. Dried, unripe fruit is the part used. During pregnancy, avoid excessive use; moderate culinary use is permitted.

ALOE VERA *(Aloe vera, A. barbadensis, A. ferox)* is a member of the Liliaceae (lily) family. The gelatinous substance in the stalks is the part used. Aloe should not be used internally during pregnancy.

ANISE *(Pimpinella anisum)* is a member of the Apiaceae (parsley) family. The seed is most often used medicinally. Avoid therapeutic doses during pregnancy except under the direction of a health-care professional. Culinary use during pregnancy is fine.

ASTRAGALUS *(Astragalus membranaceus, A. hoangtchy, A. mongolicus)* is a member of the Fabaceae (pea) family. The root is the part used. Astragalus is not recommended in cases of severe congestion, extreme tension, or an overactive immune system. It is generally not recommended in cases of fever and inflammation or extreme dryness (as evidenced by persistent thirst, dry skin, and constipation). It is best to avoid its use in cases of hot, toxic skin lesions and at the onset of cold and flu symptoms. It tends to hold infection in the body, so if you use astragalus during cases of infection, combine it with diaphoretic herbs.

BIRCH *(Betula alba, B. lenta, B. pendula, B. nana)* is a member of the Betulaceae *(birch)* family. The leaf bud, leaf, and inner bark are the parts used. Birch is considered safe when used appropriately.

BLACK COHOSH *(Actaea racemosa, formerly Ciimicifuga racemosa)* is a member of the Ranunculaceae (buttercup) family. The rhizomes and roots are the parts used. Excess use can cause nausea, vomiting, headache, and low blood pressure. If pregnant or nursing, use only upon recommendation of a competent health professional. It is generally not recommended during pregnancy. Avoid with heart conditions.

BLUE COHOSH *(Caulophyllum thalictroides)* is a member of the Berberidaceae (barberry) family. The rhizome is used. Use only the dried root as the fresh plant may cause dermatitis and the berries are toxic. Avoid its use during pregnancy until the onset of labor or until labor is overdue and then use only under the guidance of a qualified healthcare professional.

BONESET *(Eupatorium perfoliatum)* is a member of the Asteraceae (daisy) family. The aboveground plant is used. Large doses can cause vomiting, trembling, weakness, drooling, stiffness, and diarrhea. It is best to use boneset for no more than five days in a row.

BUCHU *(Agathosma betulina, formerly Barosma betulina, Diosma betulina)* is a member of the Rutaceae (citrus) family. The leaf is used. Avoid buchu during acute inflammatory conditions, as well as during pregnancy and while nursing. Large amounts can cause nausea and vomiting. It is not unusual for a person who has been drinking buchu tea to have his or her urine become scented like buchu, although this is not harmful in any way.

BUGLEWEED *(Lycopus virginicus, L. americanus, L. europaeus)* is a member of the Lamiaceae (mint) family. The aboveground plant is used. Avoid bugleweed during pregnancy.

BURDOCK *(Arctium lappa, A. minus)* is a member of the *Asteraceae* (daisy) family. The root and seed are used. Take care to avoid the sharp spines when working with the seeds. If you are collecting in the wild, avoid confusing burdock with rhubarb, which has similar-looking but toxic leaves.

CALENDULA *(Calendula officinalis)* is a member of the *Asteraceae* (daisy) family. The flower is used. Calendula is generally regarded as very safe.

CARAWAY *(Carum carvi)* is a member of the *Apiaceae* (parsley) family. The seeds are used. Caraway is safe when used appropriately.

CARDAMOM *(Elettaria cardamomum)* is a member of the *Zingiberaceae* (ginger) family. The seeds are used. It is considered very safe, but avoid it if you have an ulcer.

CATNIP *(Nepeta cataria)* is a member of the *Lamiaceae* (mint) family. The leaves are used. It is not recommended for use during pregnancy,

CAYENNE PEPPER *(Capsicum frutescens, C. annuum, C. species)* is a member of the *Solanaceae* (nightshade) family. Keep away from eyes. Wash hands after any contact with any loose form of cayenne. Avoid large doses when pregnant and nursing. Seeds can be especially hot and in some varieties are best avoided.

CELERY *(Apium graveolens)* is a member of the *Apiaceae* (parsley) family. The seed and stalks are used therapeutically. Large amounts of celery seed may increase photosensitivity, so avoid using the essential oil topically when going out in the sun. Use only in moderation during pregnancy, as large amounts could have an abortifacient effect. Avoid celery seed in cases of kidney inflammation.

CHAMOMILE *(Matricaria recutita)* (German chamomile; formerly *Chamomilla recutita*; syn. M. chamomilla), *Chamaemelum nobile* (Roman chamomile; syn. *Anthemis nobilis*) is a member of the *Asteraceae* (daisy) family. The flowers are used. Some people may be severely allergic to chamomile, especially those sensitive to ragweed. It can cause contact dermatitis in some individuals. Roman chamomile is more likely to cause an allergic reaction than the German variety. On the other hand, chamomile is sometimes used to treat allergies. Use the herb with caution the first time you try it. Otherwise, chamomile is considered very safe. It is not recommend during pregnancy.

CHICKWEED *(Stellaria media, S. graminea, S. alsine)* is a member of the *Caryophyllaceae* (pink) family. The aboveground plant is used. Excess use may cause diarrhea.

CINNAMON *(Cinnamomum cassia, C. zeylanicum,)* is a member of the *Lauraceae* (laurel) family. The inner bark is used. Avoid cinnamon during hot feverish conditions. Avoid large amounts during pregnancy (culinary use is okay) and large amounts can decrease mother's milk. Avoid large doses for long periods of time.

CLEAVERS *(Galium aparine, G. verum)* is a member of the *Rubiaceae* (madder) family. The aboveground plant is used. Cleavers is not recommended in cases of diabetes as it will increase urination. Contact dermatitis from the fresh juice is a rare occurrence.

CLOVE *(Eugenia aromatica)* is a member of the *Myrtaceae* (eucalyptus) family. The dried flower bud is used. Avoid large amounts during pregnancy or in cases of fever. Prolonged contact of the essential oil with gum tissue can be irritating.

CODONOPSIS/DANG SHEN *(Codonopsis pilosula)* is a member of the *Campanulaceae* (bellwort) family. The root is used. It is generally regarded as safe when used appropriately.

COLLINSONIA *(Collinsonia canadensis)* is a member of the *Lamiaceae* (mint) family. The rhizome is used. Avoid during pregnancy. Beware the aboveground portion of the plant, which can be emetic even in small amounts.

COMFREY *(Symphytum officinale)* is a member of the *Boraginaceae* (borage) family. Comfrey is recommended only for short-term use of less than six weeks and is not recommended for use during pregnancy or while nursing. Herbalists debate about the safety of using herbs containing pyrrolizidine alkaloids, and more research needs to be conducted to determine whether comfrey is safe for internal use. But there is no problem with using it topically. Because comfrey causes rapid wound healing, make sure a wound is clean of any dirt before applying comfrey. Also be sure of your species; poisonings have occurred from novices collecting toxic foxglove, mistaking it for comfrey.

CORIANDER *(Coriandrum sativum)* is a member of the *Apiaceae* (parsley) family. The seed is used. There have been rare reports of allergic reactions to coriander.

CORNSILK *(Zea mays)* is a member of the *Poaceae* (grass) family. The stigmas from the female flowers are used. When used appropriately, it is considered very safe.

CORYDALIS *(Corydalis formosa)* is a member of the *Papaveraceae* (poppy) family. The rhizome is used. Use corydalis only as needed and do not take more than is needed. Large amounts can be toxic. Avoid during pregnancy.

COUCH GRASS *(Elytrigia repens, also known as Agropyron repens)* is a member of the *Poaceae* (grass) family. The rhizome and roots are used. Couchgrass is generally regarded as safe.

CUMIN *(Cuminum cyminum)* is a member of the *Apiaceae* (parsley) family. Cumin is generally regarded as safe.

DAMIANA *(Turnera aphrodisiaca, T. diffusa)* is a member of the *Turneraceae* (turnera) family. The aboveground plant is used. Damiana is generally considered safe, but avoid using it in cases of urinary tract disease and during pregnancy.

DANDELION *(Taraxacum officinale)* is a member *Asteraceae* (daisy) family. All parts are used. Dandelion is generally regarded as safe, even in large amounts and even during pregnancy. However, as is the case with any plant, there is always a possibility of an allergic reaction. There have been a very few cases reported of abdominal discomfort, loose stools, nausea, and heartburn associated with dandelion. The fresh latex of the plant can cause contact dermatitis in some sensitive individuals.

DEVIL'S CLAW *(Harpagophytum procumbens)* is a member of the *Pedeliaceae* (sesame) family. The secondary tubers are used. There are no known harmful side effects from long-term use of devil's claw. It may take a couple of weeks to notice results. Use devil's claw in combination with demulcent herbs to avoid irritating the digestive tract and avoid it during pregnancy.

DILL *(Anethum graveolens)* is a member of the *Apiaceae* (parsley) family. The seed is used medicinally. Avoid therapeutic doses during pregnancy, but culinary use is fine.

DONG QUAI *(Angelica sinensis, A. polymorpha)* is a member of the *Apiaceae* (parsley) family. The root is used. Avoid dong quai during pregnancy except under the supervision of a qualified health-care practitioner. Avoid in cases of diarrhea, poor digestion, abdominal distention, heavy menstrual flow, or high fever with a strong fast pulse or when using blood-thinning medications. Use of dong quai can increase photosensitivity.

ECHINACEA *(Echinacea purpurea, E. angustifolia, E. pallida)* is a member of the *Asteraceae* (daisy) family. The root, rhizome, leaf, flower, and seed are used medicinally. Excessive use of echinacea can cause throat irritation, nausea, dizziness, and excessive salivation. Rare cases of allergic reactions have been reported. Those with a compromised immune system, such as might result from lupus, should use echinacea only under the advice of a qualified health-care professional. Echinacea can be taken frequently (every couple of hours) during acute infection, but this sort of dosing should be undertaken only for a few days. Echinacea commonly produces a slightly tingly sensation on the tongue, which is a harmless reaction.

ELDER *(Sambucus nigra, S. canadensis)* is a member of the *Caprifoliaceae* (honeysuckle) family. The flower and berry are used as medicine. Avoid elder in cases of fluid depletion, as elder is a diuretic. Cook or dry ripe berries before consuming large quantities of them as excess amounts can have a laxative effect. Know your species and avoid using red-berried elders as many of them are poisonous.

EUCALYPTUS *(Eucalyptus globulus, E. species)* is a member of the *Myrtaceae* (eucalyptus) family. Large amounts taken at one time can cause headache, vertigo, convulsions, and even death. The essential oil may cause irritation or burning; avoid contact of the essential oil with mucous membranes.

EYEBRIGHT *(Euphrasia rostkoviana, E. officinalis, E. americana)* is a member of the *Scrophulariaceae* (figwort) family. The aboveground plant is used. Though this herb is regarded as safe, eyebright is best used under the guidance of a qualified health-care professional in cases of serious eye disorders. Avoid during pregnancy.

FENNEL (*Foeniculum vulgare, F. officinale*) is a member of the *Apiaceae* (parsley) family. The seeds are used. Excess use of fennel seed can overstimulate the nervous system. Avoid therapeutic dosages during pregnancy, though culinary use is fine.

FENUGREEK (*Trigonella foenum-graecum*) is a member of the *Fabaceae* (legume) family. The seeds are used in medicine. Avoid fenugreek seed during pregnancy as it can be a uterine stimulant. Although fenugreek can be used to lower blood sugar levels, diabetics should use it for this purpose only with guidance from a qualified health-care practitioner.

FEVERFEW (*Tanacetum parthenium*) is a member of the *Asteraceae* (daisy) family. The flowers and leaves are used. In rare cases, feverfew can cause irritation of the gastrointestinal tract, mouth, or tongue. Taking it with food can minimize this possibility. Avoid during pregnancy and nursing. Don't use feverfew if you are on blood-thinning medications or about to have surgery within a week because it can have an effect on the rate of blood clotting. If you are very allergic to ragweed, use under supervision of a health professional.

FLAX (*Linum usitatissimum, L. lewisii, L. perenne*) is a member of the *Linaceae* (flax) family. Once flax seeds are ground or made into an oil, they can quickly go rancid.

GARCINIA (*Garcinia cambogia, G. indica, G. atriviridis*) is a member of the *Clusiaceae* (Saint-John's-wort) family. Those allergic to citric acid (citrus fruits, tomatoes) may have sensitivities to garcinia. It has been safely used as a food for many centuries. Avoid during pregnancy and nursing. Large doses can be cathartic.

GARLIC (*Allium sativum*) is a member of the *Lilliaceae* (lily) family. Garlic breath can be a problem, remaining in the body for up to ten hours. Do not apply cut garlic directly to the skin for more than a few minutes as it can burn the skin (always dilute with vegetable oil). Avoid large doses during pregnancy and while nursing as it may cause digestive distress in the mother and baby.

GENTIAN (*Gentiana officinalis, G. lutea, g. andrewsii, G. villosa, g campestris, G. macrophylla, G. scabra*) is a member of the *Gentianaceae* (gentian) family. Gentian can aggravate hyperacidic conditions and ulcers. Large doses can cause nausea and vomiting.

GINGER (*Zingiber officinale*) is a member of the *Zingiberaceae* (ginger) family. The rhizome is used. Although ginger can relieve morning sickness, pregnant women should not ingest more than 1 gram daily. Avoid in cases of peptic ulcers, hyperacidity, or other hot, inflammatory conditions. Avoid excessive amounts of ginger in cases of acne, eczema, or herpes. Ginger may cause adverse reactions when used in combination with anticoagulant drugs such as Coumadin or aspirin; if you are using such medications, seek the advice of a qualified health-care practitioner before commencing use of ginger.

GINKGO (*Ginkgo biloba*) is a member of the *Ginkgoaceae* (ginkgo) family. The leaves are the most used part. Side effects from using ginkgo leaves are rare. However, large amounts have been reported to cause gastrointestinal disturbance, irritability, restlessness, and headache. Ginkgo leaf can negatively affect the blood's ability to clot, so avoid ginkgo for at least a week before surgery; in cases of hemophilia; or in concurrence with anticoagulant drugs such as Coumadin, aspirin, or monoamine-oxidase inhibitors.

GINSENG (*Panax quinquefolium: American ginseng*) (Panax ginseng: Asian ginseng) is a member of the *Araliaceae* (ginseng) family. The root is the part used. Avoid ginseng in cases of heat and inflammation, such as fever, flu, pneumonia, hypertension, or constipation. Do not give to children for prolonged periods as it may cause early sexual maturation. Avoid during pregnancy and while nursing. Do not take ginseng in conjunction with cardiac glycosides except under the guidance of a qualified health-care professional. It is best not to take ginseng at night as it can inhibit sleep.

GOJI (*Lycium chinense, l. barbarum*) is a member of the *Solanaceae* (nightshade) family. The berries are used. Avoid buying bright red berries that may have been trested with sulfite preservatives.

GOLDENROD *(Solidago species)* is a member of the *Asteraceae* (daisy) family. The aboveground plant is used. In cases of chronic kidney disorder, consult with a qualified health-care practitioner before using. Avoid in cases of edema resulting from heart or kidney failure. Goldenrod is often accused of causing hay fever. However, its pollen is actually quite heavy and falls to the earth rather than becoming airborne. It is more likely ragweed, which blooms at the same time as goldenrod, that is culprit.

GOLDENSEAL *(Hydrastis canadensis)* is a member of the *Ranunculaceae* (buttercup) family. Avoid during pregnancy, in cases of high blood pressure, or in the week preceding surgery as it may increase blood pressure. It also can elevate blood sugar levels and blood pressure in one who is already so inclined; use only under the guidance of a qualified health-care professional in such cases. Use only for short periods (three weeks or less) as long-term use can kill off friendly intestinal flora and reduce assimilation of B vitamins. Follow a course of goldenseal with probiotics such as acidophilus.

GOTU KOLA *(Centella asiatica)* is a member of the *Apiaceae* (parsley) family. The aboveground plant is used. Avoid during pregnancy, except under the guidance of a qualified health-care practitioner. Avoid in cases of overactive thyroid.

GRAVEL ROOT *(Eupatorium purpureum, E. ternifolium, E. verticullatum, E. maculatum)* is a member of the *Asteraceae* (daisy) family. Large doses may cause vomiting. Avoid during pregnancy. Gravel root contains some pyrrolizine alkaloids and it is not recommended for use for periods of more than six weeks.

GRINDELIA *(Grindelia camporum, G. robusta, Gg. squarrosa, G. rigida)* is a member of the *Asteraceae* (daisy) family. The tops (flowers, buds, and upper leaves) and resin are used. Excessive dosages, due to all the resins can irritate kidneys. Grindelia can collect high doses of selenium from the soil, which can cause large doses of this plant to be irritating.

GUARANA *(Paullinia cupana, P. sorbilis, Cupania americana)* is a member of the *Sapindaceae* (lychee) family. The seeds are used. It contains caffeine and can cause nervousness, insomnia, and B vitamin depletion. Guarana is contraindicated for those with heart disease, ulcers, diabetes, and epilepsy. Avoid in cases of high blood pressure. Avoid guarana during pregnancy and nursing.

GUGGULU *(Commiphora mukul, C. africana)* is a member of the *Burseaceae* (frankincense) family. The resin is used. In rare cases, an allergic skin reaction can occur. It disappears when use of the herb is discontinued. In cases of bowel inflammation, liver disease, or diarrhea, consult with a competent health-care professional before using.

GYMNEMA *(Gymnema sylvestre)* is a member of the *Asclepiadeceae* (milkweed) family. The leaves are used. If you are insulin dependent, consult with your physician before using gymnema as insulin levels may need to be adjusted.

HAWTHORN *(Crataegus oxycantha, C. species)* is a member of the *Rosaceae* (rose) family. The leaf, flower, and berry are used. Using hawthorn may potentiate the effects of heart medications such as beta-blockers, digoxin, or Lanoxin. If you are using heart medication, consult with a qualified health-care professional before commencing use of hawthorn. It is generally considered safe.

HIBISCUS *(Hibiscus sabdariffa, H. rosasinensis, H.* spp.*)* is a member of the *Malvaceae* (mallow) family. Persons who are very chilled should avoid hibiscus as it is cooling.

HOPS *(Humulus lupulus)* (European hops) is a member of the *Cannabaceae* (hemp) family. The strobiles are used. Avoid during pregnancy and in cases of depression. Use in conjunction with pharmaceutical sedatives only under the guidance of a qualified health-care professional. It may exacerbate their effects.

HOREHOUND *(Marrubium vulgare)* is a member of the *Lamiaceae* (mint) family. The aboveground portions are used. Large doses may be laxative and cathartic. The juice of the fresh plant may cause dermatitis. Avoid during pregnancy.

HORSE CHESTNUT (*Aesculus hippocastanum*) is a member of the *Hippocastanaceae* (horse chestnut) family. The seeds, leaves, flowers, and bark are somewhat toxic unless processed. Use in one fourth the dosages of other herbs. Avoid using if pregnant or nursing.

HORSETAIL (*Equisetum arvense, E. species*) is a member of the *Equisetaceae* (horsetail) family. Large amounts can be toxic due to the presence of the enzyme aneurinase, which, if eaten over a long period of time, can cause B vitamin deficiency. Small amounts are fine. However, drying, cooking, and tincturing horsetail destroys that enzyme, making horsetail safe. Avoid long-term use during pregnancy.

HO SHOU WU (*Polygonum multiflorum*) is a member of the *Polygonaceae* (rhubarb) family. The processed root is used. Avoid ho shou wu during bouts of diarrhea and excessive phlegm.

HYDRANGEA (*Hydrangea arborescens*) is a member of the *Saxifragaceae* (rockfoil) family. Only the root and rhizhome are used. Excessive amounts can cause gastrointestinal distress, dizziness, and chest congestion. Hydrangea is not recommended for long-term use or during pregnancy.

HYSSOP (*Hyssopus officinalis*) is a member of the *Lamiaceae* (mint) family. Avoid during pregnancy.

IRISH MOSS (*Chondrus crispus*) is a member of the *Gigartinaceae* (gigartina) family. Because Irish moss has some blood-thinning properties, people who are on anticoagulating medications should avoid its use.

ISATIS (*Isatis tinctoria*) is a member of the *Brassicaceae* (cabbage) family. The root is primarily used. Do not use isatis for more than three weeks at a time. Long-term use can deplete the body of friendly intestinal flora, weaken digestion, and cause internal coldness.

JUJUBE (*Ziziphus jujuba*) is a member of the *Rhamnaceae* (buckthorn) family. The berries are used as food and medicine. Avoid jujube in cases of bloatedness or intestinal parasites.

KAVA KAVA (*Piper methysticum*) is a member of the *Piperaceae* (pepper) family. The root and upper rhizome are used. Avoid during pregnancy and while nursing and do not give to young children. Avoid in cases of Parkinson's disease and severe depression. Do not take in conjunction with with alcohol, sedatives, tranquilizers, or antidepressants as it can potentiate their effects. Try to avoid driving, operating heavy machinery, or other activities that require fast reaction times after taking kava kava. On the plus side, kava kava, unlike many sedatives, is not habit forming. Daily use of kava shouldn't exceed three months, though occasional use is fine for healthy people. Kava kava may cause the tongue, mouth, and other body parts to feel somewhat numb and rubbery temporarily; this is normal. However, excess amounts can cause disturbed vision, dilated pupils, and difficulty walking. Large doses taken for extended periods can have a cumulative effect on the liver, causing kawaism, a condition marked by a yellowish tinge to the skin, a scaly rash, apathy, anorexia, and bloodshot eyes.

LADY'S MANTLE (*Alchemilla vulgaris*) is a member of the *Rosaceae* (rose) family. The leaf and flowering shoot are used. Avoid during pregnancy except under the guidance of a qualified health-care professional. Do not use in conjunction with oxytocin.

LAVENDER (*Lavendula species*) is a member of the *Lamiaceae* (mint) family. The flower is used. Avoid large doses of lavender during pregnancy.

LEMON BALM (*Melissa officinalis*) is a member of the *Lamiaceae* (mint) family. The aboveground plant is used. Lemon balm is generally considered very safe and a favorite children's herb. It can lower thyroid function, however, which is beneficial in some cases but not for those with a hypothyroid condition.

LEMONGRASS (*Cymbopogon citratus*) is a member of the *Poaceae* (grass) family. The leaf is used. Avoid large doses during pregnancy as it can stimulate the uterus.

LICORICE (*Glycyrrhiza glabra: European licorice, G. uralensis: Chinese licorice, G. glandulifera: Russian licorice*) is a member of the *Fabaceae* (pea) family. The root, also known as stolen, which is an underground stem, is used. Avoid licorice in cases of edema, nausea, vomiting, and rapid heartbeat. Licorice is not recommended during pregnancy or in combination with steroid or digoxin medications. Large doses may cause sodium retention and potassium depletion and may be emetic. Prolonged or excessive use may elevate blood pressure and cause headache and vertigo. Continuous use is not recommended in excess of six weeks.

CHINESE LICORICE *(G. uralensis)* is said to be less likely to cause side effects than the European variety (G. glabra). All these precautions notwithstanding, licorice is often added in very small amounts to other herbal formulas to harmonize them and prevent undesirable side effects. Before using licorice in moderate amounts daily, for longer than six weeks, consult with a competent health-care practitioner.

LINDEN *(Tilia platyphyllos, T. americana, . cordata, T. x europea, T. spp.)* is a member of the *Tiliaceae* (tilia) family. The flower is used. Tilia americana should be consumed only in moderation as large doses may cause nausea and excess use may damage the heart. Older flowers of most species used in making tea can have a slight narcotic effect.

LOBELIA *(Lobelia inflata, L. siphilitica: blue lobelia, L. cardinalis: red lobelia, cardinal flower)* is a member of the *Lobeliaceae* (bluebell) family. The entire plant can be toxic if not used properly. Avoid during pregnancy or in cases of hypotension, hypertension, fainting, paralysis, shock, pneumonia, or fluid surrounding the heart or lungs. Avoid overdosing, as overdose can cause sweating, nausea, vomiting, pain, paralysis, lowered body temperature, rapid pulse, coma, and even death. Lobelia is best used in combination with other herbs and in small amounts, being one-fifth to one-third of a formula.

MACA *(L. Peruvianum)* is a member of the *Brassicaceae* (mustard) family. The root is used as food and medicine. It is generally regarded as safe. High doses may contribute to insomnia.

MARSHMALLOW *(Althaea officinalis)* is a member of the *Malvaceae* (mallow) family. The root is used. The mucilage in marshmallow may cause a delay in the effects of pharmaceuticals taken at the same time.

MEADOWSWEET *(Filipendula ulmaria)* is a member of the *Rosaceae* (rose) family. The aboveground plant is used. Avoid meadowsweet in cases of sensitivity to salicylates, such as those found in aspirin.

MILK THISTLE *(Silybum marianum)* is a member of the *Asteraceae* (daisy) family. The seeds are used as food and medicine. There have been occasional reports of bloating, diarrhea, and a laxative effect. Mint (Mentha spp., especially M. x piperita [Peppermint] and M. spicata [Spearmint]) is a member of the *Lamiaceae* (mint) family. The aboveground plant is used. Avoid mint in cases of coldness, such as chills or yin deficiency, and during acute gallstone attack. Pregnant women should ingest no more than 1 to 2 cups (475 ml) daily of peppermint tea. Nursing mothers should avoid large amounts of mint, which can dry breast milk.

MOTHERWORT *(Leonurus cardiaca)* is a member of the *Lamiaceae* (mint) family. The aboveground plant is used. Avoid motherwort in cases of excessive menstrual bleeding. Avoid during pregnancy (but note that motherwort can be helpful during labor, under the guidance of a qualified health-care practitioner). The plant may cause contact dermatitis in some people.

MUIRA PUAMA *(Ptychopetalum olacoides, P. uncinatum)* is a member of the *Olaceae* (olive) family. The inner bark and root are used. It may cause insomnia in some people if taken before bedtime.

MULLEIN *(Verbascum thapsus)* is a member of the *Scrophulariaceae* (figwort) family. The leaf and sometimes flower (without the calyx) are used. Mullein leaves are generally regarded as safe, though the leaf contains coumarin and rotenone, which in the past have drawn expressions of concern from the U.S. Food and Drug Administration.

MYRRH *(Commiphora myrrha, c. abyssinica)* is a member of the *Burseraceae* (frankincense) family. Use only small amounts internally and only for short periods of time as resins can be difficult for the body to eliminate. Avoid during pregnancy as myrrh can stimulate the uterus. Large amounts can be overly laxative.

NEEM *(Azadirachata indica)* is a member of the *Meliaceae* (mahogany) family. The bark, twigs, leaves, roots, seeds, and sap are used. Neem is considered safe and has a long history of use. However, long term internal use may result in anemia, weakness, appetite loss, and weight loss. It should not be used for infants, the elderly, or infirmed.

NETTLE *(Urtica dioica, U. urens)* is a member of the *Urticaceae* (nettle) family. The aboveground plant is used. All fifty species of the genus Urtica can be used medicinally, but stick with urens and dioica species unless you have consulted with local herb authorities on the safety of local varieties. Nettle is not known as stinging nettle for nothing; avoid touching or eating the fresh plant unless it is very young and/or you are very brave. Touching the fresh plant can cause a burning rash. Wearing gloves when collecting can help prevent this, but the hairs in large plants may still pierce through. A nettle sting can be soothed with a poultice of yellow dock or plantain or even the juice of the nettle plant itself (but good luck obtaining this without getting many more stings).

OAK *(Quercus alba: white Oak)* is a member of the *Fagaceae* (beech) family. The inner bark and gall (growth produced by fungus or insect) are used. Oak galls are extremely astringent; use only in small quantities. Use oak bark for no longer than a month continuously.

OAT *(Avena sativa: cultivated oat, A. fatua: wild oat)* is a member of the *Poaceae* (grass) family. The seed (unripe) and stem (also known as oat straw) are used. Those with gluten allergies should use oats with caution.

OLIVE LEAF *(Oleum europea, O. olviva)* is a member of the *Oleaceae* (olive) family. Olive leaf is used as medicine and the fruit as food. Olive leaf and oil are generally regarded as safe. "Die off" reactions have been reported from olive leaf use, where the body experiences the die off of pathogens, which can manifest as aches, sore throat, or flu like symptoms. Some have found olive leaf tea irritating to the stomach.

ORANGE *(Citrus reticulata: mandarin orange or tangerine, C. x aurantium: bitter or Seville orange, C. vulgaris: sweet orange)* is a member of the *Rutaceae* (citrus) family. The peel is used. Use bitter orange with caution during pregnancy as large doses may stimulate contractions. Use of orange peel essential oil in massage oils, baths, and other cosmetics make increase photosensitivity.

OREGON GRAPE *(Mahonia aquifolium),* (synonym) *Berberis aquifolium, Mahonia repens, m. nervosa, m. pinnata, berberis repens, b. vulgaris)* is a member of the *Berberidaceae* (barberry) family. The root, root bark, and rhizome are used. Use only the dried plant as the fresh root can be excessively purgative. Avoid during pregnancy. Avoid in hyperthyroid conditions. Don't use in cases of excessive flatulence.

OREGANO *(Origanum vulgare, O. spp.)* is a member of the *Lamiaceae* (mint) family. The aboveground portion is used. Avoid large medicinal dosages during pregnancy, though culinary use is fine.

OSHA *(Ligusticum porteri, L. canbyi, L. scoticum, L. filicinum, l. grayi, l. tenuifolium)* is a member of the *Apiaceae* (parsley) family. The root is used. Avoid during pregnancy.

PARSLEY *(Petroselinum crispum: curly leaved, p. latifolium: broad leaves, P. sativum, P. tuberosum: hamburg parsley)* is a member of the *Apiaceae* (parsley) family. The leaf is used. Large amounts are contraindicated during pregnancy, though culinary use is fine.

PASSIONFLOWER *(Passiflora incarnata, P. edulis: yellow passionflower, P. spp.)* is a member of the *Passifloraceae* (passionflower) family. The leaf, vine, and flower are used. Large doses may cause nausea and vomiting. Avoid large doses during pregnancy. Unripe fruits have some level of toxicity and should not be consumed.

P'AU D'ARCO *(Tabeuia spp., including T. impetiginosa, T. rosea, and T. serratifolia)* is a member of the *Bignoniaceae* (bignonia) family. The inner lining of the bark (known as phloem) and bark are used. Excess use may loosen bowels or cause nausea and vomiting. Avoid during pregnancy and nursing. Product adulteration is common, so be sure that your source is trustworthy.

PEPPER *(Piper nigrum: black pepper)* is a member of the *Piperaceae* (pepper) family. The dried unripe fruits are used as food and medicine. Overuse may cause hypersecretions of digestive juices, leading to a burning sensation in the digestive tract. Large amounts may elevate blood pressure.

PINE *(P.* spp., *including P. sylvestris: Scotch pine, P. tabuliformis, P. strobus: white pine, P. pinaster, P. pinea, P. nigra, P. contorta: lodgepole pine)* is a member of the *Pinaceae* (pine) family. The inner bark, needles, young buds, and pitch are used. Some may experience contact dermatitis if in contact with the wood, resins, or sawdust of some pine species.

PLANTAIN *(Plantago major: broad-leaf plantain, P. lanceolata: lance-leaf plantain, P. media: hoary plantain, sweet plantain)* is a member of the *Plantaginaceae* (plantain) Family. The leaf and seed are used. Plantain is generally regarded as safe.

PRICKLY ASH *(Zanthoxylum americanum:* Northern prickly ash*, Z. clava-herculis:* Southern prickly ash*)* is a member of *Rutaceae* (rue) family. The bark is the portion used. Avoid during pregnancy, in cases of stomach or intestinal inflammation, and in conjunction with blood-thinning medications. Prickly ash can produce a hot, tingling sensation throughout the body that is not a cause for alarm; it is as strong a stimulant as cayenne pepper but is slower acting and longer lasting.

PSYLLIUM *(Plantago psyllium, P. ovata, P. indica)* is a member of the *Plantaginaceae* (plantain) family. The seed and outer husk of the seed are used. Always use psyllium with plenty of liquids; otherwise, it can cause constipation. Psyllium can dilute digestive enzymes and is best taken between meals, especially before bed or first thing upon rising, rather than with food.

RASPBERRY *(Rubus* spp.*)* is a member of the *Rosaceae* (rose) family. The leaf is used medicinally. There are no known toxic levels. Once nursing is established, excess consumption of raspberry leaf should be avoided as its astringent properties could lessen the amount of breast milk.

RED CLOVER *(Trifolium pratense)* is a member of the *Fabaceae* (pea) family. The flower and young leaf are used. Red clover is not recommended for use during pregnancy, though it can be used prior to pregnancy as a fertility tonic. Avoid red clover for at least a week prior to surgery.

REHMANNIA *(Rehmannia glutinosa)* is a member of the *Scrophulariaceae* (foxglove) family. The root is used. Avoid excessive use in cases of loose stools or a very coated tongue.

REISHI *(Ganoderma lucidum)* is a member of the *Polyporaceae* (polypor) family. The fruiting body is used. Reishi has a very low potential for toxicity. Some may experience dry mouth, dizziness, and digestive distress from ingesting reishi after long-term use. Pregnant or nursing women should consult with a competent health-care professional before using reishi. Because reishi can inhibit blood clotting, it should be avoided at least one week before surgery, birthing, or if using blood-tinning medications.

ROSE *(Rosa* spp., *including R. canina: dog rose, R. species)* is a member of the *Rosaceae* (rose) family. The flower and hip are used. As with all herbs, avoid using rose flowers or hips that have been sprayed with toxic chemicals. Remove the irritating hairs from the rose hip seeds before eating them. When making a tea from them, use a strainer to filter out the fine hairs.

ROSEMARY *(Rosmarinus officinalis)* is a member of the *Lamiaceae* (mint) family. The aboveground plant is used. Avoid therapeutic doses during pregnancy (though moderate culinary use is ok). Though rosemary is generally considered so safe that it is a common kitchen herb, extremely large doses can cause convulsions and death.

SAINT-JOHN'S-WORT *(Hypericum* spp., *including H. perforatum)* is a member of the *Clusiaceae* (Saint-John's-wort) family. The flowering tops are used. Saint-John's-wort should not be combined with anti-depressant pharmaceuticals (for example, Celexa, Eldepryl, Marplan, Nardil, Parnate, Paxil, Prozac, or Zoloft), protease inhibitors, or organ antirejection drugs (such as cyclosporine), except under the guidance of a qualified health-care practitioner. In fact, because Saint-John's-wort cleanses the liver, it is best to use it with caution in conjunction with any pharmaceutical drug. Saint-John's-wort is not recommended during pregnancy, while nursing, or for children under the age of two. It may cause photosensitivity, especially in fair-skinned individuals. There have been rare reports of dizziness, nausea, fatigue, and dry mouth from its use. Some people may experience contact dermatitis from the plant.

SARSAPARILLA *(Smilax aristolochiifolia, S. aspera, S. officinalis, S. ornata, S. papyracea, S. regelii: Jamaican sarsaparilla)* is a member of the *Smilacaceae* (smilax) family. The rhizome is used. Avoid during pregnancy.

SAW PALMETTO *(Serenoa repens)* is a member of the *Arecaceae* (palm) family. The berry is used. Avoid during pregnancy and while nursing, at least until further research has been done to ascertain its safety during these times. Mild gastrointestinal disturbances are a rare side effect.

SCHIZANDRA *(Schisandra chinensis)* is a member of the *Schisandraceae* (magnolia vine) family. The berry is used. Avoid schizandra in cases of excess heat (such as fever), overly acidic conditions, cough, epilepsy, intracranial pressure, or in the early stages of rash. Schizandra is not recommended during pregnancy. Do not give to children under the age of two, except under the guidance of a qualified health-care practitioner.

SENNA *(Senna alexandrina, S. spp.)* is a member of the *Fabaceae* (legume) family. The leaf, pod, and seed are used. Avoid senna during pregnancy, while nursing, and in children under age twelve. Avoid in cases of colitis or conditions of inflammation of the digestive tract. Do not use in conjunction with cardiac glycoside pharmaceuticals, except under the guidance of a qualified health-care practitioner. The seeds have a gentler effect than the leaves and are more appropriate for the young, the elderly, and those prone to stomach cramps. To prevent gripe, combine senna with carminative herbs such as cinnamon, cardamom, coriander seed, fennel seed, ginger, or peppermint. Overuse may cause laxative dependency, so do not use senna for more than ten days in a row. Large doses or overuse can cause bloody diarrhea, intestinal cramps, nausea, vomiting, and nephritis. Long-term use can cause dehydration and can deplete the body of electrolytes, including potassium, worsening constipation and weakening the muscles. Senna may cause the urine to become reddish, which is no cause for concern.

SHEPHERD'S PURSE *(Capsella bursa-pastoris)* is a member of the *Brassicaceae* (mustard) family. The aboveground plant is used. Use shepherd's purse only in moderate doses, as large doses may be toxic. Avoid during pregnancy, except during labor, and then only under the guidance of a qualified health-care professional.

SHIITAKE *(Lentinus edodes)* is a member of the *Polyporaceae* (polypor) family. The cap of fruiting mushroom body is used. Shiitakes are considered nontoxic and generally safe. Avoid in cases of extreme weakness or diarrhea. There have been rare reports of allergic reactions affecting the throat, lungs, or skin.

SKULLCAP *(Scutellaria californica, S. canescens, S. galericulata, S. lateriflora, S. pilosa, S. tuberosa, S. versicolor)* is a member of the *Lamiaceae* (mint) family. The aboveground plant is used. Avoid during pregnancy. Large doses may cause confusion and giddiness.

SLIPPERY ELM *(Ulmus rubra; syn. U. fulva)* is a member of the *Ulmaceae* (elm) family. The inner bark is used. Slippery elm is regarded as one of the safest herbs. When consuming slippery elm in capsule form, be sure to take in plenty of fluids as it absorbs moisture in the body and can be dehydrating.

SPILANTHES *(Spilanthes acmella)* is a member of the *Asteraceae* (daisy) family. The aboveground plant is used. Spilanthes is nonpoisonous to humans though toxic to cold-blooded organisms. Eating the plant can cause numbness in the mouth. The volatile isothio-cyanates cause an intense pungent sensation in the mouth.

STEVIA *(Stevia rebaudiana)* is a member of the *Asteraceae* (daisy) family. The leaf and flower are used. It is generally considered safe. Too much stevia can leave an aftertaste.

TEA *(Camellia sinensis)* is a member of the *Theaceae* (tea) family. The leaf bud and young leaf are used. Excessive use of tea may cause nervous irritability and digestive distress such as ulcers. Some believe tea to be addictive. Avoid tea in cases of hypertension and insomnia; avoid large doses during pregnancy and while nursing.

THYME *(Thymus spp., including T. vulgaris: garden thyme, T. serpyllum: wild thyme)* is a member of the *Lamiaceae* (mint) family. The aboveground plant is used. Avoid therapeutic doses during pregnancy, though culinary use is fine.

TRIBULUS *(Tribulus terrestris, T. cistoides)* is a member of the Zygophylaceae (caltrop) family. The sharp fruit is used. Avoid during pregnancy except under the guidance of a qualified health-care practitioner. Avoid in cases of dehydration or blood or chi deficiency.

TURMERIC *(Curcuma longa)* is a member of the *Zingerberaceae* (ginger) family. The rhizome is used. Some people have experienced skin rashes from using turmeric. It may cause photosensitivity in some individuals. Therapeutic dosages should be avoided during pregancy (though culinary use is fine).

USNEA *(Usnea barbata, U. species)* is a member of the *Parmeliaceae* (usnea) family. The mycelia (of the thallus), which is technically the tissue of the plant, is used. There have been rare cases of contact dermatitis from applying the herb directly to the skin. It is best avoided during pregnancy.

UVA-URSI *(Arctostaphylos uva-ursi, A. species)* is a member of the *Ericaceae* (heath) family. The leaf is used as medicine. Use for ideally no longer than one week. (Take a one-week break and then resume, if needed.) Large or frequent doses may be irritating to the stomach mucosa and can cause nausea and vomiting. Long-term use may be constipating. It can be beneficial to combine uva-ursi with a demulcent herb such as cornsilk, marshmallow root, or licorice. Avoid during pregnancy as uva-ursi may decrease circulation to the uterus. Arbutin inhibits the breakdown of insulin and should be used cautiously by those who are hypoglycemic. It can turn urine a greenish color, due to the hydroquinone, though this effect is not harmful.

VALERIAN *(Valeriana officinalis, V.* spp.*)* is a member of the *Valerianaceae* (valerian) family. The root or rhizome is used. Large doses of valerian can cause depression, nausea, headache, and lethargy. Some individuals, especially those who are already overheated, may find valerian stimulating rather than sedating. Do not use large doses for more than three weeks in a row. Avoid during pregnancy except in very small doses. Do not give to children under the age of three. Avoid in cases of very low blood pressure or hypoglycemia; avoid long-term use in cases of depression. Use with caution if you are going to be driving, operating heavy machinery, or undertaking other activities that require fast reaction times. Valerian may potentiate the effects of benzodiazepine and barbiturates. Those taking sedatives, antidepressants, or anti-anxiety medications should use valerian only under the guidance of a qualified health-care professional.

VIOLET *(Viola odorata)* is a member of the *Violaceae* (violet) family. The leaf and flower are used. Violet is not recommended in cold conditions such as chills. Otherwise, violet leaf tea is safe and gentle; it even can be used as a substitute for baby aspirin. Do not substitute African violets as a medicine plant.

VITEX *(Vitex agnus-castus)* is a member of the *Verbenaceae* (vervain) family. The berry is used. Discontinue if diarrhea, nausea, or abnormal menstrual changes occur. Large doses can cause formication, a strange symptom, where one feels as if ants are crawling on their skin. To improve hormonal problems with vitex, the herb should be taken for at least six months.

WALNUT *(Juglans regia: English walnut, Persian walnut, J. nigra: black walnut, J. cinerea: butternut)* is a member of the *Juglandaceae* (walnut) family. The leaf, dried inner bark, green hull of nut, and nut are used. Avoid walnut leaf, inner bark, and green hull during pregnancy; the nut is safe. The nut has caused mouth sores in sensitive individuals. The green hulls and leaves have been known to cause contact dermatitis. The inner bark should be dried for one year before use, as the fresh bark can cause intestinal gripe.

WILD CHERRY *(Prunus virens, P. aviium: wild cherry, Prunus serotina: black cherry, P. virginiana: choke cherry)* is a member of the *Rosaceae* (rose) family. The dried inner bark is used. The bark is toxic in large doses. Do not boil bark; simply steep in hot water. It may cause drowsiness. Though it helps coughs, it does not treat the infection that may be causing the cough. Do not use during severe infection.

WILD YAM *(Dioscorea villosa, D. batata, D. japonica, D. bulbifera)* is a member of the *Dioscoreaceae* (yam) family. The root and rhizomes are used. Avoid large doses during pregnancy unless suggested by a competent health-care professional. Avoid large doses in cases of constipation or with high blood pressure.

WILLOW *(Salix alba: white willow, S.* spp.*)* is a member of the *Salicaceae* (willow) family. The inner bark is used. Willow is not recommended during pregnancy. Avoid in cases of hemophilia or in others at risk of hemorrhage, and do not use in conjunction with blood-thinning medications. Avoid giving willow bark to children with a viral infection accompanied by headache to avoid the risk of Reye's syndrome. Those who suffer from tinnitus or who are allergic to aspirin should use willow with caution.

WITCH HAZEL *(Hamamelis virginiana)* is a member of the *Hamamelidaceae* (witch hazel) family. The bark, twig, and leaf are used. Because of its high tannin content, witch hazel is very astringent. Topical applications of witch hazel should use only products made from the twigs, as those made from the bark or leaves may be disfiguring. Tincture of witch hazel can be too astringent for topical skin use. Use witch hazel internally only for short periods of time as the high tannin content can be too astringent for the liver and constipating. Although distilled witch hazel does not contain tannins, it often contains rubbing alcohol, and it should not be used internally or applied close to mucus membranes, on broken skin, or in the eyes.

WOOD BETONY *(Stachys officinalis)* is a member of the *Lamiaceae* (mint) family. The aboveground plant is used. Wood betony is generally regarded as safe. However, large doses may cause vomiting. Pregnant women should avoid large doses, except during labor, and then only under the guidance of a qualified health-care practitioner. Do not confuse Stachys species with Pedicularis species, which are also known as betony, as their uses are not interchangeable.

YARROW *(Achillea millefolium)* is a member of the *Asteraceae* (daisy) family. The flowering top is used. Overuse may cause skin photosensitivity, dizziness, and headache in some people. Rare individuals may be sensitive to yarrow and experience dermatitis after use. Avoid yarrow during pregnancy.

YELLOW DOCK *(Rumex crispus)* is a member of the *Polygonaceae* (buckwheat) family. The root is used. Yellow dock leaves are high in oxalate, which can impair calcium absorption and potentially aggravate kidney stones, arthritis, gout, and hyperacidity. Large amounts of the leaves or roots may cause nausea, vomiting, or diarrhea.

YERBA MANSA *(Anemopsis californica)* is a member of the *Saururaceae* (lizard tail) family. The root and leaf are used. It is generally considered safe when used appropriately.

YERBA MATÉ *(Ilex paraguariensis, I. domestics, i. sorbilis, I. mate)* is a member of the *Aquifoliaceae* (holly) family. The leaf is used. Maté contains caffeine; however, its tannins tend to bind with the caffeine, thereby reducing the effects of both compounds. Most people who find that caffeine impairs their sleep will not experience this effect with maté. However, those suffering from anxiety, heart palpitations, or insomnia should use maté cautiously. It is best to avoid consuming maté with meals, as the high tannin content can impair nutrient assimilation.

YUCCA *(Yucca species, including Yucca baccata: banana yucca/Our Lord's candle, Y. brevifolia: Joshua tree, Y. filamentosa: Adam's needle, Y. glauca: soapweed, Y. schidigera: Mojave yucca)* is a member of the *Agavaceae* (agave) family. Use only dried yucca root. Avoid during pregnancy. The fresh leaves have been reported to be toxic to livestock and should not be consumed.

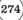

Appendix B: Herbal Education

American Botanical Council
P.O. Box 144345
Austin, TX 78714-4345
800-373-7105
www.herbalgram.org
Publishes Herbalgram; sells herbal books

American Herbalists Guild
141 Nob Hill Road
Cheshire, CT 06410
203-272-6731
www.americanherbalist.com
Offers a member directory of peer-reviewed herbal practitioners

American Herb Association
P.O. Box 1673
Nevada City, CA 95959
530-265-9552
www.ahaherb.com
Provides listing of herb schools throughout the country and an excellent newsletter

California School of Herbal Studies
P.O. Box 39
Forestville, CA 95436
707-887-7457
www.cshs.com
Provides in depth on site herbal education with many fine teachers

Herb Research Foundation
5589 Arapahoe Ave. #205
Boulder, CO 80303
303-449-2265
www.herbs.org
Clearinghouse for herbal information

The Science and Art of Herbalism Correspondence Course
P.O. Box 420
East Barre, VT 05649
802-479-9825
www.sagemountain.com
An excellent home-study program designed by beloved herbalist Rosemary Gladstar

Tai Sophia Institute
7750 Montpelier Road
Laurel, MD, 20723
410-888-9048/6620
www.tai.edu
Provides in depth herbal education and a degree program

United Plant Savers
P.O. Box 400
East Barre, VT 05649
802-476-6467
www.unitedplantsavers.org
Group that promotes awareness about rare and endangered species and offers a great newsletter

Appendix C: Resources for Buying Herbs and Supplies

Asia Natural Products
590 Townsend Street
San Francisco, CA 94103
415-522-1668/800-355-3808
www.drkangformulas.com
Sells quality Oriental herbs

Astara Cosmetics
Astara Biogenic Skincare
BachFlower.com
Los Angeles, CA
800-214-2850
www.bachflower.com
Distributers of Rescue Remedy and other Bach Flower remedies

Boiron Homeopathics
6 Campus Boulevard
Newtown Square, PA 19073-3267
800-264-7661
www.boironusa.com
Offers a complete line of homeopathic products

Bragg Live Foods, Inc.
Box 7
Santa Barbara, CA 93102
800-446-1990
www.bragg.com
Sells the best raw apple cider vinegar

Desert Essence
P.O. Box 14007
Hauppauge, New York 11788
www.DesertEssence.com
Sells quality aromatherapy and beauty products,
many based on tea tree oil

Dr. Bronner's Magic Soaps
P.O. Box 28
Escondido, CA 92033
877-786-3649
www.drbronner.com
Excellent soaps for cleaning everything on the body
and in the home

Flora Inc.
P.O. Box 73
805 E. Badger Road
Lynden, WA 98264
800-446-2110
www.florahealth.com
Makes Floradix herbal tonics

Frontier Natural Products Co-Op
P.O. Box 299
Norway, IA 52318
800-669-3275
www.frontiercoop.com
Offers mail-order herbs and herbal products

Herb Pharm
P.O. Box 116
Williams, OR 97544
541-846-6262/800-348-4378
www.herb-pharm.com
Makers of excellent quality herbal tinctures
Herbal Products

Allergy Research Group
2300 North Loop Road
Alameda, CA 94502
800-545-9960/510-263-2000
www.allergyresearchgroup.com
Sells homeopathic products for specific allergens

Honey Gardens, Inc.
P.O. Box 52
Ferrisburg, VT 05456
802-877-6766
www.honeygardens.com
Sells the best raw wildflower honey

Horizon Herbs, LLC
P.O. Box 69
Williams, OR 97544-0069
541-846-6704
www.horizonherbs.com
Offers an excellent selection of herbal seeds
and seedlings

Little Moon Essentials
2475 West Highway 40
Steamboat Springs, CO 80477
888-273-0683
www.littlemoonessentials.com
Sells excellent bath and body care products, salves,
and bug repellants

MegaFood
P.O. Box 325
Derry, NH 03038
800-848-2542
www.lovemegafood.com
Sells vitamins enhanced with super foods

Mountain Rose Herbs
P.O. Box 50220
Eugene, OR 97405
800-879-3337
www.mountainroseherbs.com
Sells herbs and herbal products such as strainers,
empty tea bags, and tincture bottles

Peaceful Mountain
5345 Arapahoe Ave, Suite B-1
Boulder, CO 80301
888-303-3388
www.peacefulmountain.com
Makes a wide selection of healing salves and balms,
including for pain, shingles, eczema, and sprains

Planetary Herbals
P.O. Box 1760
Soquel, CA 95073
800-606-6226/831-438-1700
www.planetaryherbals.com
Sells herbal remedies based on the work
of Dr. Michael Tierra

Primal Essence
1351 Maulhardt Avenue
Oxnard, CA 93030
805-981-2409/877-774-6253
www.primalessence.com
Makes excellent tea additions such as cinnamon,
chai, ginger, and peppermint essences

StarWest Botanicals
11253 Trade Center Drive
Rancho Cordova, CA 95742
800-800-4372
www.starwest-botanicals.com
Offers mail-order herbs and herbal products

Sunburst Bottle Company
4500 Beloit Drive
Sacramento, CA 95838
916-929-4500
www.sunburstbottle.com
Sells glass and plastic bottles and containers
for herbal preparations

Sunstar Dimensions, Inc/Astara Skin Care
5017 E Washington Unit 105
Phoenix, AZ 85034
602-393-1907
www.astaraskincare.com
Sells excellent natural cosmetics

Weleda North America
1 Closter Road
P.O. Box 675
Palisades, NY 10964
800-241-1030
www.weleda.com
Sells remedies and body care products including
baby care

Appendix D: Bibliography

American National Red Cross, Standard First Aid and Personal Safety. New York: C.V. Mosby, 1993.

Angier, Bradford. *How to Stay Alive in the Woods.* New York: Black Dog & Leventhal Publishers, 2001.

Blate, Michael. *First Aid Using Simple Remedies.* Columbus, NC: The G-Jo Institute, 2005.

Bragg, Paul C., ND, PhD, and Patricia Bragg. *Apple Cider Vinegar: Miracle Health System.* Santa Barbara, CA: Bragg Health Sciences, 2009.

Brown, Jude. *Aromatherapy for Travellers.* San Francisco: Thorsons Publishers, 1996.

Brown, Tom. *Tom Brown's Field Guide to Wilderness Survival.* New York: Berkley Trade, 1987.

Chamberlain, Mary. *Old Wives' Tales: The History of Remedies, Charms and Spells.* London: Tempus Publishers, 2002.

Clouatre, Dallas, PhD. *Getting Lean with Anti-Fat Nutrients.* San Francisco: Pax Publishing, 1994.

Elliot, Rose, and Carlo de Paoli. *Kitchen Pharmacy: A Book of Healing Remedies for Everyone.* New York: Orion, 1998.

Gardner, Joy. *The New Healing Yourself: Natural Remedies for Adults and Children.* Freedom, CA: The Crossing Press, 1989.

Geelhoed, Glen W., MD, and Jean Barilla, MS. *Natural Health Secrets from Around the World.* New Canaan, CN: Keats Publishing, 1997.

Greenbank, Anthony. *The Book of Survival.* Long Island City NY: Hatherleigh Press, 2003.

Harris, Ben Charles. *Kitchen Medicines: Curative Recipes and Remedies.* New York: Pocket Books, 1970.

Heinerman, John, PhD. *The Healing Benefits of Garlic: From Pharoahs to Pharmacists.* New Canaan, CT: Wings, 1994.

Igram, Cass, DO. *How to Survive Disasters with Natural Medicines.* Hiawatha, IA: Cedar Graphics, 1995.

Irons, Diane. *911 Beauty Secrets*. Naperville, IL: Sourcebooks, 1999.

Kirkwood, Byron. *Survival Guide for the New Millennium*. Grass Valley, CA: Blue Dolphin, 1993.

McIntyre, Anne. *The Herbal for Mother and Child*. London: Thorsons Publishers, England, 2003.

Maleskey, Gale, and Brian Kaufman. *Home Remedies: What Works*. Emmaus, PA: Rodale Press, 1997.

Mayell, Mark, and the editors of Natural Health Magazine. *The Natural Health First Aid Guide*. New York: Pocket Books, 1994.

Meyer, Clarence. *American Folk Medicine*. Glenwood, IL: Meyerbooks Publisher, 1985.

Newman, Bob. *Survival in the '90s*. Birmingham, AL: Menasha Ridge Press, 1996.

Nyerges, Christopher. *Urban Wilderness*. Culver City, CA: Peace Press, 1979.

Reader's Digest Staff. *Reader's Digest Action Guide: What to Do in an Emergency*. Montreal, 1989.

Sun Bear, Wabun, and Nimimosha. *The Bear Tribe's Self-Reliance Book*. New York: Simon and Schuster, 1992.

Tkac, Debora and Prevention Magazine Health Books editors. *The Doctor's Book of Home Remedies: Thousands of Tips and Techniques Anyone Can Use to Health Everyday Health Problems*. Emmaus, PA: Rodale Press, 1990.

Vogel Alfred. *Health Guide through Southern Countries*. Teufen, Switzerland: Vogel, 1975.

Werner, David. *Where There is No Doctor*. Palo Alto, CA: Hesperian Foundation, 1992.

White, Martha. *Traditional Home Remedies: The Old Farmer's Home Library Almanac: Time Tested Methods for Staying Well The Natural Way*. New York: Yankee Publishing, Inc., 1997.

Wilen, Joan, and Lydia Wilen. *Live and Be Well: New Age and Age Old Folk Remedies*. New York: Harper Books, 1992.

Wilen, Joan and Lydia Wilen. *More Chicken Soup and Other Folk Remedies*. New York: Ballantine Books, 2000.

Wiseman, John. *Survive Safely Anywhere*. New York: Crown Publishers, 1986.

COMPUTER SOFTWARE PROGRAM

The *Herbal Pharmacy: The Interactive CD-ROM Guide to Medicinal Plants*. Boulder, CO: Hale Software, 1998.

DVDS

Rawsome: Maximizing Health, Energy and Culinary Delight with the raw Foods Diet, 2007.

Healing Herbs and Wild Food, Herb TV, 2009, www.HerbTVonline.com.

AUDIOTAPES

The Herbal Renaissance: How to Heal with Common Plants and Herbs. Louisville, CO: Sounds True, 1990.

Natural Remedies for a Healthy Immune System. Louisville, CO: Sounds True, 1990.

You can order these tapes directly from Sounds True by calling their mail-order number: 800-333-9185.

About the Authors

Brigitte Mars is an herbalist and nutritional consultant from Boulder, Colorado, who has been working with natural medicine for more than forty years. She teaches herbal medicine through Naropa Universty, Omega Institute, Esalen, Hollyhock, Boulder College of Massage Therapy, and Bauman Holistic College of Nutrition. She is a professional member of the American Herbalist Guild. Brigitte Mars is also available for herbal formulations and consultations. She blogs for The Huffington Post, Care2, and My Intent. For more information, visit her website at www.brigittemars.com.

Chrystle Fiedler has written more than a hundred articles on health topics for many national publications, including *Woman's Day*, *Better Home & Gardens*, *Prevention*, *Natural Health*, *Remedy*, *Medizine's Healthy Living*, *The Health Monitor Network*, *Great Health*, *Vegetarian Times*, *Bottom Line/Women's Health*, *Heart Healthy Living* and *Health* magazine. Chrystle is also the co-author of *Beat Sugar Addiction Now!* (Fair Winds Press 2010) and *The Complete Idiot's Guide to Natural Remedies* (Alpha 2009). For more information, visit her website at www.chrystlecontent.com.

Acknowledgments

A heartfelt thank-you to Fair Winds Press: Jill Alexander, Marilyn Allen, and Shannon LeMay-Finn.

Many thanks to Rosemary Gladstar, Mindy Green, Diana DeLuca, Kathi Keville, Beth Baugh, Sara Katz, Cascade Anderson Geller, Pam Montgomery, Jane Bothwell, and Chanchal Cabrerra. Susun Weed and Amanda McQuade Crawford, you inspire! Briggs Wallis, your spirit of adventure is refreshing. Debra St. Claire, Farida Sharan, Lilja Oddsdottir, Gitte Lassen, Trish Flaster, Mark Blumenthal, and Rob McCaleb, you all make such a contribution to the herbal realm.

To Laura Lamun for joy, laughter, and song. To friends and celestial artisans Bob Venosa and Martina Hoffmann. To Steve McIntosh and Tehya Jai, always on the path of truth, beauty, and goodness. Rebecca and Robbie Gordon—such amazing friends you are. Elysabeth Williamson, Bob Ramey, Naomi Boggs, Norm Allard, Jia Gottlieb, and Kate Bullings, you have great healing gifts. Thank you my beloved friends at Pharmaca. Kimba Arem, Donelda Curren, Jirka Rysavy, and Donna Eagle, you all bring your wonderful contributions to the planet.

Matthew Becker, herbalist extraordinaire, you always comfort and heal with your kindness and wisdom. Thanks to herbalists Michael and Lesley Tierra, L.Ac., A.H.G, Christopher Hobbs, L.Ac., A.H.G., Roy Upton, Herbal Ed Smith, David Winston, David Hoffmann, Win Smith, L.Ac., Matthew Wood, James Green, Paul Bergner, N.D., Rick Scalzo, and the late and great ones: Rosemary Woodruff Leary, Jeannine Parvati Baker, William LeSassier, and Terence McKenna.

Index

CPSIA information can be obtained
at www.ICGtesting.com
Printed in the USA
LVHW02s1751020218
565079LV00005B/5/P

9 781592 336319